RESEARCH METHODS IN HEALTH PROMOTION

Second Edition

Laura F. Salazar

Richard A. Crosby

Ralph J. DiClemente

JB JOSSEY-BASS™

A Wiley Brand

Published by Jossey-Bass
A Wiley Brand
One Montgomery Street, Suite 1200, San Francisco, CA 94104-4594—www.josseybass.com

Jossey-Bass books and products are available through most bookstores. To contact Jossey-Bass directly call our Customer Care Department within the U.S. at 800-956-7739, outside the U.S. at 317-572-3986, or fax 317-572-4002.

Wiley publishes in a variety of print and electronic formats and by print-on-demand. Some material included with standard print versions of this book may not be included in e-books or in print-on-demand. If this book refers to media such as a CD or DVD that is not included in the version you purchased, you may download this material at http://booksupport.wiley.com. For more information about Wiley products, visit www.wiley.com.

Library of Congress Cataloging-in-Publication Data
Research methods in health promotion / [edited by] Laura F. Salazar, Richard A. Crosby, Ralph J. DiClemente.—Second edition.
     p. ; cm.
   Includes bibliographical references and indexes.
ISBN 978-1-118-40906-0 (pbk.)—ISBN 978-1-118-44844-1 (pdf)—ISBN 978-1-118-44842-7 (epub)
   I. Salazar, Laura Francisca, 1960- , editor. II. Crosby, Richard A., 1959- , editor. III. DiClemente, Ralph J., editor.
   [DNLM: 1. Health Promotion. 2. Biomedical Research—methods. 3. Research Design. WA 590]
   RA427.8
   613.072—dc23
                                                                                        2014046755

Printed in the United States of America
SECOND EDITION
PB Printing   SKY10033595_030222

CONTENTS

FIGURES, TABLES, AND BOXES

Figures

Tables

Boxes

The authors of this textbook have been teaching graduate students about health behavior and health promotion research for over three decades. As successful researchers, we have a love for precision and rigor in the process of scientific inquiry. Our passion in the process of using science to promote health has been conveyed to our students through countless applied examples. We believe that even the most daunting concepts can be easily learned once students make a clear connection to these concepts' utility to promote health. We also maintain that the research process is an enjoyable sequence of decision-making challenges that compose a journey. It is this journey that often creates anxiety for novice researchers. Our mission in writing this book is to alleviate that anxiety by replacing it with competence and anticipation.

Nine years ago we wrote the first edition of *Research Methods in Health Promotion*, which was widely embraced across schools of public health throughout the United States. We are always gratified to meet students who have used our book and to hear how they have progressed in their level of expertise. As satisfying as it is to receive praise from students, after using our textbook for the past eight years we realized that that there were areas for improvement. As a consequence of our continued quest to demystify and illuminate research methods in health promotion, we are pleased to offer this expanded second edition. We have reorganized the book so that the first thirteen chapters are grouped into parts and form the core of the textbook: Foundations of Health Promotion Research (Chapters One through Three), Fundamentals of Health Promotion Research (Chapters Four through Eight), and Applications of Health Promotion Research (Chapter Nine through Thirteen). The fourth part focuses solely on Data Analysis and includes chapters for observational studies, experimental studies, and qualitative research. The final part is Core Skills, which provides how-to guidance on writing a journal article and writing a grant.

Chapter One still outlines the steps necessary in undertaking research in health promotion; however, we couch these steps in an analogy of "embarking on a road trip" so that new researchers can, from the beginning, feel a sense of excitement when embarking upon a research study. Chapter Two, a solid chapter on the philosophy of science, provides the Greek and Latin origins of many of the terms we use in research and a basic foundation in science and the scientific method and highlights the different epistemologies often used to contribute to knowledge. Chapter Three has been rewritten and expanded to include more content specific to health promotion research, with less focus on the historical and federal legislation aspects of this topic and more focus on the practical approaches to preparing an IRB application. Chapter Four has been updated with new research examples—many of them global—and new figures that illustrate all of the designs, tables that describe strengths and weaknesses, and a focus on observational designs only. Chapter Five was spun off from the previous Chapter Four; this new chapter describes experimental and quasi-experimental designs. Similar to Chapter Four, Chapter Five includes global examples, new visuals depicting each of the designs, tables with strengths and weaknesses, and an expanded section on threats to internal validity. Chapter Six, on sampling, has been expanded to include two newer types of sampling methods used frequently in health promotion research: respondent-driven sampling and venue-day-time sampling. Chapter Seven, on measurement, is now more streamlined and integrates principles regarding the improved use of self-reported assessments (thereby allowing for one less chapter in this edition). Chapter Eight, on qualitative research strategies, excludes the former small section on data analysis but is expanded to include the different types of triangulation and more recent examples pulling from global health promotion. Chapter Nine begins the Applications part and provides the practical nuts and bolts of conducting observational research in the field, answering questions such as How do you gain access to a sample? and How do you recruit your sample? Chapter Ten is also a "how-to" chapter in that it provides step-by-step guidance on preparing and implementing a randomized controlled trial, a design used frequently to test health promotion interventions. Chapter Eleven, a new addition to our textbook, is dedicated entirely to methodologies that integrate community-based participatory research (CBPR) with traditional research methods. Chapter Twelve, on program evaluation, has been updated with recent examples, new visuals, and an expanded section on cost-benefit analysis. Chapter Thirteen, a new addition to the book, provides an overview of and guidance on planning and conducting large-scale survey research.

Chapters Fourteen and Fifteen, our data analysis chapters, have been updated with more recent and global examples but are still meant to provide knowledge on how to analyze the data rather than instruct on the mathematical equations or probability theory underlying statistics. Chapter Sixteen is a brand-new chapter that provides an overview of the data analytic process for qualitative research. This chapter, like the others in this textbook, is very readable, keeping the jargon to a minimum; it instructs on interpretation and how to write-up qualitative results, with examples provided throughout. The final two chapters, Seventeen and Eighteen, focus, respectively, on the publication process, with tips for writing up your results, and on writing a successful grant application for funding—two very important aspects of being a successful health promotion researcher.

Other novel additions to this second edition include:

- A brief preview of each chapter at its outset, along with specific learning objectives

- The use of photos and other visuals to help convey the concepts more clearly

- An expanded range of case studies and vignette examples, many of which are global

- A greater use of examples that transcend the individual level of health promotion research and extend to structural levels of intervention

- Added examples that integrate health promotion with environmental health

- Four new chapters that provide a greater depth and breadth of information for students who are dedicated to a successful career in health promotion practice and research

- An expanded array of examples and options that optimize advances in technology as applied to health promotion research

- Key concepts bolded and defined within the text

- Discussion and "for practice" questions to stimulate thinking and encourage application of the concepts

- The return of Mincus and Dincus, our small furried friends, who try so hard to conduct their research in four new cartoons

An instructor's supplement is available at www.wiley.com/go/Salazar2e. Additional materials, such as videos, podcasts, and readings, can be found at www.josseybasspublichealth.com. Comments about this book are welcome; please send them to publichealth@wiley.com.

We invite you to use this second edition as a primary tool of your trade and to constantly challenge yourself to find creative ways to apply science to health promotion. As you learn the methods contained in this book, please bear in mind that the future of public health is in your hands.

ACKNOWLEDGMENTS

First and foremost, we would like to acknowledge our late editor and dear friend, Andy Pasternack. As an editor he was superb. As a friend he was without equal. This second edition would not have been possible if it weren't for him. Andy was a champion of our first edition textbook, and because of his encouragement, his tenacity, and his guidance, we have produced a second edition that we hope is up to his high standards and worthy of his praise. We would also like to acknowledge each of our contributors, who took time out of their very busy schedules and put forth great effort and careful thought to their respective chapters. Furthermore, we extend our thanks to Ellie Faustino for her superb editorial wizardry, which ensured that our written words were free of non sequitur and that we avoided any grammatical faux pas; to Rachael Wendlandt, our research assistant, for her dedication in helping us find recent, relevant, and global studies to include as examples; to Monique Carry, a qualitative guru and supreme expert, for her feedback and comments on our qualitative chapters; and to Justin Wagner, once again, for his amazing original artwork and a slightly newer conceptualization of our beloved Mincus and Dincus. We want to thank the anonymous reviewers who provided wonderful feedback and helped further improve this textbook.

Also, we wish to acknowledge our new Jossey-Bass editor, Seth Schwartz, who has been very supportive and seamlessly took over to help produce this volume. He has been understanding of our needs, forgiving of deadlines, and helpful in ways too numerous to enumerate. Melinda Noack of Jossey-Bass has also been a delight to work with, as she systematically and patiently helped us wade through a voluminous number of images, permissions, and tasks. Finally, we wish to acknowledge the future, current, and retired public health researchers and practitioners for the work they have done and for the work they continue to do to improve the public's health.

We would like to thank proposal reviewers Christian Grov, Eric Jefferis, Sherryl Johnson, Ryan J. Martin, Kay Perrin, Diana Silver, and Leslie Spencer, who all provided valuable feedback on the original book proposal. Randy L. Byington, Sachiko Komagata, and Sheryl Strasser provided thoughtful and constructive comments on the complete draft manuscript.

To the stars in my universe—my children, Nicholas, Zachary, and Francesca, and my dear husband, Chuck—who are always there for me and provide much-needed perspective.

—L.F.S.

• • •

To my former students, throughout the United States and the world, who have helped shape the way this book teaches future generations of students, who will promote health and prevent disease.

—R.A.C.

• • •

To the three women in my life—Gina Maria, Sahara Rae, and Sianna Rose—who are my soul, inspiration, and motivation.

—R.J.D.

L aura F. Salazar is an associate professor and associate dean for research at Georgia State University's School of Public Health. Dr. Salazar's research has been devoted to helping prevent and ameliorate violence against women and HIV/AIDS. She was trained as a community psychologist at Georgia State University (GSU), where she received her PhD (2001). She also completed a postdoctoral fellowship in HIV/AIDS at Emory University's School of Medicine (2003). Before joining the faculty at GSU in 2011, Dr. Salazar was a member of the faculty at Emory University's Rollins School of Public Health. Her research has been funded by the Centers for Disease Control and Prevention and the National Institutes of Health and includes the use of social media marketing and web-based approaches to expand the reach of health promotion efforts. Dr. Salazar has published over one hundred journal articles in medical, public health, and social science journals and is the author of over thirty book chapters and coauthor of two other public health textbooks. Dr. Salazar teaches advanced research methods and health behavior theory for public health.

Richard A. Crosby is the Good Samaritan Endowed Professor and Chair in the College of Public Health at the University of Kentucky. He has devoted his career to preventing HIV infection among minority populations and to teaching theory and research methods to students pursuing graduate degrees in health promotion/public health. Having taught several hundred graduate students, Dr. Crosby's passion for writing textbooks is an extension of his work in the classroom. He earned his Ph.D. in health behavior from Indiana University, his master's in health education from Central Michigan University, and his bachelor's in school health education from the University of Kentucky. He has published nearly three hundred journal articles related to health promotion (especially to safer sex practices for high-risk populations) and he has authored more than fifty book chapters on topics ranging from HIV prevention to behavioral and social science theory applied to health promotion, and (most important) to the practice of conducting rigorous health promotion research.

Ralph J. DiClemente is Charles Howard Candler Professor of Public Health and associate director, Emory Center for AIDS Research. He holds concurrent appointments as professor in the School of Medicine, Department of Pediatrics, in the Division of Infectious Diseases, Epidemiology, and Immunology; the Department of Medicine, in the Division of Infectious Diseases; and the Department of Psychiatry. He was recently chair, the Department of Behavioral Sciences and Health Education at the Rollins School of Public Health, Emory University. Dr. DiClemente was trained as a health psychologist at the University of California, San Francisco, where he received his Ph.D. degree (1984) after completing his master's (1978) in behavioral sciences at the Harvard School of Public Health and his bachelor's degree (1973) at the City University of New York.

Dr. DiClemente's research interests include developing decision-making models of adolescents' risk and protective behaviors. He has a particular interest in the development and evaluation of theory-driven HIV/STD-prevention programs for adolescents and young adult women. He has published over 500 peer-reviewed articles in medical, public health, and social and behavioral science journals, over 150 book chapters, and 18 books. He currently teaches a course on grant writing and research ethics and serves on numerous editorial boards and national prevention organizations, such as the Office of AIDS Research Advisory Council.

Alejandra Mijares, M.P.H., is a senior analyst in the Public Health and Epidemiology Practice at Abt Associates Inc., where she leads qualitative data collection and analysis of research and evaluation projects in the United States and abroad.

Richard R. Clayton, Ph.D., is an emeritus professor in the Department of Health Behavior of the College of Public Health at the University of Kentucky in Lexington, Kentucky.

Michelle C. Kegler, Dr.PH., M.P.H., is a professor in the Department of Behavioral Sciences and Health Education at the Rollins School of Public Health, and director of the former Emory Prevention Research Center at Emory University.

Nancy J. Thompson, M.P.H., Ph.D., is an associate professor in the Department of Behavioral Sciences and Health Education at the Rollins School of Public Health at Emory University.

• • •

Even the best textbooks benefit from the wide classroom testing of their first edition, especially in a field as fast developing, technologically wired, and interdisciplinary as health promotion, and as politically central as health promotion is to the social and economic development of health. The editors and chapter authors of this book have taken much comfort and guidance from the reception and the experience of instructors, students, and practitioners to their first edition. This second edition will be welcomed.

M uch of the published writing on research methods misses the mark for students of the health professions because academic authors tend to emphasize research methods that will meet scientific needs rather than practitioner or population health needs. They often start with theory or research questions from more basic disciplines and ask what opportunities or challenges clinical, school, or community health situations offer to test those theories. It seems too often that preprofessional students are being trained to turn their practices into community laboratories to serve the cause of science and theory testing, rather than using science and theory to solve population health needs or their problems in practice. The editors of this volume have challenged their contributing authors (and themselves, with the many chapters they have written) to show how their research methods can answer the questions that practitioners are asking. They acknowledge the growing demand for evidence-based practice and theory-based practice, but they demonstrate that these will come most effectively when we have more practice-based evidence and practice-based theory.

Rather than starting with theories and asking what practice situations can offer to test them, practice-based research starts with problems in practice and asks what research and theory can offer to solve them. It is that twist that sets this book apart from the usual emphasis of research methods textbooks used in professional preparation programs.

The other distinction between this book and many of the research methods books used in health professional training is the emphasis in this book on social and behavioral change as the intervening and dependent variables. Too often, the only texts required of students pursuing health promotion in health professional schools have been on epidemiological and biostatistical methods. In those, the complexities of social and behavioral determinants tend to be minimized in favor of the long and deep traditions of change in communicable diseases associated with the physical environment and biological processes of threats to health. Designing research and evaluation in which social and behavioral processes are the dominant determinants of today's chronic diseases has produced a range of innovations and shifts in emphases within the repertoire of research designs and methods. This book seeks to reflect those.

The chapters of this book offer applied examples from health promotion that illustrate the key concepts or research methods presented in each chapter. The chapters present a series of pros and cons for the methods presented as well as case studies that challenge readers to apply what they have learned. Another added value of this book, as distinct from the numerous textbooks available on research methods for each of the cognate disciplines (for example, epidemiology, psychology, sociology, anthropology, political science, economics) underpinning health promotion practice, is that this book seeks the multidisciplinary blending of methods necessary to understand, predict, and address the several ecological levels at which causation happens and change must occur. Any of the excellent research methods books from other disciplines deal with only a relatively narrow slice of the multilayered reality that health promotion must address. Research methods in health promotion must blend approaches from psychology and sociology, for example, to encompass the ecological reality of reciprocal determinism between individual behavior and environment. Health promotion research must also accommodate anthropological and economic methods to probe the culture differences that account for many of the problems of inequity and underserved populations.

Notwithstanding the differences and complexities of mixed methods and multiple levels of analysis, the authors have strived to give cohesiveness to varied research methods by maintaining a consistent theme that "research involves a predetermined series of well-defined steps." They revisit these steps throughout in a common sequential format. They seek to present a cohesive understanding of the role of science in public health and, more specifically, in health promotion. Even as they are ecumenical in their admission of the methods from various disciplines, they are also critical in evaluating their use and their limitations in health promotion research, and the ethical issues and problems of external validity surrounding some methods of experimental design, sampling, and randomization in the health promotion context.

The authors of this book have drawn on both their considerable academic experience in teaching students of health promotion and their field experience in practice-based research in HIV/AIDS, school health, reducing health disparities, and numerous other areas of public health, to represent the research methods most relevant and specific to the work ahead for students in health promotion.

Lawrence W. Green
Professor, Department of Epidemiology and Biostatistics
School of Medicine and Comprehensive Cancer Center
University of California at San Francisco

CHAPTER 1

KEY STEPS IN THE RESEARCH PROCESS

Richard A. Crosby
Laura F. Salazar
Ralph J. DiClemente

Health promotion has become a cornerstone of efforts designed to prevent morbidity and premature mortality (Smedley and Syme, 2000). Indeed, many nations have embraced health promotion as an approach to enriching and extending the lives of their people. Core tasks of health promotion include the primary and secondary prevention of disease and health-compromising conditions. These tasks are reflected in two overarching goals established by the United States Department of Health and Human Services: to "increase the quality and years of healthy life" and to "eliminate health disparities" (Department of Health and Human Services, 2010). Of course, the broad scope of these tasks presents an enormous challenge to the discipline of health promotion. This challenge demands that the efforts and resources of health promotion practitioners be firmly grounded in the context of research findings.

To begin, it is important to state that health promotion research is the harbinger of effective health promotion practice. Accordingly, a great deal of time and attention should be devoted to research agendas before health promotion programs are designed and widely implemented. Moreover, successful research endeavors must ensure rigor, which is the hallmark of scientific inquiry. Rigor is properly thought of as a quantity—it exists (or fails to exist) in varying degrees. Although no study can be "perfect" in rigor, studies can have a high degree of rigor. As rigor increases, confidence in the findings also increases.

LEARNING OBJECTIVES

- Understand how the health promotion discipline constitutes a paradigm shift in terms of its emphasis on preventing disease.

- Understand the nine-step model and be able to apply this to your own research project.

- Understand the importance of rigor in health promotion research and how to achieve greater rigor.

- Consider issues in scholarship, grantsmanship, and ethics that are part of the research process.

Therefore rigorous studies have great potential to shape health promotion practice.

Although this book focuses on the application of research methods to health promotion, there are at least two frameworks that address the broader set of issues relevant to the conceptualization, design, implementation, and evaluation of programs. In particular, one framework, the RE-AIM model (Glasgow, Vogt, and Boles, 1999) can be used as both a design and an evaluation tool for health promotion planning. The acronym stands for five stages. The first is Reach, which represents the level of spread or diffusion of a health promotion program within a given population. The second is Effectiveness, which represents the utility of the program to make a difference when used in ordinary circumstances. The third is Adoption, which is the uptake of the program by health promotion professionals. The fourth is Implementation, which describes the fidelity of program use among those adopting it. The final stage is Maintenance, which represents the ongoing and correct use of the program such that substantial changes to morbidity and mortality can occur.

The second framework, the PRECEDE-PROCEED model (Green and Kreuter, 2005), is a comprehensive model for organizing the health promotion planning process from its inception to its widespread implementation and ongoing evaluation. This planning model is one that should be firmly understood by anyone engaged in health promotion and, by extension, anyone engaged in health promotion research. The two models are depicted in Figures 1.1 and 1.2, which provide overviews of their logic and utility for health promotion.

Without question, the rewards of health promotion research are the excitement generated by evidence-based conclusions along with the associated implications for widespread implementation and ultimately the effects on public health. We may think of health promotion research as a journey down the research highway that reveals insights into human behavior pertaining to health and wellness. This exploration into people's lives should never be taken for granted; indeed, the opportunity provides health promotion practitioners a partial blueprint for the design, implementation, and justification of behavioral and structural interventions.

As with any journey, however, there are many decisions to make and myriad options from which to choose. Each leg of this research journey will have consequences (both good and bad) and, depending on the path taken, may result in reaching a crossroads or even a dead end, so it is important to consider each decision point and plan your journey carefully. Because you may not have been on this type of journey before, you won't be expected to travel alone. We will be your tour guide for this journey, walking you through the research process, helping to identify salient points of interest, and warning you of any potential dangers.

> **RE-AIM (Reach, Efficacy/Effectiveness, Adoption, Implementation, and Maintenance)**
>
> **Brief Description:**
>
> RE-AIM is a conceptual model to help identify key factors to implementation. It is a systematic way for evaluating public health interventions that assesses five dimensions: Reach, Efficacy/Effectiveness, Adoption, Implementation, and Maintenance.
>
> **Reach** is the absolute number, proportion, and representativeness of individuals who participate in a given program.
>
> **Efficacy/Effectiveness** is the impact of an intervention on important outcomes. This includes potential negative effects, quality of life, and costs.
>
> **Adoption** is the absolute number, proportion, and representativeness of settings and staff who are willing to offer a program.
>
> **Implementation,** at the setting level, refers to how closely staff members follow the program that the developers provide. This includes consistency of delivery as intended and the time and cost of the program.
>
> **Maintenance** is the extent to which a program or policy becomes part of the routine organizational practices and policies. Within the RE-AIM framework, maintenance also applies at the individual level.

Figure 1.1 The RE-AIM Model

In this journey, the mode of transportation will be the methodological *paradigm* applied to your research. From the Greek word *paradeigma,* **paradigm** literally means model, pattern, or example; however, this rather simple definition can be expanded to encompass a "worldview" that may be influential in shaping the development of a discipline. A methodological paradigm is a discipline's view of which research techniques and practices are promoted and should be practiced. A discipline's methodological paradigm has strong implications for how the discipline as a whole will progress. Thomas Kuhn, a twentieth-century professor in philosophy and the history of science, is credited with popularizing the term *paradigm*. He wrote a provocative book, *The Structure of Scientific Revolutions,* in which he describes the history of science as being composed of "a series of peaceful interludes punctuated by intellectually violent revolutions" (Kuhn, 1970, p. 10), which can change profoundly the existing worldview and result in a paradigm shift. He articulated the importance of paradigms in shaping and guiding a scientific discipline:

paradigm
a way of viewing the world around you; this includes the way in which disciplines conduct research

> A shared commitment to a paradigm ensures that its practitioners engage in the paradigmatic observations that its own paradigm can do most to explain. Paradigms help scientific communities to bind their discipline, in that they help the scientist create avenues of inquiry, formulate questions, select methods with which to examine questions, define areas of relevance, and establish or create meaning. A paradigm is essential to scientific inquiry [Kuhn, 1970, p. 142].

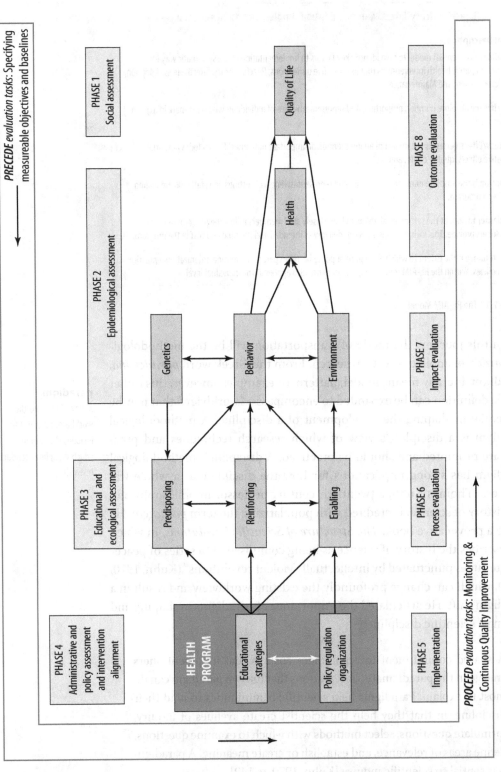

Figure 1.2 The PRECEDE-PROCEED Model

Source: Green & Kreuter (2005), with permission.

The establishment of health promotion as a discipline can be viewed as a paradigm shift in that health promotion researchers and practitioners place an emphasis on improving health and well-being and preventing disease, where previously the focus had been on treating disease. To truly have an impact on the health of the public, prevention requires a body of knowledge generated by rigorous research to help inform its efforts. As was ancient Rome, rigor is built "one brick at a time." Fortunately, clear blueprints exist for building rigorous studies. In fact, successful research can be characterized by a series of well-defined steps, all of which are essential. Following the steps sequentially is equally important. In this chapter, we provide an overview of the research process (the "journey") beginning with discovery of the idea; we then illustrate each of the essential and sequential steps in detail. We also emphasize the importance of the context in which the research process takes place. The result should be a keen understanding of the research process so that your journey will be a successful one.

Discovery

The research process in health promotion can be viewed as a process of discovering new ideas that can ultimately help improve the health and well-being of the public. This process of discovery is an **iterative process**, which means that each time a research question is addressed successfully, several new questions emerge. The diversity of potential research questions in any one aspect of health promotion creates an unending challenge (see Chapter Four for more detail regarding potential research purposes and questions). Research questions may appear quite humble yet demand rather complex and intense investigation efforts. Consider, for example, a question as simple as determining why people consume large amounts of saturated fats despite widespread awareness that these fats cause heart disease. An investigator could pursue cognitive reasons (for example, "those foods taste really good" or "those foods are satisfying"), social reasons (such as "most party foods are not healthy, but having fun is more important"), cultural reasons (for instance, "those foods are a tradition in our house"), or economic reasons ("fatty foods are usually more filling and less expensive than healthy foods"). An investigator could also approach the question based on perceived vulner-ability of the study participants to the multiple forms of disease associated with a diet high in saturated fats (such as heart disease, stroke, obesity, and some forms of cancer). Obviously, then, the seemingly humble research question is actually an entire research career. In fact, successful researchers typically devote themselves to only one or two areas of inquiry. This focus enables them to use the findings from one study as a platform to formulate subsequent research questions for the next study, and so on.

iterative process
one in which a cycle of discovery and revision occurs several times

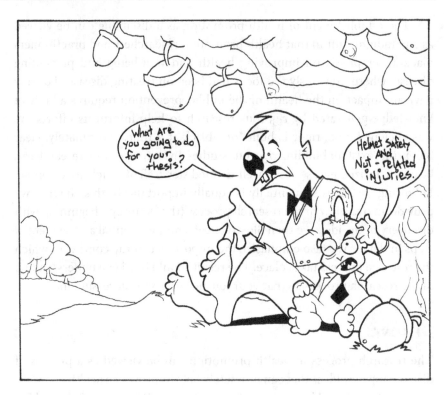

Mincus "Discovers" His Research Idea

Copyright 2005 by Justin Wagner; reprinted with permission.

In addition to being a discovery process, health promotion research is also a public venture. Conclusions from health promotion research often have a direct impact on public health. For example, health promotion studies have shown that raising on alcohol and cigarettes reduces consumption, which has led many states to adopt raising taxes as a form of public health intervention. Other studies have identified the individual and social determinants that contribute to vaccine acceptance (for example, flu, human papilloma virus), leading public health efforts to focus on reducing barriers such as cost or inconvenience to increase uptake of vaccines. Further, evidence suggests that people in malaria-affected countries are more likely to use bed nets if social marketing programs work to influence perceived risk and change cultural norms. As a public venture, then, discovery through health promotion research makes indispensable contributions to maintaining

IN A NUTSHELL

As a public venture, then, discovery through health promotion research makes indispensable contributions to maintaining the health and well-being of society.

the health and well-being of society. In the following section, we illustrate this discovery process using tobacco use as the public health issue.

VIGNETTE: PREVENTING TOBACCO DEPENDENCE

Globally, the use of tobacco is a behavior that leads to multiple forms of **morbidity** (incidence of disease in a given population) and premature **mortality** (incidence of death due to a particular disease in a given population). Thus health promotion programs designed to prevent tobacco dependence among young people are strongly warranted. A substantial number of these programs seek to prevent youths from initial experimentation with tobacco. These approaches certainly have value; however, research suggests that among young people tobacco dependency may be an extended process, which may be amenable to intervention even after their initial use of the substance. Imagine, then, that you have been asked to determine the effectiveness (that is, the capacity to produce the desired effect) of providing structural interventions to youths who have recently begun to use tobacco but have yet to develop a physical dependence. A **structural intervention** is one that alters environmental factors such as policies and laws regulating tobacco rather than trying to alter individuals' knowledge, attitudes, and beliefs with a small group intervention. Ultimately both methods should shape tobacco use behavior, but they differ in their approach.

morbidity
the incidence of disease in a given population

mortality
the incidence of death in a given population

structural intervention
one that alters the environment to foster improved health

The Nine-Step Model or "A Journey Down the Research Highway"

The research process can easily become unwieldy. Even seemingly simple research questions may lead an investigator to wonder if he or she is on the right track with regard to the process. The process is very much analogous to a long road trip—one that can start out with a straightforward path (see Figure 1.3) but later may take some turns or detours and be fraught with dan-

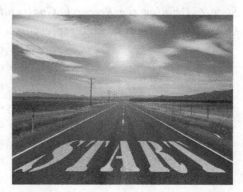

Figure 1.3 Road Image

ger, but nonetheless reach a desired destination. To streamline the thinking and actions involved in rigorous research, we have created a nine-step model.

Choosing Your Destination

Step 1: Defining the Research Population. Given that the elimination of health disparities is a priority, health promotion research typically seeks solutions to problems that disproportionately exist among members of a defined population. Because population is a broad term and can be defined in many different ways, it is up to the researcher to specify the parameters that will describe the target population. For example, the researcher may define the population as "adolescents residing in low-income households, thirteen to nineteen years of age, residing in areas of dense tobacco sales." Thus, as with any journey you ever take by driving, having a clear goal in mind before you get behind the wheel is essential. Deciding on the exact population that will become the recipient of your work is the equivalent of selecting where your destination will be when your journey comes to a successful end.

The process of defining the target population is far from arbitrary. Ideally, selecting the target population should be based on known *epidemiology* (the scientific discipline studying the distribution of disease in human populations) of the disease or health risk behavior under consideration. As shown in Figure 1.2, the PRECEDE-PROCEED model refers to this step as the Epidemiological Diagnosis and suggests that, generally speaking, health promotion programs should be delivered to epidemiologically defined populations on a prioritized basis. In other words, those with the greatest degree of burden—often expressed as the rate of disease per hundred thousand people—are served first.

Mapping Your Route

Step 2: Defining the Research Goal and Specifying the Exact Research Questions. This second step represents a turning point for the remainder of the research process. As a rule, narrow and precisely defined goals and questions are far more amenable to rigorous research designs than broadly defined goals and questions. At times, new researchers propose goals and questions that are far too broad to be addressed with ample rigor. An effective strategy to avoid this pitfall is to thoroughly review the recent and relevant empirical literature. This can be a time-consuming process, but it is nonetheless time well spent. Engaging in this process will yield a clear picture of gaps in the

IN A NUTSHELL

As a rule, narrow and precisely defined goals and questions are far more amenable to rigorous research designs than broadly defined goals and questions.

existing research. For new investigators, these gaps represent an opportunity to build on and extend the research literature, and they should be a logical focus of their subsequent research. Just as the process of thoughtfully planning and mapping out your journey can be time-consuming but well worth the investment, so too is the process of ensuring that your research question is firmly grounded in the existing literature. Once you have established a precisely defined research question, you can map out your ideal pathway of research.

Although conventional standards do not exist, from a practical standpoint many researchers restrict their review of the literature to the past five years. Online search engines such as Medline® and PsychInfo® are invaluable resources for the literature review process. A thorough review should include both articles directly related to the topic and those that are related tangentially. Directly related articles could include those that report findings from research designed to prevent tobacco dependence in new smokers, for example. Indirectly related articles could include those involving different populations and address broader issues such as use of other substances like alcohol or marijuana. When interpreting your review, it is important to assign a higher priority to directly related articles, whereas articles that are indirectly related should be applied judiciously.

Once the literature review is complete, a research goal can be formulated. The research goal is a general statement that conveys the purpose of the planned study. The research goal as stated in the vignette is "to determine the effectiveness of structural interventions for adolescents aged 13 to 19 residing in areas with high-density tobacco sales." The goal provides an overview of purpose and scope, but it lacks precision and specificity. Therefore we must go further by formulating research questions that provide the precision and specificity. Research questions are based on the research goal. In the given vignette, examples of a few appropriate research questions may include

Do laws prohibiting tobacco sales to adolescents effectively decrease their use?

How do adolescents view the risks of smoking?

What is the impact on adolescent tobacco use of an intervention that is meant to increase compliance among convenience store owners dispensing tobacco and located in these high-density tobacco sales areas?

Note that each question is a derivative of the overarching research goal. Each research question should provide information that serves the research goal. This derivative approach to research questions ensures that research efforts are accurately directed. Research questions should be centered on a common purpose: the research goal. This practice sets the stage for the next step.

Choosing Your Ride

Step 3: Determining Whether the Research Should Be Observational or Experimental. Briefly stated, *observational research* refers to research in which variables are observed as they exist in nature—no manipulation of variables occurs. Observational research asks questions pertaining to "why people do what they do." This form of research *does not involve* treatment or intervention, and in general, it is less involved and requires less time to implement and complete. Thus observational research is like driving a Ferrari as opposed to driving a semitruck pulling a heavy load. The journey for experimental research will be slower because this type of work involves implementing a health promotion program for a time period ample enough to yield changes in behavior or even disease incidence. However, this protracted journey is well worth the added time and investment. Once you arrive at your destination with the heavy load, the products of your trip will be valuable to the people in your chosen population.

Experimental research *does involve* manipulation of a variable (this could include education, policy changes, or changes in the environment). It builds on observational research by asking, "How can we help people achieve positive change?" and is the culmination of several observational studies. Developing and implementing effective interventions that serve the population of interest takes enormous time and effort, and, given the inevitable complexity, researchers should proceed at a slower pace. Experimental research is the type of research used to evaluate the effectiveness of interventions and is always concerned with the essential question of whether a given intervention program can produce outcomes of statistical significance and, even more important, practical significance.

Which Lane Are You In?

Step 4: Selecting a Research Design That Provides a Rigorous Test of the Research Questions. The choice of research designs is similar to choosing which lane you will be driving in and ranges from simple observational studies requiring relatively little time and generally manageable resources (think in terms of driving that Ferrari in the fast lane for this journey and arriving quickly at your destination) to complex experimental studies, which typically require several years to complete. Experimental studies require the use of extensive resources in addition to more time; thus the semitruck chosen for this design must "stay to the right"—once you select your research design, you are committed to a given lane (and speed) in your journey.

The guiding principle in making the selection is parsimony. Parsimony implies that the need (that is, investigating the research questions) is met by a tool (that is, research design) that does the job well, without going beyond that which is necessary.

Figure 1.4 shows a graph of research designs that describes the time and resource requirements of various forms of health promotion research. These designs are described in greater detail in Chapter Four (observational designs) and Chapter Five (experimental designs). At the Y-intercept, relatively simple research designs can be seen. Examples include qualitative studies and cross-sectional studies. As the level of complexity increases, the time and resource requirements increase linearly and include designs that necessitate the maintenance of a *cohort* (a **cohort** being a sample of research participants) over multiple assessment periods. A *cohort study* is synonymous with the terms *panel study, longitudinal study,* or *prospective study* and is located mid-level along the trajectory of increasing complexity. Similarly, various levels of complexity exist among experimental designs, which are located toward the upper right end of the trajectory. The phrase "randomized controlled trial (RCT)" denotes a true experimental design located near the peak of the trajectory. Figure 1.4 also shows that

cohort
a sample of study participants being followed over time

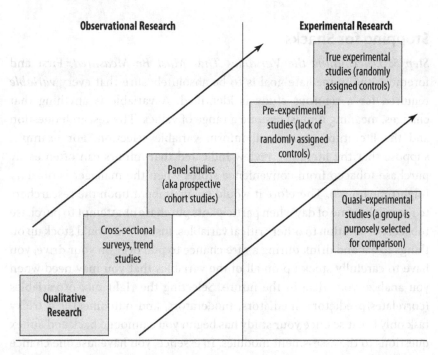

Figure 1.4   Research in Health Promotion: Resource Requirements

quasi-experimental designs are located at the peak, as these experimental designs are often necessary in health promotion involving structural-level or community-level interventions. For instance, in the research study targeting convenience store compliance with tobacco policies, only the quasi-experimental design is appropriate for determining effectiveness, because randomizing convenience stores to the intervention group within the high-density areas might create a form of contamination, a threat to internal validity. **Internal validity** refers to the degree of control an investigator exercises over the condition of an experimental design. In other words, adolescents residing in these high-density areas might learn that some stores are "cracking down" on the sale of tobacco while others are not, thereby affecting the outcomes.

internal validity
the degree of control an investigator exercises over the condition of an experimental design

As a rule, research should be constructed with designs that approximate the trajectory shown in Figure 1.4. That is, designs located to the left end of the trajectory serve as the building blocks for subsequent research questions that can then be addressed by progressively more complex designs.

IN A NUTSHELL

Designs located to the left end of the trajectory serve as the building blocks for subsequent research questions that can then be addressed by progressively more complex designs.

Stopping for Snacks

Step 5: Determining the Variables That Must Be Measured. First and foremost, the immediate goal is to be absolutely sure that every *variable* required for a rigorous study is identified. A variable is anything that changes, meaning it must assume a range of values. The research question and the literature review will inform variable selection. For example, suppose that the literature review indicated that minors can often easily purchase tobacco from convenience stores when the manager is off-duty (nighttime hours). Therefore it would be incumbent upon the researchers to record the time of day when participants purchase or attempt to purchase tobacco, in addition to other critical variables. Just as you would stock up on things to eat and drink during a rare chance to pull over on your drive, you have to carefully stock up on all of the variables that you may need when you analyze your data in the future. Selecting the right mix of variables (correlates/predictors, mediators, moderators, and outcomes) is a tricky task only because once your study has begun you cannot go back and annex questions to the assessment modules. In essence, you have just one chance to gather all that you will need.

The way in which the variables are measured is equally important. Indeed, rigor is dependent on the selection of reliable and valid measurement instruments. Like research, measurement is a process. It involves identifying appropriate measures, adapting existing measures to your unique research question, or creating new measures. Chapter Seven provides further discussion of measurement issues in health promotion research.

Some variables may be measured directly using a physical instrument (for example, a sphygmomanometer for blood pressure, or a scale for weight), whereas other variables, such as level of skill applying a condom to a penile model, can be measured only through direct observation. In health promotion research, most variables are measured indirectly using participants' self-reports. A mode of administration (for example, paper and pencil, face-to-face interview, or computer-assisted self-interview) must be selected based on previous knowledge of the research population and the nature of the previously identified research questions.

The process concludes with pilot testing designed to ensure that measures are appropriate for the planned study population. The pilot test also allows researchers to evaluate the psychometric properties of the self-report measures that purport to represent a **construct**. Constructs are intangibles described as concepts representing things that are not directly observable, as opposed to tangibles such as height or mass. Therefore constructs would be considered abstractions. Examples of constructs used in health promotion research include self-esteem, depression, and self-efficacy.

construct
intangible described as a concept representing something that is not directly observable

Do You Take the Bypass or Continue?

Step 6: Selecting the Sampling Procedure. As in other aspects of the research enterprise, there are choices to be made among numerous sampling procedures as you conduct your research. Sampling exists across a continuum of complexity and rigor. The sampling procedure employed is one of the most critical determinants of *external validity*. **External validity** refers to the ability to generalize study findings to the population of individuals with similar characteristics represented in the study sample. It should be noted, however, that not all research studies need to use a sampling procedure that yields high external validity. Although taking the time to engage the use of probability sampling techniques (much like driving through a congested city) will enhance the external validity of your study, the use of non-probability methods (taking the bypass) may be far more prudent and well worth the loss of external validity.

external validity
the ability to generalize study findings to the population of individuals with similar characteristics represented in the study sample

Sampling should also include specifying the number of study participants. This number is selected based on a *power analysis*. Stated simply,

power analysis
estimate of a statistical test's capability to find true differences between variables or between groups of study participants

a **power analysis** estimates the ability of a statistical test to find true differences between variables or between groups of study participants. Although a study's power is determined by multiple factors, sample size is one of the most important determinants. Planned sample sizes that provide inadequate power are crippling to the overall study. In the vignette, for example, a power analysis may suggest that each of the three study conditions should have one hundred participants. Having fewer participants in each condition could severely jeopardize the power of the study. More detailed descriptions of sampling procedures are presented in Chapter Six.

Is Autopilot a Good Idea?

Step 7: Implementing the Research Plan. A basic requirement of *internal validity* is consistency in the implementation of all study protocols. *Internal validity* implies that the study is not confounded by design, measurement, or poor implementation of study procedures. Protocols spell out key procedures such as the sampling procedure to be used, how participants will be assigned to intervention conditions, when and where assessments will occur, who will provide the assessments, what participants will be told or not told about the research study, and how reticent participants will be enticed to return for follow-up programs or assessments. Because protocols are generally quite detailed, subtle departures from these detailed plans can be a common problem and may throw you off your planned route. Over time, however, this deviation can amount to substantial changes in the way late-entry participants are treated as compared with those enrolling earlier in the study. Based on this list of concerns, you can quickly see that a primary obligation of the researcher is to constantly ensure that the study protocols are followed in a precise manner. Far from simply waiting for the data to be collected, the best researchers avoid the temptation of placing their study on "cruise control," as doing so will inevitably lead to problems. The best researchers develop systems that constantly monitor their progress and provide periodic (such as weekly or monthly) feedback on progress, emerging issues, and clear-cut problems. These systems are comparable to using a GPS to guide your continued travel on the road to research. One key advantage of being vigilant about the journey as it progresses is especially apparent in intervention studies, in which a phenomenon known as **drift** can occur. Drift occurs when research staff make subtle (unauthorized) changes to the intervention procedures. These small changes may become magnified over time and therefore cause the original intervention plan to morph in a substantial way.

drift
a phenomenon that occurs when research staff make subtle (unauthorized) changes to the intervention procedures

As an example of drift, consider the study of preventing tobacco dependence outlined in this chapter. The protocol specifies that convenience store owners in an entire geographic area will be the recipients of an intervention designed to enforce laws regarding tobacco sales to minors. Conversely, the comparison area will not receive this program. As one might imagine, however, the program may be applied inconsistently in the intervention area, and it may even be used to some degree in the comparison area by a staff member who is well-intended but less than committed to study rigor. The inconsistency in the intervention area is especially problematic, as this threatens the external validity of the study. Other common forms of drift include deviations in how assessments are administered (perhaps research assistants change the way they perform interviews) and departure from sampling protocols. Fortunately, drift can be averted by vigilant attention to an established set of quality-assurance procedures. Ultimately, then, the principal investigator is the one person who must be accountable for implementing these procedures, thereby ensuring that drift does not occur.

Arriving at Your Destination

Step 8: Analyzing the Data. Your journey, even if it occurred in a Ferrari, has not been an easy one, so when you finally reach the destination (a complete dataset), you'll want to be sure that you will benefit from your work. In other words, do what you came to do—fulfill the goal of the trip. Once all the assessments have been conducted, a dataset can be established. The dataset consists of the variables measured for each participant. The dataset is, of course, quite valuable, as it can subsequently be used to answer the research questions that were formulated in step 2. After the data are checked for logical inconsistencies (called "cleaning"), the research process becomes dependent on the statistical skills of the research team. Again, parsimony is important at this step—the goal is to perform an analysis that provides a rigorous and fair test of the research questions while avoiding the introduction of artificially imposed procedures.

In the tobacco study vignette, a parsimonious analysis would be to simply compare the mean number of cigarettes sold in defined geographic areas, before and after making the interventions designed to enforce a no-purchase law for minors. If the intervention was successful, then a noticeable drop in sales should occur for that geographic area, whereas the same drop should not occur for the location designated as the comparison area. Suppose, for example, the means are 15,769 cartons sold in the intervention area before the program began and 12,234 after it had been in place for 3 months. This precipitous drop suggests that the program worked. However, to rule out a trend caused by something other than your program, you then must look at sales for the comparison area. Those figures are 15,234 and 14,993, respectively. The decline in means can be compared using a very simple test (a one-way analysis of co-variance), which answers an essential question: Are the declines in means a function of the interventions or are they a function of chance? Chapters Fourteen through Sixteen provide more detailed discussion of data analysis.

Creating Your Slideshow and Sharing with Family and Friends

Step 9: Disseminating the Findings. Although memories from your trip will stay with you forever, it is important to document your journey for others. Just as you would want to show family members and friends where you went on your trip (and how you got there), a research journey deserves equal attention. In fact, the process of historically chronicling your journey is a longstanding tradition when it comes to research. Rigorous research clearly warrants widespread dissemination, and this is achieved through oral presentation of findings (at professional meetings) and through peer-reviewed publications. Indeed, this step elevates the project from a work in progress to a lasting scientific contribution. Like each of the previous eight steps in this chapter, step 9 is also a process unto itself. The rudimentary starting point in this process is transforming the analytic results into carefully articulated findings.

> **IN A NUTSHELL**
>
> The rudimentary starting point in this process is transforming the analytic results into carefully articulated findings.

Findings are answers to the research questions that are generated by the data analysis. The findings must be considered in the context of related research by showing how they strengthen or extend previous work. At this juncture, it is important to know that null findings or statistical analyses that were nonsignificant can be just as important as significant findings with respect to building the research base. Regardless, the study should have a high degree of rigor.

Moreover, the findings may raise additional questions that bring the research process back to its origin. Figure 1.5 illustrates this point. Inspection of the figure shows that research is an iterative process. Every time a research question is asked and answered, another question or set of questions becomes apparent. New researchers should be aware that their research debut (initial entry into this iterative process) is likely to be difficult, but that repeated cycles become progressively less difficult. In fact, this observation may explain why health promotion researchers often tend to specialize in a narrowly defined field of study (such as prevention of adult-onset diabetes, prevention of HIV infection among women, or promoting Pap testing among Latinas), as doing so enables them to

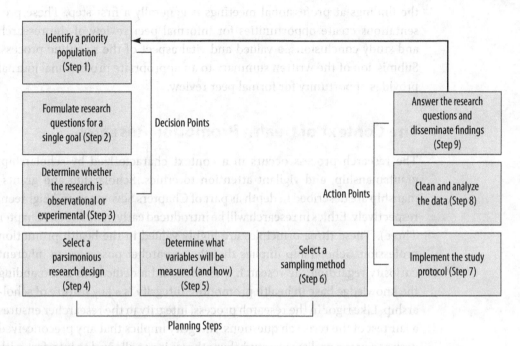

Figure 1.5 Schematic Illustration of the Nine-Step Research Process

develop a body of research and make significant contributions to the knowledge base in their area.

After the researcher (or research team) has successfully answered the research questions, the remaining task is to prepare written and visual (that is, tables and figures of study results) summaries of the research process (steps 1 through 8)—not unlike the infamous slideshow or photo album. Recall from step 2 that research is a collective process; therefore, disseminating the results adds to the larger empirical knowledge base. Fortunately, the preparation of written and visual summaries does not have to be a daunting task. In fact, when rigor is high, this task can be very satisfying and enjoyable. The task is primarily a historical account of the rationale underlying the research questions and the protocols used to answer these questions. Researchers customarily bring the task to a close by suggesting subsequent research questions that could be investigated to further strengthen and expand the research base.

Dissemination of the research findings is a key part of the scientific process. The written and visual records can be disseminated through multiple channels. Oral presentation of

IN A NUTSHELL

Dissemination of the research findings is a key part of the scientific process.

the findings at professional meetings is generally a first step. These presentations create opportunities for informal peer review of the research and study conclusions, a valued and vital aspect of the scientific process. Submission of the written summary to an appropriate professional journal provides opportunity for formal peer review.

The Context of Health Promotion Research

The research process occurs in a context characterized by scholarship, grantsmanship, and vigilant attention to ethics. Scholarship and grantsmanship are described in depth as part of Chapters Seventeen and Eighteen, respectively. Ethics in research will be introduced early in this book (Chapter Three). These three principles are highly valued in the health promotion profession. Scholarship implies that the researcher possesses an inherent curiosity regarding the research questions and a dedication to expanding the knowledge base in health promotion. Integrity is a key feature of scholarship. Like rigor in the research process, integrity in the researcher ensures a fair test of the research questions. Integrity implies that any preconceived desire to prove or disprove study hypotheses is not allowed to interfere with the research process. The research process is quite eloquent in that it forces objectivity; however, adherence to the process is based on the self-report of the researcher, making integrity vital.

Grantsmanship is also a vital part of the research process (see Chapter Eighteen for more details on the grant process). Rigor is often expensive, and obtaining funds for health promotion research is typically a competitive process. In addition to other factors (for example, quality of the research proposal, the relevance of the topic and the population, and so on), grant awards, to some extent, are given based on the current degree of engagement in the iterative process shown in Figure 1.5.

Vigilant attention to ethics is the most critical of the three concerns briefly described here (see Chapter Three). Just as practitioners of medicine take the Hippocratic Oath, health promotion researchers must adopt the principle, "First, do no harm." Moreover, health promotion research is highly regulated by local and federal organizations that protect the rights of research participants. The nature of health promotion research demands studies of humans, and these studies are oftentimes directed at very personal (and therefore protected) behaviors.

Summary

Health promotion practice and policy should be based on rigorous research. This chapter has provided a sketch of the research process as it applies to health promotion. This sketch can be used as a platform to gain competence and proficiency in each of the nine steps described. Competence and proficiency in scholarship, grantsmanship, and ethics should be an equally high priority. The remainder of this volume is devoted to expanding this sketch into a more complete primer of health promotion research methods.

KEY TERMS

Cohort	Morbidity
Construct	Mortality
Drift	Paradigm
External validity	Power analysis
Internal validity	Structural intervention
Iterative	

For Practice and Discussion

1. Read a journal article that reports original findings from an empirical investigation of a research question of interest to you. Be sure to read this from cover to cover, very carefully. As you read, please make notes regarding whether the article reports information pertaining to each of the nine steps described in this chapter. Which, if any, of the nine steps was not described in this article? Of the information provided, please briefly describe (a) the study population, (b) the research question, (c) whether this was observational or experimental, (d) the research design that was used, (e) the measures employed, and (f) the sampling plan that was used.

2. Find a colleague who is also learning from this same textbook and discuss with him/her the following question: Is it more important to identify the study population first or the research question first? A bit of background to this question may help—some researchers maintain that the choice of a population is subservient to the larger choice of the research question (which implies that steps 1 and 2 in the nine-step model are reversed). Conversely, other researchers contend that the goal of public health is to rectify disparities experienced by identified populations. With this background in mind, attempt to come to a consensus with the colleague and then compose a one-paragraph justification for your answer.

3. The ninth step of the model may well be the most critical. With this in mind, use the Internet to search for the key term *publication bias*. Learn all that you can about this form of bias and then answer the following two questions.

    a. What are journals currently doing to avert this problem?

    b. For studies that are not acceptable by reputable journals, what obligations do the researchers have relative to step 9, and how can these be met?

4. As you have learned by reading Chapter One, research is a complex undertaking, fraught with pitfalls and barriers to success. Given this reality, consider the question of whether a single study should be used to create a shared dataset (one that—with permission—can be used by other investigators). Then prepare a one-page opinion on this question that may be read in class (or posted online) for your course colleagues (and professor) to consider. In your written opinion, please include possible drawbacks of shared datasets and potential issues that may arise as a result of this practice. It will be equally important to expound on the advantages of shared datasets and the obligation to disseminate findings.

References

Department of Health and Human Services. (2010). *Healthy people 2010*. Available online at www.health.gov/healthypeople. Accessed June 30, 2001.

Glasgow, R. E., Vogt, T. M., and Boles, S. M. (1999). Evaluating the public health impact of health promotion interventions: The RE-AIM framework. *American Journal of Public Health, 89*, 1322–1327.

Green, L. W., & Kreuter, M. W. (2005). *Health program planning: An educational and ecological approach* (4th ed.). Boston: McGraw-Hill.

Kuhn, T. S. (1970). *The structure of scientific revolutions*. Chicago: University of Chicago Press.

Smedley, B. D., and Syme, S. L. (Eds.). (2000). *Promoting health: Intervention strategies from social and behavioral research*. Washington, DC: National Academy Press.

CHAPTER 2

PHILOSOPHY OF SCIENCE AND THEORY CONSTRUCTION

Laura F. Salazar
Ralph J. DiClemente
Richard A. Crosby

Health promotion research, in general, comprises nine steps that are used to investigate health-related behaviors, as described in Chapter One. The overarching goal of health promotion research is to better understand the ways in which we can influence health behaviors and ultimately health by first identifying the behavioral risk factors for a particular disease. By understanding and then affecting behaviors that contribute to health, health promotion researchers can have a substantive impact on the associated morbidity and mortality. In addition to knowing the research process, it is equally important to understand the underlying philosophy when conceptualizing and undertaking health promotion research.

Derived from the Latin word *scientia,* the literal meaning of *science* is knowledge. Yet science can also be viewed as the process of arriving at knowledge. This process entails systematically gathering seemingly disparate facts and then organizing them into an interconnected whole. Science is the process of acquiring knowledge for the purpose of having knowledge. Why is science important, and why do we hold science in such reverence? Because science is knowledge, and knowledge is the source of empowerment. Creating a body of knowledge regarding myriad subjects—such as the properties of matter and energy (physics), the structure of matter (chemistry), living organisms (biology), human behavior (psychology),

LEARNING OBJECTIVES

- Understand what constitutes scientific inquiry and be able to differentiate it from other ways of knowing.

- Understand the health promotion researcher's obligation to employ scientific inquiry for acquiring and evaluating knowledge.

- Learn to critique information that is presented and identify fallacies in arguments.

- Understand how scientific theories are generated and integrate this understanding into your own research

IN A NUTSHELL

Derived from the Latin word *scientia,* the literal meaning of science is knowledge. Yet science can also be viewed as the process of arriving at knowledge. This process entails the systematic gathering of seemingly disparate facts and then organizing them into an interconnected whole. or human societies (sociology), to name a few scientific disciplines—can greatly benefit the human experience and provide insight into how nature works and how we as human beings function within nature and with each other. Think of science as an indispensable tool, much like the wheel, that can take us where we want to go by aiding us in our understanding of, and in our attempt to control, our environment.

In Chapter One, we referred to health promotion research as a discovery process that is analogous to embarking on a journey. If health promotion research is the process through which knowledge of health-related behaviors is "discovered," and science equals knowledge, then health promotion research must be considered a science, right? To answer this question fully and accurately, we first provide an overview of what constitutes science and describe key concepts from its related discipline—the philosophy of science. The word **philosophy** is from the Greek word *philosophia,* meaning love (*philo*) of the pursuit of knowledge (*sophia*). Philosophy of science pertains to the structure, principles, and components of the scientific process—the framework used for the pursuit of knowledge.

Another important and related term used often when discussing the philosophy of science is **epistemology**. Epistemology attempts to answer the basic question: what distinguishes true (adequate) knowledge from false (inadequate) knowledge? René Descartes, referred to as "the father of modern philosophy," embraced **rationalism** in his writings as a way of acquiring knowledge. He is well-known for the philosophical statement "*Cogito ergo sum,*" meaning "I think, therefore I am," and Descartes is considered an epistemologist. Yet in addition to rationalism, there are many other ways of acquiring knowledge, some of which will be described in more detail later in this chapter. As a health promotion practitioner or researcher, you may be called upon to evaluate different types of health information. Learning to distinguish valid health-related information from false information will be an important skill.

The goals of this chapter are to introduce the various epistemological positions taken in pursuit of knowledge, such as authority, tenacity, logic, and, of course, scientific inquiry. Once you have built a solid foundation in epistemology, you may then be in a position to ascertain whether or not specific instances of health promotion research constitute science. Of course, you will also be able to ascertain whether other fields' inquiries can

philosophy
the study of the nature of knowledge

epistemology
a branch of philosophy concerned with distinguishing true knowledge from false knowledge

rationalism
the belief that reason is a fundamental source of knowledge

be considered science, **junk science**, or neither. Consequently, you will also acquire insight about how scientific knowledge is generated.

Epistemology: Ways of Acquiring Knowledge

The way in which knowledge is generated determines whether or not it should be deemed science and therefore added to an overall scientific body of knowledge. Given that science is a process in which we gather knowledge and organize that knowledge systematically, just because an effort is conducted "in the name of science" does not necessarily make it science. Second, although *science* literally means knowledge, in the modern sense it refers to a process that adheres to specific standards and methods of generating knowledge. We come by knowledge about the world in many different ways. Some of these ways of gathering knowledge may contribute to science; other ways may appear to be scientific but are not science in the technical sense. Regardless of the method, knowledge is conveyed (although the value of that knowledge will vary depending on the context in which it is presented). Thus not all knowledge is created equal. It is most important to know the different ways or methods in which we accrue knowledge so that the quality of the knowledge can be judged appropriately and the implications for choosing one method over another can be determined.

In the following section, we describe various ways we acquire knowledge, such as through **authority** or **tenacity** (sometimes called tradition) and **logic** and reason, which are not considered scientific in the modern sense but nevertheless provide new ideas and suggestions. We also describe **scientific inquiry** as a way of generating knowledge. The former methods (authority, tenacity, and logic) are ways in which knowledge is derived, so they are important to know. By understanding these alternative epistemologies you will better understand science. Consequently, you may embrace scientific inquiry as the most important way of knowing. As you will see, these epistemologies must be evaluated rather subjectively and contrast sharply with scientific inquiry as a way of knowing, because science is able to provide both a body of knowledge and a specific method in which to evaluate that knowledge.

Unfortunately, in some instances science may not yet have contributed to a specific research goal, so it may not be an available source of knowledge. For example, in the early 1980s, before the etiologic cause of compromised immune systems—later deemed *acquired immune deficiency syndrome* (AIDS)—was discovered, researchers were unsure exactly what was causing the syndrome or how it was being transmitted. Epistemologies such as authority, tenacity, and logic were first called upon to formulate theories,

junk science
data, research, or analysis that is spurious or fraudulent

authority
acquiring knowledge from experts or from those in power

tenacity
acquiring knowledge from myths, superstitions, or other cultural means

logic
acquiring knowledge through reasoning or inference

scientific inquiry
acquiring knowledge regarding the nature of the universe through testing ideas, evaluating questions, and determining how things work

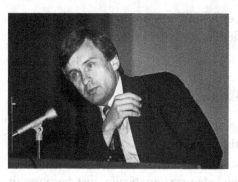

Figure 2.1 Dr. Jim Curran

which were used to explain the phenomenon and were later tested as hypotheses using scientific inquiry. In fact, one of the key researchers at the Centers for Disease Control and Prevention, Dr. Jim Curran (Figure 2.1), who was on the task force to understand the disease, was purported to ask, "What do we think, what do we know, and what can we prove?" In essence, scientific inquiry is the only epistemology that requires data-driven conclusions and provides answers to the question "What can we prove?" Other epistemologies exist regardless of whether data are available or whether people choose to consider the data. The challenge in those instances is to examine the underlying source of the knowledge and make the best possible determination regarding its accuracy.

Authority

Albert Einstein dubbed the renowned mathematician and scientist Galileo "the father of modern physics—indeed of modern science altogether" (Sobel, 1999, p. 326). Most everyone is familiar with the historical account of Galileo and his quest to advance the field of science, which up to that point in history was based mostly on the philosophy of Aristotle. Galileo sought to move beyond an understanding of *why* **phenomena** *(things or events that are difficult to explain but can be observed)* occur to *how* they occur. For Galileo, mathematics was one of his scientific tools. According to Galileo:

> Philosophy is written in this grand book the universe, which stands continually open to our gaze. But the book cannot be understood unless one first learns to comprehend the language and to read the alphabet in which it is composed. It is written in the language of mathematics, and its characters are triangles, circles, and other geometric figures, without which it is humanly impossible to understand a single word of it; without these, one wanders about in a dark labyrinth. [quoted in Drake, 1957, p. 237]

Although most scientists agree that Galileo's greatest contribution to **science** is his application of mathematics to the study of motion, he has been immortalized for his defense of Copernicus's theory that posited the sun rather than the Earth as the center of the cosmos. This sun-as-center-of-the-universe perspective was not only contrary to the Aristotelian

phenomena
events or circumstances evident to the senses and possible to describe scientifically

science
knowledge generated about the world and universe based on experiments and observation

perspective (Aristotle believed that the Earth was the center of the cosmos), but more important, it contradicted the teachings and beliefs espoused by the Catholic Church, which based its views on the Aristotelian perspective.

During this period in history, the Catholic Church was for many the moral and philosophical authority. If the Catholic Church said it was so, then most people accepted it for fact. Most people did not understand the order of the universe at this time. Hence it was easier for people to defer to some authority, one who held some degree of knowledge regarding an issue. People during this era mostly obtained their knowledge through authority because there were not many other sources. This approach has a major shortcoming, however; the authority in question can be wrong, as was the case with the Church's adherence to the Aristotelian perspective. Unfortunately, because Galileo went against the most powerful authority of his time, he was "tried by the Church" in front of the Inquisition. Refusing to recant his beliefs, Galileo was sentenced to life imprisonment, which was later reduced to house arrest (Sobel, 1999).

In his search for knowledge, Galileo truly believed that "the authority of a thousand is not worth the humble *reasoning* of a single individual" (Redondi, 1987, p. 37). Even in our contemporary times this attitude should still apply. Failing to evaluate the validity of an authority's ideas, suggestions, or comments is problematic. Of course, an evaluation of the knowledge transferred by authority would require knowing what evidence (if any) the authority is using. For example, when the United States president describes the current "state of the union," we should consider whether or not the description is based on scientific evidence (such as gathering of key economic indicators, scientific surveys, archival data, and so on) or on anecdotal evidence from a few people or, even worse, is not based on any evidence at all but is simply rhetoric. Furthermore, when a physician instructs a patient to drink eight eight-ounce glasses of water per day, the patient should consider whether this recommendation is based on scientific evidence or on tenacity with no real basis (see Box 2.1, which describes an investigation into the origins of the health recommendation to drink eight glasses of water per day). Even with your professors (including the one teaching this course), you should question knowledge presented in class and inquire about the epistemology being applied. These are only a few ways in which to question authority, but as health promotion researchers and purveyors of knowledge, you should learn to question the knowledge that is presented to you. Moreover, you have an obligation to employ scientific inquiry regardless of the prevailing epistemologies of the day. As with Galileo, however, be warned that your research may not be popular or readily accepted by society. Yet as Albert Einstein stated, "A foolish faith in authority is the worst enemy of truth" (quoted in Calaprice, 2000, p. 303).

BOX 2.1. THE "8 × 8" RECOMMENDATION

Valtin (2002) conducted a review of the scientific literature to determine the origin of the advice to "drink at least eight eight-ounce glasses of water per day." He found no scientific studies in support of the "8 × 8" health recommendation, and he could not find its origins in the scientific literature. In fact, he found evidence to suggest that such large amounts of water are not necessary in *healthy* adults who live in temperate climates and are largely sedentary. Moreover, his review of a large body of related research suggested that the human body's osmoregulatory system maintains water balance naturally. Thus it would appear that the ubiquitous "8 × 8" recommendation is without scientific merit, but it persists as a modern myth that is viewed as medically beneficial.

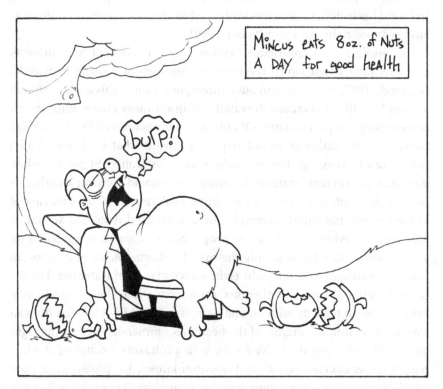

Mincus Takes Dr. Dincus's Advice for Good Health

Tenacity or Tradition

Even in this postmodern age of technology, many health beliefs that have been around for a very long time and are sometimes even referred to as "old wives' tales" still remain firmly entrenched in our culture and continue to influence our health behaviors. For example, were you told that it is dangerous to swim unless you wait an hour after eating? Were you scolded for going outside as a child with wet hair because it would cause you to catch a cold? Did your mother tell you that you should eat all of your carrots because it will improve your eyesight? Certainly you have heard the expression, "An apple a day helps keep the doctor away." Do you still believe that chocolate causes acne? Are you familiar with the notion that oysters are an aphrodisiac? Many young women maintain that they cannot get pregnant while breastfeeding or the very first time they have vaginal intercourse. A more recent health belief that has become somewhat entrenched in modern society is that the flu vaccine will cause you to get the flu. Not surprisingly, some of these health beliefs may be rooted in truth, which may explain their longevity. For example, eating vegetables high in vitamin A (for example, carrots) *is* good for maintaining healthy eyesight; however, having more than the recommended daily requirement will not improve your eyesight. Also, the flu vaccine takes a full two weeks to afford protection, so it is possible to contract the flu shortly after getting vaccinated. What is surprising is that some of these health beliefs continue to persist despite the fact they have been proven false, hence the term "*tenacity*." For example, many people still believe that going out in cold weather with wet hair will cause them to catch a cold, even though science has shown it is exposure to a virus that causes a cold. Also, the flu vaccine uses inactivated or dead viruses, so it cannot cause you to get the flu.

Why do these beliefs persist even though they are false? Many have been handed down from one generation to the next through storytelling and printed material, and presently through other forms of media. For many cultures, these beliefs become part of their tradition, and as tradition they tend to provide people with an acceptable way of seeming to exert control over certain unavoidable events. Hence accepting traditional beliefs as a way of knowing at a very basic level serves to help people feel that they understand and have some measure of control over their environment.

Health beliefs based on tradition, whether true or not, may also contribute to the cohesiveness of a cultural group. Unified cultures are grounded in their acceptance of similar beliefs and traditions. Female genital mutilation (FGM) is one example of a cultural tradition that has absolutely no scientific health benefit and in fact has severe long-term physical consequences. In many communities where it is practiced, it is believed to reduce a woman's libido and help her to resist sexual opportunities. According to the World Health Organization (WHO), FGM is most common in the western, eastern, and north-eastern regions of Africa, in some countries in Asia and the Middle East, and among migrants from these areas. Unfortunately, about 140 million girls and women worldwide are living with the consequences of FGM. Surprisingly, 18 percent of FGMs are performed by health care providers, and this number is increasing (World Health Organization, 2013). It is for these reasons that using only tenacity as a valid way of knowing can be problematic: if the beliefs are erroneous, then there will be great difficulty in changing or discrediting them once they have been accepted widely and are entrenched within a culture. It may be useful for you to think about different health beliefs you have accepted and consider whether they are based on tradition or evidence.

Logic and Reasoning

The term *logic* is derived from the Greek word *logos*, which can mean "word," "thought," "principle," or "speech." The term *logos* has been used by both philosophers and theologians and embodies both human reason (that is, intellect, the capacity to discern and distinguish) and universal intelligence (that is, the Divine). Although philosophers are undoubtedly concerned with both aspects of *logos*, as health promotion researchers we are concerned mainly with the human-reason aspect for this construct. Reason, along with its cousin term *logic*, is the foundation of philosophy and is still in use today as a way of knowing.

In modern terms, *logic* can be defined as the science of reasoning, proof, thinking, or inference. Logic is useful in that it allows you to analyze arguments or a piece of reasoning and determine whether or not they are accurate or "illogical." Having a foundation in logic and reasoning can assist you in spotting the arguments that are invalid and conclusions that are false.

As previously stated, the Catholic Church based much of its beliefs and knowledge on another authority—Aristotle. Because Aristotle concerned himself with the investigation of natural phenomena, he was able to make many observations about the world. He then used logic and reasoning to define, analyze, and systematize his observations to make sense of what he observed. Logic and reasoning were his tools; in the absence of science, logic and reasoning were the accepted standards of the time.

syllogism
an argument of a very specific form, consisting of two premises and a conclusion

More specifically, Aristotle used an approach called a **syllogism**—an argument of a very specific form consisting of two premises and a conclusion—to amass his knowledge. Generating knowledge regarding the Earth and the cosmos, Aristotle used the following syllogism:

Again, everything that moves with the circular movement, except the first sphere, is observed to be passed, and to move with more than one motion. The earth, then, also, whether it move about the centre or as stationary at it, must necessarily move with two motions. But if this were so, there would have to be passings and turnings of the fixed stars. Yet no such thing is observed. The same stars always rise and set in the same parts of the earth [Aristotle, 350 B.C., part 14, paragraph 1].

Using this syllogism, Aristotle concluded that "the earth, spherical in shape, is at rest in the centre of the universe" (Aristotle, 350 B.C., part 14, paragraph 4). Of course, it was later ascertained that Aristotle's conclusion was inaccurate. His syllogism contained a **fallacy**. In logic, the term *fallacy* has a very specific meaning: a fallacy is a technical flaw that makes an argument unsound or invalid. In this instance, the premises of Aristotle's argument were not true. Although his conclusion was sound, it was based on false premises and was therefore false. There are many other types of fallacies that occur quite frequently, such as a fallacy called *cum hoc ergo propter hoc* ("with this, therefore because of this"), which is to assert that because two events coincide, they must be causally related. An example for this type of fallacy would be

fallacy
a technical flaw that makes an argument unsound or invalid

> *Roosters tend to crow when the sun rises; therefore, the crowing of the roosters causes the sun to rise.*

Another example would be

> *Teenagers tend to eat a lot of chocolate and also tend to have acne; therefore, eating chocolate causes teen acne.*

Another fallacy is called *"converse accident"* or *"hasty generalization,"* which is the reverse of the fallacy deemed *"accident."* Converse accident or hasty generalization is the fallacy associated with prejudicial beliefs and occurs when you generalize to an entire group based on a few specific cases (hence "hasty"), which are not truly representative of all possible cases. The following statement is an example of converse accident: "Professor Dincus is eccentric. Therefore *all* professors are eccentric."

In contrast, the fallacy "accident" is referred to as a "sweeping generalization" and occurs when a general rule is applied to a specific situation, though the features of that particular situation indicate that an exception to the rule should be made. For example, "College students generally like junk food. *You* are a college student, therefore you must like junk food." Finally, another type of fallacy is called *post hoc ergo propter hoc* (after this, therefore because of this), which occurs when a cause-and-effect relationship is assumed because one factor occurred temporally before the other factor. For example, "After receiving his flu vaccine, Rick came down with the flu; therefore, we must avoid the flu vaccine because it *caused* him to get the flu."

Currently people still rely on information that is derived from logic and reasoning, especially if there are no alternative ways of knowing. Yet much information derived from logic and reasoning is based on arguments that may contain fallacies. Another issue with this way of knowing is that arguments cannot determine whether a statement is correct. Thus, as a way of knowing, logic and reasoning are useful, but only if the arguments presented do not contain fallacies and if there are alternative ways to verify the conclusions. The challenge is to critique any arguments or information presented to you and to attempt to uncover any fallacies.

Scientific Inquiry as Epistemology

Scientific inquiry or research is conducted as a means to test ideas, to evaluate questions, and to determine how things work. Generally speaking, the goal is to generate knowledge regarding the nature of our universe. Understanding the nature of our universe can range from knowing and understanding weather patterns to knowing and understanding people's exercise patterns. Scientific inquiry is simply another way of knowing, but as you will discover, it is quite different from the other epistemologies described previously. For one thing, "research is a disciplined way we come to know what we know" (Bouma and Atkinson, 1995, p. 9). It involves a process as described in Chapter One, but it also posits certain structures or components to that process. Concepts and structures such as *empiricism, data, theory, inductivism, hypothetico-deductivism,* and *falsification* are the main building blocks of scientific inquiry and constitute the foundation of modern science. The scientific process is depicted in Figure 2.2. Furthermore, it is because of these concepts and structures that scientific inquiry as an epistemology is considered more reliable and valid than other methods of inquiry.

> **IN A NUTSHELL**
>
> Concepts and structures such as empiricism, data, theory, hypothetico-deductivism, and falsification are the main building blocks of scientific inquiry and constitute the foundation of modern science.

Empiricism. From its inception, science has been a process that is objective and *empirical.* Derived from the Greek word *émpeiria,* meaning experienced or skilled, empiricism is a theory of knowledge that posits true knowledge is a product of sensory perceptions gleaned from observation, meaning that our understanding or awareness of phenomena is derived from direct experiences considered as evidence. Within the philosophy

empiricism
a theory of knowledge that suggests true knowledge is a product of sensory perceptions gleaned from observation

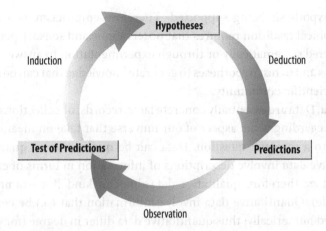

Figure 2.2 The Scientific Process
Source: Explorable.com (Sep 21, 2009). Empirical Research. Retrieved September 17, 2014 from https://explorable.com/empirical-research.

of science, empiricism denotes observation and experimentation and is therefore linked literally to the concept of scientific inquiry. As such, empiricism is considered a foundation of research in that all hypotheses and theories must be tested against observations of the natural world rather than resting solely on **a priori** logic, reasoning, or intuition. The strength of adopting this position is that many important research questions can be answered objectively through the collection of empirical *data*.

Because empiricism relies on sensory perceptions, observations, and evidence, it is important to distinguish how empirical evidence is collected and ultimately used to generate knowledge and draw conclusions when scientific inquiry is involved versus other epistemologies. For example, referring back to our previous example of a *post hoc ergo propter hoc* fallacy wherein Rick incorrectly concludes that the flu vaccine caused him to get the flu, it is true that Rick's conclusion was based on his sensory perception and direct experience of having the flu after he was vaccinated. By this definition, Rick used empirical evidence; however, he did not gather the evidence to test a hypothesis. Rather, Rick used logic and reasoning—albeit **a posteriori**—rather than scientific inquiry to try and understand why he got the flu even though he received the vaccine. In contrast, if the "flu vaccine causes one to get the flu" hypothesis were to be tested scientifically, it would require a sample of people who had been vaccinated and then multiple observations made and expanded on to also include the date the vaccine was administered, the date when flu symptoms began, known allergies, the strain of flu contracted, and so on. These observations would constitute empirical evidence and, combined with statistics, we could use them to determine with some degree of confidence the likelihood

a priori
literally "from the earlier," refers to knowledge that stems from deduction rather than experience

a posteriori
literally "from the later," refers to knowledge obtained through direct observation or empirical evidence

of our hypothesis being supported. Therefore empiricism as a scientific philosophical tradition requires that observations and sensory perceptions be collected systematically or through experimentation to answer research questions and to test hypotheses to generate knowledge that can be accepted by the scientific community.

Data. Data are essentially concrete facts, records, or collections of information regarding some aspect of our universe that take on meaning when applied to a research question. Data can be **qualitative** or **quantitative**. Qualitative data involve descriptions of information in terms of categories or qualities; therefore qualitative data differ in kind (for example, male vs. female). Quantitative data involve information that can be counted or expressed numerically; thus quantitative data differ in degree (for example, an IQ of 150 is greater than an IQ of 100). Whether qualitative or quantitative, empirical data can be used to answer many types of research questions in health promotion. For example, "Does a low-saturated-fat diet reduce LDL cholesterol?" is a research question for which there is an answer that can be derived from empirical data. In this instance, empirical data collected to answer this question would be LDL cholesterol levels of people prior to changing their diet and after changing their diet, as well as cholesterol levels of people who did not change their diets. It is important to note one limitation of strictly adopting empiricism: some research questions cannot be answered using this method alone because the answers cannot be derived from empirical data. For example, "Is Brand X cholesterol drug's *name* better than Brand Y cholesterol drug's name?" is a question for which there are no empirical data available. Of course, we could modify the question into an empirical question by asking, for example, do women aged forty-five to seventy-five who have high cholesterol judge Brand X's name to be better than Brand Y's name? We could then survey women in this age category who have high cholesterol and ask them which name they like better. The women's survey responses would constitute the empirical data.

data
concrete facts, records, or collections of information regarding some aspect of the universe that takes on meaning when applied to a research question

qualitative
descriptions of information in terms of categories or qualities

quantitative
information that can be counted or expressed numerically

Other types of data commonly used in health promotion research are presented in Table 2.1. As shown, these data are integral to the research process and help us answer many empirical research questions in health promotion such as "Are teens smoking at a lower rate in 2010 than in 2000?," "Is there a difference in alcohol consumption rates among Whites, Blacks,

IN A NUTSHELL

Data are essentially concrete facts, records, or collections of information regarding some aspect of our universe that take on meaning when applied to a research question. Data can be qualitative (that is, differ in kind) or quantitative (that is, differ in degree).

Table 2.1   Types of Data Used in Health Promotion Research

Data Collected	Sample items for Assessment
Qualitative	
Gender	What is your gender? 1 Male 2 Female 3 Transgender
Race	What is your race? 1 American Indian or Alaska native 2 Asian 3 Black or African American 4 Pacific Islander 5 White
Hispanic origin	Are you of Hispanic origin, such as Mexican-American, Puerto Rican, Cuban, or South American? 1 Yes 2 No
Education level	What is the highest grade you completed in school? 1 Grade school or less 2 Some high school 3 High school graduate 4 Some college 5 College graduate 6 Post-graduate or professional degree
Smoking behavior	How would you describe your cigarette smoking habits? 1 Never smoked 2 Used to smoke 3 Still smoke
Quantitative	
Height	What is your height? _____Feet _____Inches
Weight	What is your weight (without shoes)? _____Pounds
Alcohol use behavior	How many drinks of an alcoholic beverage do you have in a typical week? ____Bottles or cans of beer ____Glasses of wine ____Wine coolers ____Mixed drinks or shots of liquor
Diet and nutrition	During the past month, not counting juice, how many times per day, week, or month did you eat fruit? Count fresh, frozen, or canned fruit 1 _ _ Per day 2 _ _ Per week 3 _ _ Per month 4 _ _ Never
Physical Activity	In an average week, how many times do you engage in physical activity (exercise or work which lasts at least twenty minutes without stopping and which is hard enough to make you breathe heavier and your heart beat faster)? 1 Less than 1 time per week 2 1 or 2 times per week 3 At least 3 times per week

and Latinos?" and "Are adults in the Midwestern United States eating five servings of fruit and vegetables each day following a social marketing campaign to encourage five a day?" When conducting research to answer a health-related question, it is critical that the research question is constructed so that it is an empirical question, verifiable and falsifiable from the beginning, and can be answered by collecting appropriate and relevant data.

theory
an idea based on observations that guides the research question and provides order and structure to sets of relationships

Theory. If science were a movie, then theory would be the screenplay. No matter how talented the actors are, a good screenplay is still necessary to provide the framework in which the actors showcase their talents. Without the screenplay, they are simply improvising. For some talented actors, improvisation may work; however, for the majority of actors, a cohesive and intriguing plot coupled with realistic dialogue is critical. In science, theories play a major role as well because they provide a basis for understanding phenomena. In other words, they organize relationships among "characters" (that is, observations) into a coherent picture of what it all means. They provide a starting point for making future predictions as well. Furthermore, theories guide the research question.

> **IN A NUTSHELL**
>
> If science were a movie, then theory would be the screenplay.

hypothesis
a statement that specifies the nature of the relationships between variables

What exactly constitutes a scientific theory? How are theories generated? And how does a theory contrast with a **hypothesis**? Many people use the term *theory* interchangeably with *hypothesis*; however, theory expands on simple hypotheses and considers sets of relationships. *Hypotheses* are statements that specify the nature of the relationships between variables, whereas a *theory* is much more involved and provides order and structure to sets of relationships. For example, the statement "Obesity is related to increased risk of breast cancer among postmenopausal women" is a hypothesis that could be tested by comparing incidence of breast cancer among postmenopausal women who are not obese to incidence among postmenopausal women who are obese. A theory, however, would account for differences in breast cancer rates by describing the causative interaction of physiological, environmental, and psychological variables.

phenomenological
a theoretical explanation that describes and generalizes phenomena without specific reference to causal mechanisms

explanatory
a theoretical explanation that identifies and explains the underlying causal mechanism of phenomena

It is important to note that the phenomena involved in a theory must also be verifiable, meaning we can measure them or observe them either directly or indirectly. Once phenomena are measured or observed, understanding them translates into two types of theoretical explanations: **phenomenological** and **explanatory**. In a phenomenological theory, phenomena are described and generalized, but without specific reference to causal mechanisms. Newton's third law ("For every action there is an equal and opposite reaction") is one example. In contrast, an explanatory theory identifies and explains the *why* or underlying causal mechanism. An example of an explanatory theory would be the theory of general relativity, which explains that the force known as gravity arises from distortions in the space-time continuum caused by massive objects such as planets.

Most theories used in health promotion research are phenomenological theories that describe factors related to or influencers of health-related behaviors. For example, the health belief model (HBM) is a theory of behavior developed in the 1950s by a group of social psychologists who wanted to better understand the widespread failure of people to participate in programs to prevent or to detect disease (Janz, Champion, and Stretcher, 2002). The HBM, depicted in Figure 2.3, posits that individual perceptions, certain modifying factors, and a likelihood of action are related to health behavior. The HBM has been applied to the description of various health behaviors for which much research has generated support for the theory. Such behaviors include flu inoculations, breast self-examination, blood pressure screening, seatbelt use, exercise, nutrition, smoking, and regular checkups. Other types of behavior that have been tested include compliance with drug regimens, diabetic regimens, and weight loss regimens.

Given the critical role of theory in science, how are theories generated initially before they are widely implemented? In the case of the HBM, the theory grew out of the academic backgrounds of the theorists and the other theories to which they were exposed. Although there are several strategies for developing theories, such as using intuition,

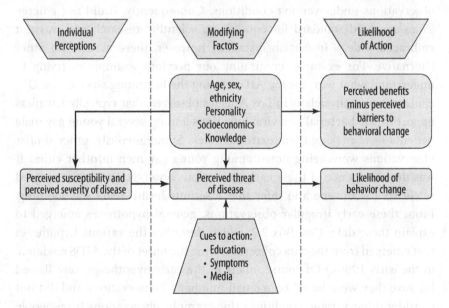

Figure 2.3 Health Belief Model Components and Linkages

Baconian inductivism
a method developed by Francis Bacon based on empirical and inductive principles and the active development of new arts and inventions, with the ultimate goal of producing practical knowledge

hypothetico-deductivism
a method developed by Isaac Newton that entailed beginning with a hypothesis and using deduction to make predictions for a specific event that could be tested through empirical observation

previous knowledge, and personal observation, only two main strategies will be described in this section: **Baconian inductivism** and **hypothetico-deductivism**. Both methods were conceptualized centuries ago and are still in use today. Each has its own strengths and weaknesses, but determining which method to use depends greatly on the domain or scope in which the theory will apply.

During the time Galileo was honing new methods to study phenomena, Francis Bacon (1561–1626) "proposed an entirely new system based on empirical and inductive principles and the active development of new arts and inventions, a system whose ultimate goal would be the production of practical knowledge for 'the use and benefit of men' and the relief of the human condition" (Internet Encyclopedia of Philosophy, n.d., paragraph 1). His system or method, later called Baconian inductivism, comprised four steps:

1. Observation and classification of relevant facts
2. Generalization by means of inductive reasoning
3. Construction of a theoretical framework that allows one to deduce predictions from its laws and postulates
4. Verification of the predictions

Although a great improvement over other nonscientific methods for generating knowledge, Baconian inductivism has two major flaws: it cannot be used to derive theories regarding phenomena that are unobservable (for example, gravity), and its validity depends on a large number of observations under varying conditions. Consequently, it did not emerge as an accepted standard for conducting scientific research and was not embraced widely. In certain instances, however, there may be no other alternative. For example, continuing our previous example of trying to understand what was causing AIDS during the beginning stage of the U.S. epidemic, two physicians in Los Angeles observed that typically harmless opportunistic bacterial and viral infections among several young gay male patients were making them extremely sick. Simultaneously, other similar observations were being noted among young gay men in other cities. It was the emergence of these early anomalous observations that prompted scientists to convene and infer that a serious health issue was looming. From these early irregular observations, general hypotheses emerged to explain these data. (See Box 2.2, which describes the various hypotheses that emerged from the data collected during the onset of the AIDS epidemic in the early 1980s.) Of course, many of the early hypotheses were flawed because they were based on a small number of observations and did not consider other varying conditions (for example, observations from people who contracted the syndrome but were not gay).

BOX 2.2. EARLY AIDS HYPOTHESES

In the beginning of the epidemic, AIDS was referred to as GRID—Gay-related immunodeficiency disease. The name was not changed to Acquired Immune Deficiency Syndrome until 1982. These are some of the early AIDS hypotheses (note, not "theories") that were inferred from the available data (Garrett, 1994).

- A virus called "cytomegalovirus" or "CMV superinfection" is the root, where repeated exposures to the virus result in the deadly syndrome.

- Gay men have been exposed to too many microbes and have "microbial overload," causing the immune system to self-destruct.

- The recreation drug called "poppers" (amyl nitrites) plays a critical role in the deadly syndrome, along with other gay lifestyle practices such as "fisting," "rimming," or steroid skin creams.

- AIDS is caused by some new variety of the HTLV virus, a virus that causes immune system disruptions and cancer.

- AIDS is an opportunistic infection, causing disease only in persons who are already immunocompromised from other microbes or conditions.

- AIDS is a new manifestation of the hepatitis B virus.

- AIDS is caused by an unknown contaminant of the hepatitis vaccine (early experimental trials of the vaccine had been conducted with gay men).

- AIDS is caused by African swine fever.

Following Bacon in the late 1600s, Sir Isaac Newton (1642–1727) developed a scientific method, later termed "hypothetico-deductivism," which is essentially the opposite of Baconian inductivism. His method entailed beginning with a hypothesis or statement of general principles and subsequently using deduction to make predictions for a specific event. The predictions could be tested through empirical observation and in this way verified, modified, or rejected.

The strength of hypothetico-deductivism lies in the ability to test any hypothesis and confirm its validity through empirical observation. For example, using this method, Newton was able to test his theory of gravitation, which he used to guide him in deducing specific predictions for which he was then able to make observations that supported or verified his theory. Thus, as a method, hypothetico-deductivism was a great improvement over inductivism and emerged as the new method for generating reliable and valid knowledge.

IN A NUTSHELL

Research conducted with the main purpose of confirming a theory may, over time, become irrelevant as the theory is modified and perhaps rejected. Moreover, a set of data cannot irrevocably confirm or prove that a theory is valid, because different theories can be supported by the same set of data.

However, hypothetico-deductivisim is not without its problems. Research conducted with the main purpose of confirming a theory may, over time, become irrelevant as the theory is modified and perhaps rejected. Moreover, a set of data cannot irrevocably confirm or prove that a theory is valid, because different theories can be supported by the same set of data. Such was the case for Newton's theory of gravitation. Although it withstood the test of time for over two hundred years because the data collected perfectly supported its predictions, Newton's theory was eventually displaced by Einstein's theory of gravity—general relativity—as general relativity was able to provide clarification and refinement that allowed predictions to hold true in a greater range of observable circumstances.

falsification

the idea that scientists must begin with hypotheses that can be refuted before observations are made

Falsification. Sir Karl Popper (1902–1994), considered one of the most influential twentieth-century philosophers of science, asserted that for a theory to be scientific, a necessary condition is that the theory consist of hypotheses that can be falsified For example, *all monkeys like to eat bananas* is a statement that can be supported through confirmatory evidence in the form of observing "lots of monkeys eating bananas"; however, the statement can also be falsified because of the possibility that one could potentially observe at least one monkey who doesn't like to eat bananas. Therefore in order for a theory or hypothesis to be falsified it must be verifiable, and it must *allow for* the collection of observations that could potentially refute it. Thus the statement *God exists*, although a strong religious belief held by many around the world, can neither be verified nor refuted.

demarcation criterion

the necessity for a scientific theory to be falsifiable

Because falsification asserts that theories must allow for its assertions to be refuted with empirical evidence, Popper advocated that *falsification* rather than verification alone is the best approach for testing scientific theories. This necessity for a scientific theory to be falsifiable is known as the **demarcation criterion**. Advocating the use of falsifiability as a scientific method to test theories, Popper therefore rejected inductivism, because falsification dictates that you must begin with falsifiable hypotheses before observations are made. Then you collect data to refute them—not to verify them. As noted earlier, it is easy for the same set of data to support or verify many different theories simultaneously. Hence falsification provides more rigor and confidence in the conclusions.

Integration with the Research Process

Integrating the research process with these underlying scientific principles will provide a better understanding of health phenomena. To accomplish this integration, health promotion researchers should undertake the nine steps delineated in Chapter One while interjecting scientific structure to those steps. For example, theory should be used to aid in the development of the research question (step 2) and in the choice of variables to be measured (step 5). The research questions should be empirical questions formulated from theory and verifiable through empirical observation. Moreover, the research design should allow for the falsification of the proposed hypotheses (step 4). The variables chosen also have to allow for empirical measurement. And finally, data analysis (step 8) should go beyond whether or not the data confirm or support the hypotheses to include falsification. If health promotion research incorporates these scientific principles, then health promotion as a field will continue to expand as a true scientific discipline.

Summary

Over the centuries, science has revolutionized its sources of knowledge, moving from authority, tenacity, and logic and reason to an elegant arrangement encompassing principles of empiricism, data, theory, deduction, and falsification. As science is considered a process that aids in our understanding of our world, throughout time, numerous scientific disciplines pertaining to specific aspects of our world have emerged. Health promotion can be considered one of the more modern scientific disciplines, but only if it adheres to sound scientific principles. In this chapter, we reviewed the philosophy of science from its origins to better understand the underlying concepts and the importance of science to health promotion research. We noted that one of the most critical scientific principles is the generation and rigorous testing of theory. As we are health promotion researchers investigating health-related behaviors, most of what we do should be grounded in theory. Theory constitutes the basic structure of our scientific inquiries for two reasons: theory guides the design of basic research studies, and theory can be used to design a health promotion program that targets risk factors deemed modifiable and that are related to health-related outcomes.

KEY TERMS

A posteriori	Junk science
A priori	Logic
Authority	Phenomena
Baconian inductivism	Phenomenological
Data	Philosophy
Demarcation criterion	Qualitative
Empiricism	Quantitative
Epistemology	Rationalism
Explanatory	Science
Fallacy	Scientific inquiry
Falsification	Syllogism
Hypothesis	Tenacity
Hypothetico-deductivism	Theory

For Practice and Discussion

1. Write a statement that you feel is true regarding the cause(s) for a specific public health issue, such as HIV/AIDS, obesity, type 2 diabetes, or cardiovascular disease. For each cause, try and identify the source of your knowledge and what epistemologies you applied. Try to create a syllogism that describes the logic on which your conclusion is based. Can you identify any fallacies? If so, what are they?

2. Choose a public health issue of interest and develop a research question that would help contribute to the knowledge base regarding the issue. What types of data would you collect to answer the question? Is the question an empirical question—meaning is it verifiable and falsifiable—and can it be answered by collecting appropriate and relevant data? Discuss why you consider your question to be an empirical question.

3. Identify a theory or theories that you are familiar with which is related to public health and/or health promotion. Discuss the type of theory it is (phenomenological or explanatory). Also, state whether it is verifiable, and describe the type of data or evidence you would need to collect to verify the theory.

4. Read a journal article of interest that involves an empirical study in public health. Discuss the hypotheses tested in the study. What were the hypotheses based on? What types of data were collected during the course of the study? What was the theoretical framework for the study? Did the study seek to verify the hypotheses or falsify them? Were the hypotheses supported? What conclusions did the investigators reach? Can you identify possible alternative explanations for the findings?

References

Aristotle. (350 B.C.). *On the heavens*. J. L. Stocks (trans.). Retrieved November 19, 2004, from http://classics.mit.edu/Aristotle/heavens.2.ii.html

Bouma, G. D., and Atkinson, G.B.J. (1995). *A handbook of social science research*. New York: Oxford University Press.

Calaprice, A. (Ed.). (2000). *The expanded quotable Einstein*. Princeton, NJ: Princeton University Press.

Drake, S. (1957). *Discoveries and opinions of Galileo*. Garden City, NY: Doubleday Anchor Books.

Garrett, L. (1994). *The coming plague: Newly emerging diseases in a world out of balance*. New York: Farrar, Straus, and Giroux.

Internet Encyclopedia of Philosophy. (n.d.). Francis Bacon. Retrieved November 19, 2004, from www.iep.utm.edu/b/bacon.htm

Janz, N. K., Champion, V. L., and Stretcher, V. J. (2002). The health belief model. In K. Glanz, B. K. Rimer, and F. M. Lewis (Eds.), *Health behavior and health education* (3rd ed., pp. 45–66). San Francisco: Jossey-Bass.

Redondi, P. (1987). *Galileo: Heretic*. R. Rosenthal (trans.). Princeton, NJ: Princeton University Press.

Sobel, D. (1999). *Galileo's daughter: A historical memoir of science, faith, and love*. New York: Walker and Co.

Valtin, H. (2002). "Drink at least eight glasses of water a day." Really? Is there scientific evidence for "8 × 8"? *American Journal of Physiology—Regulatory Integrative and Comparative Physiology, 283*(5), R993–R1004.

World Health Organization. (2013). Female genital mutilation. Fact sheet No. 241. Updated February 2013. Accessed April 24, 2013, from http://www.who.int/mediacentre/factsheets/fs241/en/

CHAPTER 3

ETHICAL ISSUES IN HEALTH PROMOTION RESEARCH

Richard A. Crosby
Laura F. Salazar
Ralph J. DiClemente

Health promotion research commonly involves biomedical or behavioral research; health promotion practice involves implementing biomedical or behavioral interventions. Protections for human subjects and program participants are essential to minimize risk and maximize benefit in both research and practice. In the United States, federal guidelines are in place to ensure that researchers adhere to core ethical principles such as respect for persons, beneficence, and justice. Moreover, professional associations have developed ethical codes of conduct for health promotion practitioners. Ultimately, the protection of human beings in the context of health promotion research and practice is dependent on informed and conscientious researchers and practitioners.

Ethical conduct should be fundamental to any type of research, particularly research involving human subjects; however, history indicates that this has not always been the case. Egregious and unethical conduct in the past, ranging from the atrocities committed by the Nazis during World War II on concentration camp inmates to the United States Public Health Service's deceptive and harmful research with African-American men in Tuskegee, Alabama (the "Tuskegee Syphilis Study") eventually led to significant changes in policy regarding the conducting of both biomedical and behavioral research on humans. Today, research involving human subjects is bound by

LEARNING OBJECTIVES

- **Understand the historical precedent for the federal regulations governing human subjects.**

- **Learn the basic ethical principles underlying the federal regulations.**

- **Apply the principles to health promotion research and practice.**

- **Know which populations are considered vulnerable and are afforded special consideration in research.**

- **Learn the different categories of research.**

- **Understand the role of and oversight by Institutional Review Boards.**

a specific code of federal regulations (CFR) with strong ethical underpinnings and designed to protect human subjects, commonly referred to as 45 CFR 46. It is important to note that when we refer to research, it has a very specific meaning: a "systematic investigation, including research development, testing and evaluation, designed to develop or contribute to generalizable knowledge." Researchers conducting federally funded research must comply with these federal regulations; however, research institutions responsible for overseeing the conduct of researchers usually extend these protections to participants in nonfederally supported research as well. Although unanticipated adverse events or **iatrogenesis** may still occur during the course of a research study, having these federal regulations in place minimizes the potential for harm and reduces the likelihood of ethical misconduct.

iatrogenesis
inadvertent consequence of medical treatment

Because most health promotion research and practice involves biomedical and behavioral research and interventions, ethical considerations should be paramount and a priority. To assist in the process of making good ethical decisions involving research, 45 CFR 46 can be used; however, health promotion practice, because it is not defined as research, is not governed by these federal regulations. Thus there is more room for ethical error. In fact, one author has questioned the philosophy and corresponding ethical issues underlying the practice of health promotion (Buchanan, 2000). Others have written about ethical concerns in very specific areas of health promotion practice. For example, several journal articles discuss **libertarian paternalism** in the context of health promotion efforts and the specific ethical issues involved in "nudging" people into making better, healthier choices (such as placing apples more conspicuously and within easy reach at a lunch counter so that customers are more likely to choose an apple than a piece of cake) (Ménard, 2010; Vallgarda, 2012). Another article highlights the ethical issues relevant to health promotion practice in the context of an anti-obesity social marketing campaign (Carter et al., 2011), questioning whether inducing fear, playing on parental guilt, contributing to the stigma of being overweight or obese, or teaching viewers with a body mass index of more than 25 to perceive themselves negatively might be overly coercive or unethical. Clearly, just because health promotion practice is not considered research does not mean that its activities cannot be equally harmful; therefore it must be given the same ethical consideration as research activities.

libertarian paternalism
a policy perspective that seeks to influence people to make better, healthier choices that they would regard as better while providing the option for them to opt out

Health promotion practice relies on a professional code of ethics that has been promulgated by several health promotion associations. Although not as legally binding as the federal regulations, this code provides some oversight and ethical guidance. For example, the Society for Public Health Education and the Association for the Advancement of Health Promotion both use the same code of ethics for their practitioners (see Box 3.1). The

International Union for Health Promotion and Education, which represents health promotion professionals internationally, is currently considering a code of ethics. Recently, health promotion professionals in Australia have proposed a new ethical framework that expands on codes of ethics to also incorporate evidence to guide health promotion practice (Carter et al., 2011). Thus health promotion practice as a field continues to develop new ethical standards and promote dialogue that guide practitioners in the design and implementation of their programs to ensure protection for their program participants.

BOX 3.1. CODE OF ETHICS FOR THE HEALTH EDUCATION PROFESSION BY THE SOCIETY FOR PUBLIC HEALTH EDUCATION AND THE ASSOCIATION FOR ADVANCEMENT OF HEALTH PROMOTION

Article I: Responsibility to the Public

A Health Educator's ultimate responsibility is to educate people for the purpose of promoting, maintaining, and improving individual, family, and community health. When a conflict of issues arises among individuals, groups, organizations, agencies, or institutions, health educators must consider all issues and give priority to those that promote wellness and quality of living through principles of self-determination and freedom of choice for the individual.

Article II: Responsibility to the Profession

Health Educators are responsible for their professional behavior, for the reputation of their profession, and for promoting ethical conduct among their colleagues.

Article III: Responsibility to Employers

Health Educators recognize the boundaries of their professional competence and are account-able for their professional activities and actions.

Article IV: Responsibility in the Delivery of Health Education

Health Educators promote integrity in the delivery of health education. They respect the rights, dignity, confidentiality, and worth of all people by adapting strategies and methods to the needs of diverse populations and communities.

Article V: Responsibility in Research and Evaluation

Health Educators contribute to the health of the population and to the profession through research and evaluation activities. When planning and conducting research or evaluation, health educators do so in accordance with federal and state laws and regulations, organizational and institutional policies, and professional standards.

Article VI: Responsibility in Professional Preparation

Those involved in the preparation and training of Health Educators have an obligation to accord learners the same respect and treatment given other groups by providing quality education that benefits the profession and the public.

Federal regulations must be adhered to, as they provide oversight of research involving human subjects so that human subjects are protected from harm and risk is minimized. Health promotion practice encourages observance of its ethics code to ensure that program participants are protected not just in research but also in practice. Ultimately, though, compliance depends on researchers and practitioners being informed of the policies, regulations, and codes, and being up to date on best evidence-based practices while also being conscientious and dutiful professionals. Even though this chapter cannot teach you how to be conscientious or dutiful, we provide examples from history that illustrate flagrant unethical biomedical research and that will, we hope, serve as a moral foundation. In fact, it is vital to be familiar with this history of research abuse because such knowledge helps to explain the stringent regulation of research and why these policies have been put in place.

This chapter will help you to become informed and knowledgeable so that you can maintain rigorous ethical standards whether you engage in research or practice. First, we review the reasons for safeguarding the integrity of research involving human subjects (more properly referred to as study participants) and why taking multiple precautions to avoid physical, mental, or emotional harm to volunteers is paramount. Next, you will learn about the three principles of the Belmont Report, a landmark document that largely shaped modern-day practices and research procedures with human subjects. Then you will learn about key issues that apply to research with minors and other vulnerable populations. As a matter of applied knowledge, you will learn about the three different types of review under the Internal Review Board (IRB) as well as applicable points to bear in mind when composing an IRB application. Finally, you will learn about your obligations as a researcher, including those obligations that transcend your local IRB. The chapter includes practical suggestions for working with your IRB and, more important, ensuring that research subjects are protected.

The Origin of Research Ethics

As is so often the case, history has a profound influence on current practices. In public health this is particularly true of a town in Alabama located in Macon County and known as Tuskegee. The "shadow of Tuskegee" is quite prominent even today, signaling an unfortunate history lesson. In 1966, a private physician treated an African-American man for neurosyphilis. Penicillin was used to treat what had become syphilitic insanity in a man who had not previously been diagnosed with the disease. Syphilis is a sexually transmitted disease (STD) caused by the bacterium *Treponema pallidum*. Syphilis is transmitted primarily through sexual contact and can cause long-term complications and/or death if not adequately treated. As it turned out, the man had enrolled in a research study begun in 1932 that was designed to observe the natural history of syphilis (meaning that investigators wanted to learn how the untreated bacterial infection progressively damaged the body). The private physician who treated this case in 1966 was chastised by a county and a regional medical society for "spoiling one of our subjects" (Meyerson, Martich, and Naehr, 2008). As much of a tragedy as this appeared to be based on this one case, it became greatly magnified as the public learned that the study had been initiated by the U.S. Public Health Service (PHS), was then transferred to the Centers for Disease Control and Prevention in 1957, and ultimately included hundreds of men. Let's pause for a moment and consider: this means that the U.S. government conducted this study and it continued for forty years! Although when the study began there was no effective treatment available for syphilis, in 1945 penicillin was found to be an effective and readily available cure. Nevertheless, study investigators withheld treatment from subjects in order to continue the study. Even more alarming, because the Tuskegee study enrolled only poor African-American men, it was clear that this case was not only about unethical and abhorrent research practices, but also about racial injustice (Figure 3.1). It is important to further note that the physician treating the man in 1966 was not able to gain the sympathetic ear of the press until six years

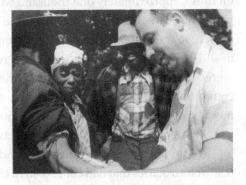

Figure 3.1 Tuskegee Syphilis Study: Doctor Injecting Subject

later. On July 26, 1972, the *New York Times* published a story highlighting these atrocities. Finally the study was officially ended, but it had become the longest-running observational study in U.S. history. Records indicated that about four hundred African-American men with syphilis had been followed during the course of the study and were purposively and sur-reptitiously denied treatment. It was revealed later that deliberate efforts were made on the part of the United States PHS investigators to deceive the human subjects and the wider community. The aftermath of Tuskegee continues and resonates today: in the African-American community there is profound and warranted distrust of government-sponsored research and researchers. This has been particularly evident in the era of HIV/AIDS prevention research.

In 1997, sixty-five years after Tuskegee, President Clinton issued a formal apology to the remaining survivors: ". . . on behalf of the American people what the United States Government did was shameful, and I am sorry." So it seemed that an ugly chapter of U.S. history was closed; however, on October 1, 2010, President Obama found himself in a similar position of having to issue a formal apology—he made a telephone call to President Álvaro Colom of Guatemala to apologize to the people of Guatemala for medical research supported by the United States and conducted in Guatemala between 1946 and 1948 (Presidential Commission for the Study of Bioethical Issues, 2011). As horrific and infamous as the Tuskegee syphilis study was and still is, some of the research conducted in Guatemala was deemed worse, as it involved deliberate infection of people with sexually transmitted diseases without their consent. The study involved some of the same researchers who were involved in the Tuskegee study and the same disease—syphilis. Over 5,000 people—including children, elders, prisoners, soldiers, psychiatric patients and commercial sex workers—were enrolled. Of those, approximately one thousand were actively infected with syphilis, gonorrhea, or chancroid. Although the study took place over 60 years earlier, it was intentionally hidden from the public until its discovery in 2010. Following an investigation, President Obama expressed "deep regret" for the research and affirmed the U.S. government's "unwavering commitment to ensure that all human medical studies conducted today meet exacting" standards for the protection of human subjects (Presidential Commission for the Study of Bioethical Issues, 2011).

In conjunction with Tuskegee and other numerous examples of research atrocities that had come to light (Santelli, 2006), federal protections for persons volunteering to take part in future research studies were devel-oped and put in place. The National Commission for the Protection of Human Subjects in Biomedical and Behavioral Research was formed and wrote the Belmont Report, a key document in research ethics, and created many of the current federal regulations on research (see Box 3.2).

BOX 3.2. FEDERAL REGULATION OF HUMAN RESEARCH

In the United States, research is regulated by the Department of Health and Human Services through the Office of Human Research Protection (OHRP) (http://www.hhs.gov/ohrp/about/index.html). The OHRP, in turn, regulates through their Division of Compliance Oversight (DCO). The DCO "evaluates, at OHRP's discretion, written substantive indications of noncompliance with HHS regulations—Title 45, Part 46, Code of Federal Regulations (45 CFR 46). OHRP asks the institution involved to investigate the allegations and to provide OHRP with a written report of its investigation. The Office then determines what, if any, regulatory action needs to be taken to protect human research subjects. DCO also conducts a program of not-for-cause surveillance evaluations of institutions, and receives, reviews, and responds to incident reports from Assured institutions." An Assured institution is one that is given authority by the OHRP to convene an Internal Review Board (IRB) and therefore can confer or deny IRB approval to investigators based on their proposed research protocols and consent forms. Specifically, OHRP confers this privilege through a Federal Wide Assurance (FWA) number, granted to each institution (usually a university) that has a need to review and approve research protocols involving human participation.

Principles of the Belmont Report

Published in 1979, the Belmont Report is perhaps the single most important document pertaining to the conduct of research on human subjects (U.S. Department of Health and Human Services, 1979). Before learning about the three primary principles outlined in this landmark report, however, it is worth noting that the term "subjects" should be replaced with alternate phrasing whenever possible. Subjects are typically people who are subjected to something—this is not at all consistent with the tenets of the Belmont Report, which advocates for respect of individuals' autonomy and their right to full disclosure as they participate in research, as opposed to their unwilling or unknowing subjection to experimental conditions. Several alternate terms are preferable, such as "participants," "volunteers," or simply "persons." If your sample will consist of men, then the term "men" can be used, and if all women, the term "women" can be used as a replacement for "subjects." Of note, this same attention to avoiding the word "subjects" should be used when preparing manuscripts that report research findings.

The first principle of the Belmont Report is **respect for persons**. Specifically, this principle demands that people be provided with full disclosure of all possible risks and benefits that may conceivably be associated with study participation. This principle has multiple implications for the conduct of

respect for persons
the principle that states that individuals should be treated as autonomous agents and that persons with diminished autonomy are entitled to protection in the course of research

human researchers, but the cornerstone of these is *written informed consent*. Obtaining consent is the assurance that respect for autonomy has been met, at least in the enrollment stage of the study. Obtaining consent is a process rather than an outcome—a process that involves a verbal exchange between two parties: the person obtaining consent and the potential study volunteer. This process should not be rushed and must be conducted based on the needs of the potential volunteer. It is not fair to assume that all potential volunteers are highly literate or that they may even take the time to read a consent form even if literacy is not problematic. Consequently, the research assistant authorized to obtain informed consent has an obligation to conduct a paragraph-by-paragraph review of the entire document. This review needs to be concise yet complete, highlighting key risks and benefits to the potential volunteer should he or she decide to participate. The review must also provide ample opportunity for the potential volunteer to ask questions. This may be easily and systematically achieved by asking, after the concise oral summary of each paragraph in the consent form, "What are your questions at this point?"

A key implication of respecting a person's autonomy is that the person can decline study participation without any need for justification. This means that it is not an acceptable practice to challenge (or even inquire about the reasoning behind) a person's decision not to participate in a research study. In other words, the person's response of "no" must be unquestionable. Further, great caution should be used to ensure that the context in which consent is obtained is not coercive and allows for potential participants to comfortably decline as opposed to being awkward or problematic. A few examples are instructive:

- Example One: Young adults are often a critical study population in health promotion. Consequently, research on convenience samples of university or college students and high school students is quite common. In many studies, questionnaires are administered to student volunteers

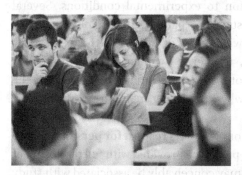

in a classroom setting. This mass administration procedure is very easy for the researcher but it may be problematic ethically. Classrooms are essentially a social environment where peers interact and can yield strong influence on behavior (Figure 3.2); as such, a person's decision to enroll in a study could be unduly influenced by these social

Figure 3.2 Classroom Social Environment

factors. Solutions to this problem are not readily apparent, but should be considered as part of the research protocol. Perhaps we need to change the practice itself.

• Example Two: Clinic attendees are another important population in health promotion research. As such, studies often seek volunteers from waiting rooms or even during or after the normal course of the clinical encounter (Figure 3.3). The provider-patient relationship that characterizes medical care is one that places power in the hands of the providers and requires at least some degree of subservience on the part of the patients (for example, a healthcare worker asks a patient, "Please undress now and wait here until someone comes back

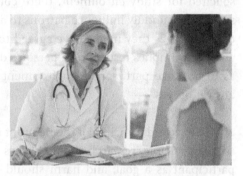

Figure 3.3 Healthcare Provider and Patient Interaction in Clinic Setting

to see you"). Although this imbalanced power dynamic is perhaps useful in the medical setting, it is not conducive to making sure that there is no coercion and that saying "no" to participating is a comfortable answer when asking attendees to take part in a research study. The solution is to create a clear separation between the research staff and the medical providers. For example, research staff should not wear scrubs or other medical attire, and they should not be entering exam rooms. In circumstances when the medical providers are the ones conducting the research, a separate research assistant should be hired to interface with potential volunteers, and that person should be identified as being disconnected from the medical care that people will be receiving (or have received) that day. When the research assistant first interacts with a potential volunteer, the fact that the research study and the medical care being provided are not linked should be emphasized in terms that are clear to patients.

• Example Three: Street-based outreach to locate and enroll research participants is a common strategy used in health promotion research, especially when the targeted population is hidden or hard to reach (such as injection drug users), a convenience sample is not available, or there is no **sampling frame** from which to sample. A sampling frame is generally an existing list of some sort (such as a university directory of all matriculated students from registrar's office) that essentially represents the entire population under study. Thus data collection often occurs in everyday settings

sampling frame
an existing list of some sort that essentially represents the entire population under study

such as city parks, cafes, bars, and street corners. Compared to classrooms and clinics, these venues provide a much more comfortable environment for potential volunteers to express an answer of "no" to the offer of joining a research study. Nonetheless, an important concern is approaching people in a way that respects their current social situation. For example, people typically go to a bar to have fun with friends. If bar patrons are being solicited for study enrollment, there could be a concern that the social setting may unduly influence patrons to answer "no" when under different circumstances they might have agreed to enroll in the study. Respect for autonomy implies respecting a person's desire to be part of a study as well as to not take part, so the environment should also be conducive to an answer of "yes."

beneficence
the principle that states that persons are treated in an ethical manner not only by respecting their decisions and protecting them from harm, but also by making efforts to secure their well-being

The second principle of the Belmont report is **beneficence**. According to this principle, research should always have the welfare of the research participant as a goal, and harm should be avoided and risk minimized. The treatments (research) must be helpful and benefits must outweigh any risks. A key here is to avoid harm. Indeed, anyone schooled in the history of medicine and public health knows that a cornerstone of the Hippocratic oath is "first, do no harm." Avoiding harm is a simple principle but not always evident. One way to translate this principle is through the common requirements of IRB-approved consent forms. Beneficence suggests that the risks of study participation must be less than the benefits. Researchers are therefore obligated to provide potential volunteers with any and all information that may add to this mental calculation or cost-benefit analysis. In fact, the consent form must provide an exhaustive description of all possible risks (regardless of likelihood) and benefits to the person. Moreover, when an IRB evaluates a consent form, the primary consideration must be whether the language provides a balanced and comprehensive treatment of the risk-versus-benefits equation.

psychosocial risk
refers to any negative social consequences that may occur if a person's private medical information—for example, diagnosis of a disease such as AIDS or a mental illness such as major depression—or information about the person's illicit behaviors becomes public

Unlike biomedical research, which often involves invasive procedures (for example, collecting blood or tissue samples, administering new drugs, testing new medical devices for efficacy), most health promotion research presents mostly **psychosocial risk** rather than physical risk. Psychosocial risk refers to any negative social consequences that may occur if a person's private medical information—for example, one's diagnosis of a disease such as AIDS or a mental illness such as major depression—or information about one's illicit behaviors (for example, injecting drugs, performing commercial sex work) becomes public. Psychosocial risk should never be underestimated in terms of the potential to cause harm. Again, a few examples are helpful to come to a better understanding of the principle.

- Example One: A study is testing the efficacy of a behavioral intervention designed to help young Black men stay HIV-negative. Keep in mind that HIV infection is still associated with a great deal of stigma. In this behavioral trial men are tested for HIV once every 3 months for one year. Their test results are protected data—stored in password-protected computers that are, in turn, stored in locked offices. Furthermore, the test results are recorded in the dataset by study identification (ID) number only rather than by name or other personal identifying information (for example, email address, address, birth date). These types of assurances create a strong set of protections; however, the possibility of improper disclosure cannot be ruled out entirely. It is possible that a malicious individual could locate the list of names that links men to their study ID and then use that information to find out that a particular study volunteer recently tested positive for HIV. Clearly, several breaches in security would have to occur to allow this unfortunate event to take place, but as we all know, security breaches do happen. The consequence of having unauthorized people know about their HIV-positive test result is certainly life-changing for most people, and thus study participation has the potential to lead to harm. Whether the odds of this happening are significant enough to avoid study participation is not a decision that can be made objectively. It is a guess, and as such this subjective judgment can be made only by the potential volunteer. This subjective judgment also embodies the principle of respect for autonomy.

- Example Two: A study is being conducted to determine whether female adolescents in a long-term sexual relationships with a male partner are more likely to use hormonal contraception than those in short-term sexual relationships. Hence an inclusion criterion is that the female adolescent must report being in a current sexual relationship with a male partner. The study was approved by the IRB with a waiver of the need for parental consent for the specific purpose of protecting sexually active female adolescents from parental retribution in the event that their sex lives had previously been kept a secret. This study involves monthly phone contact between enrolled teen females and the research assistant. By protocol, the research assistant never identifies himself or herself to the person answering the phone until he or she has firmly established that the person is indeed the enrolled participant. Although this is a fairly typical study procedure, it is certainly not without its limitations. A girlfriend of the study participant, for instance, may innocently answer her friend's cell phone while the study participant is in the bathroom. If the research assistant forgets to follow the protocol or fails to follow it perfectly, it may become clear to the friend that her friend is enrolled in a "sex study." For a vast majority of teen females, having a friend find out that they are in a sex study may not be devastating, but that is a judgment in risk and consequence that cannot be made by anyone except the potential study volunteer. In this case, the risk of inadvertent disclosure of study participation must be listed on the consent form as a possibility. In separate paperwork submitted by the investigator, the IRB application for this study would have to include protocols and assurances that guard against such inadvertent disclosure of study participation and maintain the confidentiality of the participants. Despite the assurances, the principle of beneficence requires that this risk be counted in an overall determination of risk versus benefit. Ultimately, if the potential risks are viewed as outweighing the benefits, then the IRB will most likely not approve the protocol unless the investigator can somehow put procedures in place that will minimize the risks thereby "tipping the scale."

randomized controlled trials
are a type of scientific (often medical) experiment, in which people are randomly allocated to one of the different treatments under study and one of the treatments is considered as a control group

• Example Three: **Randomized controlled trials** (RCTs) are as important to health promotion research as they are to medical research. A consummate dilemma in the design of RCTs is beneficence for persons randomly assigned to the control condition. Presumably the treatment condition offers some benefit to the person even though that benefit may not be well established (as is the case for any treatment or program in an experimental phase). Although scholars could debate the actual value of being in the treatment condition of an RCT, the debate would often be quite one-sided regarding the control condition because this treatment often is designed only to provide equivalent attention to study volunteers rather than substantive education, assistance, or support for change. Thus when an IRB determines whether risk of harm is amply counterbalanced by benefits, the members are compelled to consider benefit in the "worst-case scenario" (that is, being randomized to the control condition). Even though risk may be minimal, if there is a complete absence of clear benefit it is unlikely that an IRB will approve the study.

justice
the principle that states research should ensure that reasonable, nonexploitative, and well-considered procedures are administered fairly and equally

The third principle of the Belmont report is **justice**. This principle states that the study population should be likely beneficiaries of the study findings. At first blush this seems to be common sense. Upon reflection, however, you will realize that this principle is often violated. Drug trials are perhaps the single best example. For instance, from 2005 through 2011 investigators from the CDC conducted efficacy trials of tenofovir (and other drugs) used as preexposure prophylaxis against HIV infection (Thigpen et al., 2012). This daily-dose drug is estimated to cost approximately $1,500 per month (USD). Now that it has been approved by the Food and Drug Administration (Food and Drug Administration, 2012), a problem becomes apparent as we learn that the study occurred in Botswana, one of the poorest nations on earth. This is an excellent teaching case because the question of whether the study population (whose very existence led, in part, to FDA approval of preexposure prophylaxis drugs) is reasonably likely to benefit from the findings produces a problematic answer. Clearly, it could be argued that IRB approval for this study should not have been granted simply because the likelihood of the study population being able to afford the drug is quite low.

The principle of justice also implies that a given population should not be excluded from study participation when the study findings have potential to provide benefits to that population. An all-too-common example of studies that violate justice in this regard is the practice of conducting behavioral intervention research studies, designed to develop efficacious programs to avert sexually transmitted diseases (STDs), with populations of persons over the age of 17. Although it is quite convenient to recruit only persons 18 and older (as they can give consent), the epidemiology of STDs suggests that a substantial portion of the annual cases occur in persons younger than 18. Thus excluding a 17-year-old from a study designed to test an STD prevention program is a direct violation of justice. Indeed, grant applications submitted to the National Institutes of Health require applicants to specifically justify the exclusion of women, minorities, and persons under 21 (defined by the NIH as "children").

In defense of the studies that do exclude persons classified as children and/or minors (those under 18 years of age) when these youth do indeed stand to benefit, it is often considered problematic to gain informed consent from a minor. When a minor is involved, because they are not of legal age, they can provide only their **assent** or agreement to participate. In determining whether children are capable of assenting, the ages, maturity level, and psychological state of the children involved must be considered. This is a good teaching example because it blends two of the Belmont Principles: respect for autonomy and justice. From the perspective of justice, minors should be involved in research that can directly benefit them or whose results can provide generalizable knowledge that holds the potential to improve whatever condition is being studied. When considering respect for autonomy, however, it becomes clear that minors are not autonomous, because they are far more likely to be influenced by their peers or by adults in their assent. Thus respect for autonomy is often confused with parental autonomy, meaning that the parent(s) will have the right to decide whether a child should take part in a given research study. In fact, 45 CFR 46 states that adequate provisions must be made for soliciting the permission of each child's parent(s) or legal guardian. Depending on the research, at times only one parent is required.

Because so much of modern public health practice involves prevention programs for youth (DiClemente, Santelli, and Crosby, 2009) there is often tension between the two Belmont principles of justice and respect for autonomy. Two solutions exist. First, investigators can apply for a waiver

assent
refers to persons who are not of legal age providing their agreement to participate in a research study

of parental consent if it can be determined that parental or guardian permission is not a reasonable requirement, in order to protect the children (for example, if they are neglected or abused) and provided that an appropriate mechanism for protecting the children is substituted, and provided further that the waiver is not inconsistent with federal, state, or local law. Moreover, in some instances, even if the children are not neglected or abused, getting parental consent may result in subsequent physical or emotional harm to the child, so a waiver might be warranted. For example, a study might involve the participation of children who are lesbian, gay, bisexual, transgender, or questioning (LGBTQ) but who may not have told their parents about their sexual orientation. If the study was targeted to LGBTQ youth, this information would be in the parental informed consent form and would essentially "out" the child. A second solution would be for investigators to obtain verbal assent from minors and then seek written consent from parents. One caveat is important here: the minor providing assent to participate in the study must also provide assent for the research assistant to contact the parent(s). In studies that address highly sensitive topics, such as homosexuality or substance use, it may also be prudent to protect assenting minors by requesting a waiver of parental consent, thereby avoiding inadvertent disclosure of potentially inflammatory information about the minor to the parent. Studies that seek parental consent for the participation of minors are prone to slow rates of enrollment, as finding parents who agree to these conditions may be difficult. These studies are also prone to low participation rates because many parents may be inaccessible and even those who are accessible may refuse to provide consent. Hence there are often cases for which the principle of justice demands the enrollment of minors but the actual enrollment process, using parental consent, makes the study impractical. Hence the option of applying for a waiver of parental consent is a valid compromise between the two opposing principles. The operative term here is "applying," as the local IRB overseeing the conduct of the research will ultimately determine whether there is sufficient basis for granting such a waiver.

As you might expect, many IRBs err on the side of being conservative regarding granting waivers of parental consent. Although the aim of this extreme caution on the part of IRBs is to protect potential volunteers, the unfortunate result is that obtaining parental consent may sometimes end up placing a potential volunteer at risk of harm—exactly the opposite of what an IRB intended. Consider another example, a study of teen pregnancy that is designed to understand why teen females may begin and continue using Depo-Provera (a hormonal contraceptive given by injection every three months). To achieve the study goals, teen females who are sexually active will be enrolled. Imagine, then, the issues that may surface when a research assistant contacts a parent or guardian of a teen girl (potential study enrollee) who has concealed her sexual activity from that person. In this example, a would-be study participant may be emotionally or even physically harmed as a consequence of a research study. Clearly, such disclosures may occur even without the expressed confirmation of the research assistant. For instance, the study may take place at a clinic that is widely known to dispense contraceptives to teens (such as a Planned Parenthood clinic). The conversation, by phone, might go something like this:

Research Assistant:	I am calling from the Planned Parenthood clinic here in town; I would like to speak with the parent of Ashley Tremont.
Parent:	Speaking
Research Assistant:	I met Ashley today, and I have invited her to be in a research study.
Parent:	Where did you meet my daughter?
Research Assistant:	At the clinic.
Parent:	Why would she be going to that place?
Research Assistant:	I do not know exactly, I only know that she was here earlier today.
Parent:	My daughter is not having sex, and I have no idea why you are asking her to be in a study. Is there something wrong with her?
Research Assistant:	Not that I am aware of.
Parent:	I will deal with her soon. My answer to you is no.

With infinite variations on this sample conversation, you can easily imagine that teen girls like Ashley would experience issues at home, to say the least, after the parent or guardian spoke with the research assistant. Therefore, to protect minors and to ensure that the principle of justice is preserved with respect to minors, the Society of Adolescent Health and Medicine (SAHM) issued the following guidelines (which are consistent with federal guidelines) (Santelli et al., 2003). A waiver of parental consent should be granted under these conditions:

- The study is anonymous.
- The study is minimal risk.
- The intervention is consistent with standard of care prevention activities (such as condom use).

- The presence of a parent or guardian is likely to obscure the accuracy of information that can be collected, or the presence of a parent or guardian may even create a situation that puts the subject at risk, if behaviors or intentions considered socially undesirable are disclosed.

- The subjects under study will be seeking care for diseases that represent conditions (such as STDs and HIV) that are allowable to be treated without parent or guardian consent, so discussion of these topics is similarly permitted for research purposes (with the permission of the IRB).

Regulation of Research Involving Vulnerable Populations

Because history has shown that in the course of several U.S. government research studies certain populations have been exploited and harmed, the federal regulations provide special protection for populations considered vulnerable, including children (45 CFR 46 Subpart D), prisoners (445 CFR 46 Subpart C), pregnant women, human fetuses, and neonates (45 CFR 46 Subpart B). These special protections commonly require a higher level of scrutiny by the IRB, restrictions or prohibitions on particular kinds of research (for instance, research involving greater than minimal risk), and alternative procedures for obtaining informed consent, such as requesting the permission of a parent or guardian. Certain research with pregnant women requires the permission of both the pregnant woman and the father of the fetus.

Federal Oversight of Local IRBs

Enforcement of the principles described in the Belmont Report is controlled at the local level. To ensure that local control is uniform across the United States and also effective, all IRBs are authorized and regulated by the U.S. Department of Health and Human Services. Figure 3.4 displays this process in greater detail.

Three Categories of IRB Approval

Research was defined previously as an activity designed to create generalizable knowledge. This short definition contains two critical words: generalizable and knowledge. Let's begin with knowledge. As you might expect, knowledge is born of new findings. Knowledge is rarely universal; however, it must apply to more than an isolated case, place, or community to be consistent with what our society values as "textbook knowledge." For example, finding out that students in a freshman-level college algebra class

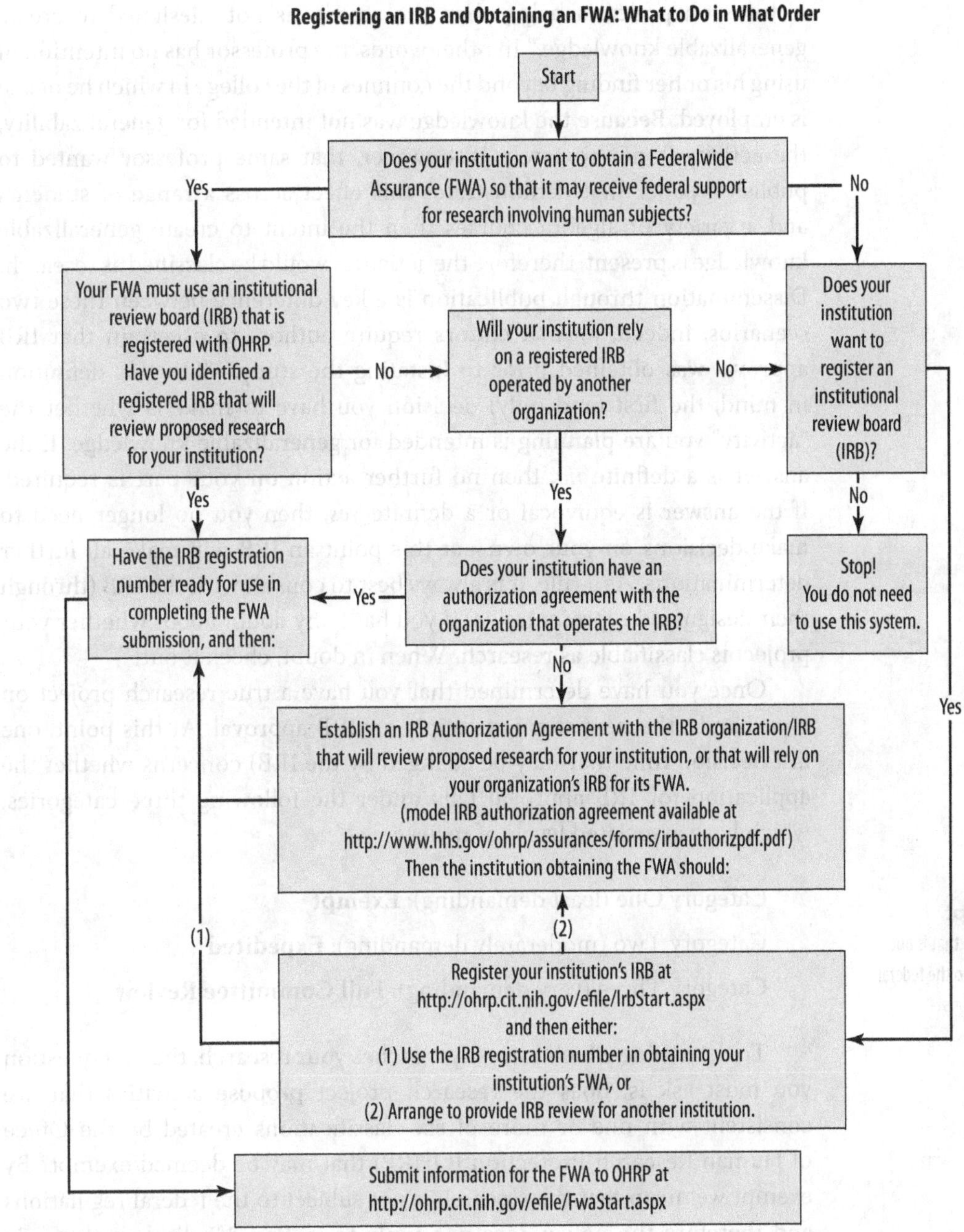

Registering an IRB and Obtaining an FWA: What to Do in What Order

Start

Does your institution want to obtain a Federalwide Assurance (FWA) so that it may receive federal support for research involving human subjects? — Yes / No

Your FWA must use an institutional review board (IRB) that is registered with OHRP. Have you identified a registered IRB that will review proposed research for your institution?

Will your institution rely on a registered IRB operated by another organization?

Does your institution want to register an institutional review board (IRB)?

Have the IRB registration number ready for use in completing the FWA submission, and then:

Does your institution have an authorization agreement with the organization that operates the IRB?

Stop! You do not need to use this system.

Establish an IRB Authorization Agreement with the IRB organization/IRB that will review proposed research for your institution, or that will rely on your organization's IRB for its FWA.
(model IRB authorization agreement available at http://www.hhs.gov/ohrp/assurances/forms/irbauthorizpdf.pdf)
Then the institution obtaining the FWA should:

(1)   (2)

Register your institution's IRB at
http://ohrp.cit.nih.gov/efile/IrbStart.aspx
and then either:
(1) Use the IRB registration number in obtaining your institution's FWA, or
(2) Arrange to provide IRB review for another institution.

Submit information for the FWA to OHRP at
http://ohrp.cit.nih.gov/efile/FwaStart.aspx

Figure 3.4 Institutional Review Board Approval Process

learn faster when the lectures are made available as podcasts may be informative to professors teaching algebra at that college, but the "finding" may not be generalizable to all college freshmen taking algebra. This is where generalizability comes into the picture. If the question is local (meaning the algebra professor doing the study wants to know whether lectures on podcasts help), then the activity is not "designed to create generalizable knowledge." In other words, the professor has no intention of using his or her finding beyond the confines of the college in which he or she is employed. Because the knowledge was not intended for generalizability, the activity is not research. If, however, that same professor wanted to publish a paper that demonstrates this effect across a range of students and a variety of algebra courses then the intent to create generalizable knowledge is present; therefore the activities would be classified as research. Dissemination through publication is a key difference between these two scenarios; indeed, journal editors require authors to ascertain that IRB approval was obtained prior to instating the study. With this definition in mind, the first (and only) decision you have to make is whether the "activity" you are planning is intended for generalizable knowledge. If the answer is a definite *no*, then no further action on your part is required. If the answer is equivocal or a definite *yes*, then you no longer need to make decisions on your own—at this point an IRB will make all further determinations. As a rule, it is always best to consult with the IRB (through their designated representative) if you have any doubt about whether your project is classifiable as research. When in doubt, check it out!

Once you have determined that you have a true research project on your hands, the next step is to apply for IRB approval. At this point, one last decision (one that may be changed by the IRB) concerns whether the application for IRB approval falls under the following three categories, which have associated levels of review:

exempt

research that is not subject to the federal regulations

Category One (least demanding): **Exempt**

Category Two (moderately demanding): **Expedited**

Category Three (very demanding): **Full Committee Review**

To determine which category matches your research, the first question you must ask is, does the research project propose activities that are consistent with one or more of six classifications created by the Office of Human Research Protection (OHRP) that may be deemed exempt? By exempt we mean that the research is not subject to the federal regulations and therefore the policy does not apply to it. Box 3.3 displays these six categories. If your answer to this question is "yes" after you have carefully considered the six classifications for exempt status, *and* if you are not proposing to study a vulnerable population (such as pregnant women, prisoners, or children), then you may ask that your protocol be considered exempt. However, the local IRB ultimately makes this determination, and after examining your research protocol the IRB could determine that it is not in fact exempt and a more rigorous review is needed.

BOX 3.3. SIX CATEGORIES OF RESEARCH ACTIVITIES THAT MAY QUALIFY A STUDY FOR EXEMPT STATUS

1. Research conducted in established or commonly accepted educational settings, involving normal educational practices, such as:

    (i)   research on regular and special educational instructional strategies, or

    (ii) research on the effectiveness of or the comparison among instructional techniques, curricula, or classroom management methods

2. Research involving the use of educational tests (cognitive, diagnostic, aptitude, achievement), survey procedures, interview procedures or observation of public behavior, unless:

    (i)   information obtained is recorded in such a manner that human subjects can be identified, directly or through identifiers linked to the subjects; and

    (ii) any disclosure of the human subjects' responses outside the research could reasonably place the subjects at risk of criminal or civil liability or be damaging to the subjects' financial standing, employability, or reputation

3. Research involving the use of educational tests (cognitive, diagnostic, aptitude, achievement), survey procedures, interview procedures, or observation of public behavior that is not exempt under category (2) of this section, if:

    (i)   the human subjects are elected or appointed public officials or candidates for public office; or

    (ii) federal statute(s) require(s) without exception that the confidentiality of the personally identifiable information will be maintained throughout the research and thereafter

4. Research involving the collection or study of existing data, documents, records, pathological specimens, or diagnostic specimens, if these sources are publicly available or if the information is recorded by the investigator in such a manner that subjects cannot be identified, directly or through identifiers linked to the subjects. PLEASE NOTE: According to the Office for Human Research Protections (OHRP), "to qualify for this exemption, the data, documents, records, or specimens must be in existence before the project begins. The principle behind this policy is that the rights of individuals should be respected; subjects must consent to participation in research."

5. Research and demonstration projects which are conducted by or subject to the approval of department of agency heads, and which are designed to study, evaluate, or otherwise examine:

    (i)   public benefit or service programs;

    (ii)   procedures for obtaining benefits or services under those programs;

    (iii) possible changes in or alternatives to those programs or procedures;

    (iv)   possible changes in methods or levels of payment for benefits or services under those programs;

   (v)   projects for which there is no statutory requirement for IRB review;

   (vi)   projects that do not involve significant physical invasions or intrusions on the privacy interests of participants;

   (vii)   authorization or concurrence by funding agencies that exemption from IRB review is acceptable

6.   Taste and food quality evaluation and consumer acceptance studies:

   (i)   if wholesome food without additives are consumed or

   (ii)   if a food is consumed that contains a food ingredient at or below the level and for a use found to be safe, or agricultural chemical or environmental contaminant at or below the level found to be safe, by the Food and Drug Administration or approved by the Environmental Protection Agency or the Food Safety and Inspection Service of the U.S. Department of Agriculture.

Source: The Office for Human Research Protections (OHRP), 45 CFR 46, §46.101 (b).

This leads to the second question: Does the research pose no more than minimal risk? If the answer is yes, regardless of the intended research population, then your study may be eligible for expedited review. This simply means that the IRB will assign your application to one reviewer who will make a recommendation without the proposal being reviewed by the full committee of twelve or more IRB members. To be eligible for expedited review, the research must be described by one or more of seven categories (see Box 3.4).

BOX 3.4. CATEGORIES OF RESEARCH THAT MAY BE REVIEWED BY THE INSTITUTIONAL REVIEW BOARD (IRB) THROUGH AN EXPEDITED REVIEW PROCEDURE

1.   Clinical studies of drugs and medical devices only when condition (a) or (b) is met: (a) Research on drugs for which an investigational new drug application (21 CFR Part 312) is not required. (Note: Research on marketed drugs that significantly increases the risks or decreases the acceptability of the risks associated with the use of the product is not eligible for expedited review.) (b) Research on medical devices for which (i) an investigational device exemption application (21 CFR Part 812) is not required; or (ii) the medical device is cleared/approved for marketing and the medical device is being used in accordance with its cleared/approved labeling.

2. Collection of blood samples by finger stick, heel stick, ear stick, or venipuncture as follows: (a) from healthy, nonpregnant adults who weigh at least 110 pounds. For these subjects, the amounts drawn may not exceed 550 ml in an 8 week period and collection may not occur more frequently than 2 times per week; or (b) from other adults and children, considering the age, weight, and health of the subjects, the collection procedure, the amount of blood to be collected, and the frequency with which it will be collected. For these subjects, the amount drawn may not exceed the lesser of 50 ml or 3 ml per kg in an 8 week period and collection may not occur more frequently than 2 times per week.

3. Prospective collection of biological specimens for research purposes by noninvasive means. Examples: (a) hair and nail clippings in a nondisfiguring manner; (b) deciduous teeth at time of exfoliation or if routine patient care indicates a need for extraction; (c) permanent teeth if routine patient care indicates a need for extraction; (d) excreta and external secretions (including sweat); (e) uncannulated saliva collected either in an unstimulated fashion or stimulated by chewing gumbase or wax or by applying a dilute citric solution to the tongue; (f) placenta removed at delivery; (g) amniotic fluid obtained at the time of rupture of the membrane prior to or during labor; (h) supra- and subgingival dental plaque and calculus, provided the collection procedure is not more invasive than routine prophylactic scaling of the teeth and the process is accomplished in accordance with accepted prophylactic techniques; (i) mucosal and skin cells collected by buccal scraping or swab, skin swab, or mouth washings; (j) sputum collected after saline mist nebulization.

4. Collection of data through noninvasive procedures (not involving general anesthesia or sedation) routinely employed in clinical practice, excluding procedures involving X-rays or microwaves. Where medical devices are employed, they must be cleared/approved for marketing. (Studies intended to evaluate the safety and effectiveness of the medical device are not generally eligible for expedited review, including studies of cleared medical devices for new indications.) Examples: (a) physical sensors that are applied either to the surface of the body or at a distance and do not involve input of significant amounts of energy into the subject or an invasion of the subject's privacy; (b) weighing or testing sensory acuity; (c) magnetic resonance imaging; (d) electrocardiography, electroencephalography, thermography, detection of naturally occurring radioactivity, electroretinography, ultrasound, diagnostic infrared imaging, Doppler blood flow, and echocardiography; (e) moderate exercise, muscular strength testing, body composition assessment, and flexibility testing where appropriate given the age, weight, and health of the individual.

5. Research involving materials (data, documents, records, or specimens) that have been collected, or will be collected solely for nonresearch purposes (such as medical treatment or diagnosis). (NOTE: Some research in this category may be exempt from the HHS regulations for the protection of human subjects (45 CFR 46.101[b][4]). This listing refers only to research that is not exempt.)

6. Collection of data from voice, video, digital, or image recordings made for research purposes.

7. Research on individual or group characteristics or behavior (including, but not limited to, research on perception, cognition, motivation, identity, language, communication, cultural beliefs or practices, and social behavior) or research employing survey, interview, oral history, focus group, program evaluation, human factors evaluation, or quality assurance methodologies. (NOTE: Some research in this category may be exempt from the HHS regulations for the protection of human subjects. 45 CFR 46.101(b)(2) and (b)(3). This listing refers only to research that is not exempt.)

As indicated, only five of these categories are applicable to health promotion research, and of those, only number seven is truly common: research that involves individuals or groups to learn about behaviors, cognitions, perceptions, and so on. Two of the other four categories that may be used in health promotion research both involve the collection of biological specimens through noninvasive procedures. The remaining two categories are: (1) analyzing data, records, or documents that were not collected for the initial purpose of research and (2) using voice or video recordings for research purposes. If your proposed research project is not described by one or more of these categories, then it is quite likely that your protocol will be subjected to full committee review. This means that a fully convened panel of IRB members will consider the ethical issues, merits, and risk-benefit ratio of your potential study. All three forms of review are ultimately equivalent in that they typically result in a letter granting IRB approval for a period of 6 months to 1 year. Before the first approval period expires, the IRB will prompt you (the investigator) to file a continuation review that will be far less demanding than the original application. Continuing reviews of protocols that were initially approved by a full committee are typically handled as expedited reviews.

The key term in this entire process is protocol—this is the language used to refer to your research plan in its entirety. Protocols should include all aspects of the planned research, including specific plans for recruitment, retention (if applicable), randomization (if applicable), intervention (if applicable), and compensation for the time that volunteers give to the study. Protocols should include plans for data analysis, and these plans should show that adequate statistical power is available to provide a fair test of all proposed study hypotheses. At first blush, this requirement may seem to be involved less with ethics than with science. However, upon reflection you will understand that studies planned without attention to adequate statistical power are actually meaningless in that they do not have a fair chance of rejecting the null hypothesis. Thus volunteers who join a research study with good intent (that is, to benefit science) are misled when the science is compromised before the study even begins. The protocol must also include detailed plans for assessment (including a copy of questionnaires that will be used) as well as a complete description of exactly how the data will be collected and how they will be protected. Indeed, "collection and protection" are key features of an IRB-approved protocol, as both must be considered to vigilantly guard the privacy of study participants. As a rule, collection and protection procedures should optimally guard against even remotely possible conditions (such as theft of records, compromise of privacy while responding to questions, loss of privacy for protected medical records) that could conceivably lead to emotional, social, financial, or physical harm of even one study participant.

Your Obligations as a Researcher

Again, your IRB will guide you in all that you need to do in the service of guarding the ethics of health promotion research. For emphasis, however, we wish to highlight three obligations that apply to all research projects.

Obligation One: Certification in Human Subjects Research

As a researcher you must complete a course in human subjects research such as the one offered by the Collaborative Institutional Training Initiative (CITI) that teaches you a great deal more detail about ethics in research than you will gain from reading this chapter. Other courses are also available, so we recommend you check with your local IRB to see which ones are acceptable. This certification process will also require periodic renewals, usually occurring every 3 years. On successful completion of this course, you will be given a certificate that becomes known to your IRB; without this certification in place, your applications will not be considered. Successful completion of this course requires about four hours of uninterrupted study time, so the "investment" is quite modest in contrast to the time you have spent (or will soon spend) earning degrees in health promotion/public health. As a word of encouragement, the goal of taking this course is not simply to pass the course; rather, it is to refine your knowledge of the ethics of research. With that point firmly in mind, we suggest that you take this course and learn as much as possible, as doing so represents your commitment to the overarching principle that the protection of study participants is the first and foremost concern of all researchers.

Obligation Two: Storing Consent Forms

The epitome of ethics in research is the consent form. As we've discussed, the signed consent form is the result of a process occurring between the researcher and the study participant. As such, this document is critical to all persons engaged in the research project, as it provides tangible evidence of an agreement between parties. It seems easy enough to say that these signed forms should be safely stored; however (as you might expect), some caveats exist.

First, signed consent forms should not be stored in the same filing cabinet as any accumulated study records that provide personal information about the participants. For instance, consider a hard copy document that displays test results for a person's scores on measures of depression, self-image, coping styles, and perceptions of body image. These measures are all private, and their release would therefore compromise the ethics and integrity of the research and possibly cause harm to volunteers. As long as these hard copy records are identified only by a number (a study ID code) and not by name, then the odds of any breaches in confidentiality greatly diminish. This is a common practice. But the security of this practice can be compromised when the consent form (a document with a full name) also contains the study ID code or the consent form is stored in tandem with the hard copy records. In either case, it is quite possible that a malicious person could discover private information about a study volunteer.

Second, signed consent forms are typically required (by IRBs) to be stored for a period of several years beyond the closing date of the study. This creates a management issue in that records must be kept, stating where the consent forms can be located for future reference even if the investigator leaves the institution for a position elsewhere. Therefore long-term storage records should be created and maintained by the institution as well as the investigator.

Obligation Three: Understanding HIPAA

The Health Insurance Portability and Accountability Act (HIPAA) was passed during the Clinton administration in 1996. If your research will take place as part of a partnership with any type of health care organization, you will need to ask the participants to sign a HIPAA waiver. The intent of HIPAA is simple—the law protects people's health information. Unfortunately, "health information" is quite broadly defined under this act to include even age. Thus, if your collected data include age or any other "health information," it falls under the HIPAA act. Again, this is the case only for research conducted in association with health care organizations of any kind (known as "covered entities" in the language of the HIPAA

Act). Although working under a covered entity and having a study that is regulated by HIPAA may seem daunting, the solution actually reverts to the Belmont principle of respect for autonomy. If the person enrolling in your study signs a waiver of his or her HIPAA rights (a waiver valid only for your study), then all is well! Typically IRBs request that the HIPAA waiver be included within the consent form, thereby alleviating the need for investigators to keep two sets of signed records. It is important, once again, to point out that informed consent is a verbal exchange process occurring between the researcher and the potential volunteer. That exchange should therefore include discussion of HIPAA and what it means for the potential volunteer to sign the waiver.

IRB-Associated Issues in Health Promotion Research

Unlike research in fields that study primarily cognition and attitudes, health promotion research frequently studies behaviors. Moreover, the behaviors that we study are often very sensitive and sometimes even illegal. Table 3.1 provides examples of frequently studied health behaviors that may pose issues from an ethics perspective. These are just some of the many behaviors that are generally considered highly sensitive and may require additional safeguards from an IRB perspective.

Other Considerations Beyond Your IRB

A common reason for potential study participants not to volunteer is their justified worries that the data they provide could be used (someday) against them in a court of law. This, of course, may be especially true for persons who abuse drugs, perpetrate sex crimes, drive while intoxicated, and so on. Perhaps more important, the fear of "court reprisals" may discourage those who do volunteer from providing complete and accurate information in response to questions that assess highly sensitive and possible illegal behaviors. Because health promotion research so often addresses substance abuse and issues related to sex, you should know that protections against a court subpoena of your data are available. The protection takes the form of a Certificate of Confidentiality (COC). The COC applies to studies funded by the National Institutes of Health (NIH), with NIH being the agency that issues this document to the PI of the study. Although it may be many years before you are involved in an NIH-funded study it is well worth remembering that the option of obtaining a COC is important for your research. In fact, it is often true that the IRB reviewing your research protocol will specifically request that you obtain a COC before data collection begins. Note that

Table 3.1   Example of Health Behaviors That May Pose Ethical Concerns in Research

Sexual Behaviors

Number of penile-vaginal sex partners in the past 12 months

Age of first intercourse

Frequency of anal receptive sex in the past 30 days

Oral sex with a member of the same sex

Use of contraception in the past 90 days

Sex with an unwilling partner in the past 5 years

Substance Use Behaviors

Use of marijuana in the past 14 days

Use of cocaine in the past 12 months

Ever used heroin

Frequency of binge drinking in the past 30 days

Ever too intoxicated to recall how much you drank?

Ever too intoxicated to recall if you had sex?

Mental Health Behaviors

Frequency of seeing a psychologist or psychiatrist in the past 12 months

Ever attempted suicide

Frequency of uncontrolled anxiety attacks in the past 90 days

Frequency of verbally abusing others without being provoked

Use of sedatives to sleep

Violent Behaviors

Ever perpetrated forced sex

Ever assaulted a person to show dominance

Frequency of reckless driving in the past 12 months

Sexual harassment of coworker

obtaining the COC can be a time-consuming process; you will need to begin the application as soon as a final protocol has been created and approved.

In addition to potentially having to obtain a COC, NIH-funded studies are often required to have what is known as a Data Safety and Monitoring Board (DSMB). This requirement typically applies to randomized trials enrolling three hundred or more study participants. Box 3.5 displays more information about the requirements for and the responsibilities of a DSMB. Briefly, this is typically a 5-member board of experts who monitor the progress of randomized trials. As noted previously in this chapter, progress relative to enrollment and retention is critical simply because reaching a sufficient sample size is necessary to power a study, thereby creating a fair test of the study hypotheses. In turn, the fair test of the study hypotheses equates with a reasonable belief that study participants could indeed "benefit science," as is so often stated in consent forms.

BOX 3.5. ROLES AND RESPONSIBILITIES OF A DATA SAFETY AND MONITORING BOARD (DSMB)

- The DSMB acts as an independent advisory board.
- The DSMB issues opinions from a collection of recognized experts in the relevant topic matter.
- At regular intervals, the DSMB convenes to monitor trial progress.
- Monitoring trial progress through accumulating outcome data is vital.
- All reports of adverse events must be made available to the DSMB.
- The DSMB must use trial endpoints to ensure the safety of study participants.
- When trial safety is compromised, the DSMB may close enrollment and halt study procedures.
- The DSMB may modify a study protocol to protect participants.
- Minutes from DSMB meetings are sent to federal Project Officers for review.

Source: NIH Office of Biotechnology Activities. Clinical trials monitoring. Available at: http://oba.od.nih.gov/policy/policy_issues.html

More important, the DSMB considers the gravity of any serious adverse events that may occur during the course of a randomized trial. An event can be considered serious if there is any reason at all to believe that harm may occur to even one study participant as a consequence. For example, consider a study that uses phone contact (or texting) to remind volunteers about appointed times to complete follow-up assessments. Although strict protocols may be developed that govern how staff contact volunteers via phone, it is of course possible that a staff member may deviate from the protocol, even if it is only one case. Thus a poorly conducted call may result in accidental disclosure of study participation to a person answering the volunteer's phone or text message.

In studies of sexual or drug-use behaviors, this disclosure may be problematic for the volunteer, as harm may ensue. Whether or not the degree of this harm is serious is a decision for the DSMB rather than the principal investigator (who is, of course, likely to have bias). An event may also be considered serious even if harm has not occurred. For example, consider a study that collects data on a laptop computer and uses name identifiers for those records. Imagine then that the computer is stolen! Clearly, the financial loss of the computer itself is negligible, as is the crime of theft. What is important in this situation is the potential for a malicious person to hack into the stolen computer, locate the data, and obtain sensitive information about people who have trusted the study principal investigator and staff with their protections of confidentiality. Even though no immediate reports of this malicious behavior may be obvious, the potential for betraying the confidentiality of one or more study participants (even hundreds) will exist indefinitely. Thus, once again, the DSMB is entrusted with making value judgments about the likelihood and gravity of this occurrence.

Perhaps the single most important function of the DSMB is to monitor the effect size of the trial. As you will learn in further detail later in this textbook, effect size is the difference between the intervention and control groups relative to the dependent variable (with the dependent variable being the behavior or biological measure of interest—the "target" of the intervention effort). If a trial has proceeded well beyond the halfway point and the effect size is negligible, then a condition known as futility may exist. **Futility** means that finding statistically significant differences between groups is no longer mathematically or pragmatically possible. Only a DSMB can declare futility. Box 3.6 displays the abstract of a study that ended in this declaration. As you might imagine, once the DSMB declares futility, enrollment in the study is closed and funding becomes limited to those activities necessary to ethically end the participation of those already enrolled. An intriguing corollary to futility occurs when an intervention program (or device/product) works so well that it becomes clear to the DSMB that the trial is prematurely successful; therefore, enrolling additional participants would have no value. The DSMB may recommend that the study be "unblinded" (this means that staff must inform participants whether they were in the intervention or control group) and all of those who were randomized to the control condition be immediately offered the intervention, given new evidence that the intervention is actually beneficial. Again, it bears repeating that only a DSMB can make this judgment—it is not within the purview of the principle investigator or the IRB.

futility

refers to the impossibility of finding statistically significant effects due to small effect size

---

BOX 3.6. AN EXAMPLE OF A TRIAL THAT WAS STOPPED BY A DSMB

BACKGROUND

Preexposure prophylaxis with antiretroviral drugs has been effective in the prevention of human immunodeficiency virus (HIV) infection in some trials but not in others.

METHODS

In this randomized, double-blind, placebo-controlled trial, we assigned 2120 HIV-negative women in Kenya, South Africa, and Tanzania to receive either a combination of tenofovir disoproxil fumarate and emtricitabine (TDF–FTC) or placebo once daily. The primary objective was to assess the effectiveness of TDF–FTC in preventing HIV acquisition and to evaluate safety.

RESULTS

HIV infections occurred in 33 women in the TDF–FTC group (incidence rate, 4.7 per 100 person-years) and in 35 in the placebo group (incidence rate, 5.0 per 100 person-years), for an estimated hazard ratio in the TDF-FTC group of 0.94 (95% confidence interval, 0.59 to 1.52; $P=0.81$). The proportions of women with nausea, vomiting, or elevated alanine aminotransferase levels were significantly higher in the TDF–FTC group ($P=0.04$, $P<0.001$, and $P=0.03$, respectively). Rates of drug discontinuation because of hepatic or renal abnormalities were higher in the TDF–FTC group (4.7%) than in the placebo group (3.0%, $P=0.051$). Less than 40% of the HIV-uninfected women in the TDF–FTC group had evidence of recent pill use at visits that were matched to the HIV-infection window for women with seroconversion. The study was stopped early, on April 18, 2011, because of lack of efficacy.

CONCLUSIONS

Prophylaxis with TDF–FTC did not significantly reduce the rate of HIV infection and was associated with increased rates of side effects, as compared with placebo. Despite substantial counseling efforts, drug adherence appeared to be low. (Supported by the U.S. Agency for International Development and others; FEM-PrEP ClinicalTrials.gov number, NCT00625404.)

Source: Van Damme, L., Corneli, A., Ahmed, K., et al. (2012). Pre-exposure prophylaxis for HIV infection among African women. *New England Journal of Medicine*, 367, 411–22.

Finally, with regard to the DSMB, it is also critical that a study protocol include a Data Safety and Monitoring Plan (DSMP), a set of operational procedures designed by the PI to protect the integrity and security of the data. This is also the plan that describes how the DSMB will be formed, how and when it will meet, and the role of the DSMB in relation to the study. In addition to being a standard element of ethical practice, a well-written DSMP is also an excellent addition to grant applications requesting funding.

Despite all of the protections provided by the IRB and, when applicable, the DSMB, the ultimate assurance that protections will be observed is a function of only one thing: the integrity of the principle investigators, co-investigators, and research staff. Integrity means that the investigators remain honest and faithful to the agreed protocols and that they never yield to the temptation to cover up indiscretions through lack of reporting or other acts of omission. This is challenging, because in environments that place a premium on funded studies, the fear of losing funds or having

Table 3.2   Examples of Circumstances That May Indicate Possible Breaches in Integrity

Circumstance	Possible Breach
Funding is contingent on meeting enrollment goals.	If rates of enrollment have been low, then protocol violations may occur when making efforts to be more persuasive with likely volunteers.
Prespecified hypotheses do not appear correct during interim data analysis.	Altering study hypotheses during a study is a violation of the approved protocol and the consent agreement.
Lack of "goodwill" and open communication between the PI and the IRB/DSMB.	Delay in reporting adverse events or delay in reporting protocol changes may occur. In extreme cases, delay in conducting DSMB-requested interim reviews of data may occur.
Publication is contingent on finding a significant effect size.	Alteration of randomization plan or an alteration of the intervention may occur. Worst-case scenarios involve data fabrication.

a study halted can be strong enough to overwhelm the commitment to protect study participants and honor all IRB and/or DSMB regulations.

Integrity is vital not only to the research process but also to analysis, interpretation, and reporting. Table 3.2 provides a listing of potential scenarios in which integrity may be violated.

Data Reporting, Timeliness, and Ethics

Health promotion research studies often reveal very high levels of risk behaviors for identifiable communities. For large communities, reporting the findings in professional literature may not be a problem at all. However, for small communities (or, even worse, clinic-based studies), reporting the findings as occurring specifically in an identified location or specifically among a defined population in an identifiable geographic area may pose ethical issues. The problem is not one of breaching confidentiality (given the aggregate nature of the reporting); rather, it is an issue with stigmatizing defined populations for specific behaviors (such as sexual behaviors, substance abuse, violent behaviors). Consequently, the accepted convention is to avoid revealing the name of the city and state where the data were collected. For example, rather than writing, "data collection occurred in Plains, GA" you would write, "data collection occurred in a small southern town."

A related reporting issue applies when the study sample is so small as to create groups of only one or two people. For example, imagine a study that tests for antibodies to the Hepatitis C virus. In your sample of 500 people, 496 test negative and 4 test positive. The "group" of only four people is still an aggregate report, but it comes very close to identifying individuals. What if, for example, only one of the four was female? In that case, your journal article singles out the lone positive case, albeit without naming her publicly. This practice is to be avoided, and this is why the CDC, for example, avoids reporting HIV incident rates for low-occurrence geographic areas.

A final issue concerns timeliness. Most data have a limited shelf life, and their applicability to the profession thus deteriorates over time. Consequently, the researcher has an obligation to report the findings reasonably soon (within less than one year, for example) after concluding data collection. This is particularly true with regard to intervention studies addressing the prevention of epidemic diseases. If the intervention "worked," that information can indeed benefit others (the principle of beneficence), and that process can begin as soon as the trial findings are published. If the intervention "failed," that information can indeed also benefit others as soon as the trial findings are published, in that prevention programs may know what not to do. Of course, as you can imagine, it is widely considered unethical to collect data and not attempt to publish the findings.

Summary

Ethical issues must always be the first concern in health promotion research and practice. This chapter addressed the general principles used to ensure that health promotion research will be conducted in ways that optimally protect study participants. The intent was not to provide an exhaustive review of all the ethical issues involved in conducting health promotion research; however, the most critical issues were presented. Researchers should be knowledgeable about the history of research abuse, core ethical principles, and federal inclusion policies, as well as federal regulations regarding research protections, and should incorporate such understanding into their research plans and personal conduct within the research setting.

KEY TERMS

Assent	Justice
Beneficence	Libertarian paternalism
Exempt	Psychosocial risk
Expedited	Randomized, controlled trials (RCTs)
Full committee review	Respect for persons
Futility	Sampling frame
Iatrogenesis	

For Practice and Discussion

1. The Tuskegee study is an extreme case of unethical conduct in research. Far more examples exist that are much less egregious. Based on what you have learned in this chapter, look through the published literature in health promotion until you locate an article that you suspect may be connected to a study that lacked complete ethical practices. At first, this may seem quite impossible, but please bear in mind that even seemingly minor infractions can pose harm to study volunteers. For example, what if you located an article that reported findings from a study of teens and their parents where both parties were interviewed in their own home about sex and drug use behaviors? You would, in this case, expect assurances that interviews with teens were conducted in a way that completely protected their responses from being overheard by their parents. As another example, what if you located a study that reported outstanding effects of a behavioral intervention trial but did not report that once these effects were discovered, the volunteers assigned to the treatment group were given the intervention program. Once you find your example, please cite the article and describe why you feel the researchers lacked complete ethical practices.

2. In the authors' experience as professors, we have found that students typically confuse the concepts of beneficence and justice. These are each complex and distinct from one another. Find a colleague who is also taking this course and engage in the following exercise with him/her. Each of you is to compose 3 artificial scenarios that illustrate at least one example of beneficence and at least one example of justice—but be sure not to use these terms in those scenarios. Then trade scenarios and label your partner's examples as either "B" or "J." Then discuss with one another the intended answers and, finally, rectify any disagreements experienced in this exchange.

3. Imagine that you have just been funded to conduct a study that will investigate reasons why people binge eat when they are depressed. Think this through carefully. Then use the guidance in this chapter to draft a potential consent form that could be used for that study—be sure to pay close attention to the three principles outlined in the Belmont Report and the remaining principles outlined in this chapter. As a rule, a good consent form should use plain language (sixth grade reading level or lower) and it should be quite complete—a minimum of 3 pages. Be prepared to turn this in to your course professor if asked to do so.

4. All U.S.-based research institutions require study investigators to take a free online course in research ethics (the CITI, introduced earlier in the chapter). Locate this website and take the modules relevant

to behavioral and social sciences research (you will need to do this anyway if you are conducting research for an honors thesis, master's thesis/capstone, or a doctoral dissertation). After you complete the course, respond to the following questions:

a. What part of the course was not consistent with one or more points in this chapter? Explain why.

b. What part of the course included material that you did not learn in this chapter? Elaborate.

c. Did you find that any material in the CITI course was incorrect, based on your understanding of this chapter? Explain your answer.

References

Buchanan, D. R. (2000). *An ethic for health promotion*. New York: Oxford University Press.

Carter, S. M., Rychetnik, L., Lloyd, B., Kerridge, I. H., Baur, L., Bauman, A., . . . and Zask, A. (2011). Evidence, ethics, and values: A framework for health promotion. *American Journal of Public Health*, *101*(3), 465–472. doi:10.2105/ajph.2010.195545

DiClemente, R. J., Santelli, J. S., and Crosby, R. A. (Eds.). (2009). *Adolescent health: Understanding and preventing risk*. San Francisco: Jossey-Bass Wiley.

Food and Drug Administration (FDA) (2012). Truvada for PrEP fact sheet: Ensuring safe and proper use. www.fda.gov/downloads/NewsEvents/Newsroom/FactSheets/UCM312279.pdf

Ménard, J.-F. (2010). A "nudge" for public health ethics: Libertarian paternalism as a framework for ethical analysis of public health interventions? *Public Health Ethics*, *3*(3), 229–238.

Meyerson, B. E., Martich, F. A., and Naehr, G. P. (2008). *Ready to go: The history and contributions of the U.S. public health advisors*. Research Triangle Park, NC: American Social Health Association.

Presidential Commission for the Study of Bioethical Issues. (2011). "Ethically impossible" STD research in Guatemala from 1946 to 1948. Washington, D.C.

Santelli, J. F. (2006). Ethical issues in health promotion research. In R. A. Crosby, R. J. DiClemente, and L. S. Salazar (Eds.), *Research methods in health promotion* (pp. 41–72). San Francisco: Jossey-Bass.

Santelli, J. S., Smith Rogers, A., Rosenfeld, W. D., DuRant, R. H., Dubler, N., Morreale, M., . . . Schissel, A. (2003). Guidelines for adolescent health research: A position paper of the Society for Adolescent Medicine. *Journal of Adolescent Health*, *33*(5), 396–409.

Thigpen, M. C., Kebaabetswe, P. M., Paxton, L. A., et al. (2012). Antiretroviral pre-exposure prophylaxis for heterosexual HIV transmission in Botswana. *New England Journal of Medicine*, *367*, 423–34.

U.S. Department of Health and Human Services. (1979). The Belmont Report. Available at: http://www.hhs.gov/ohrp/humansubjects/guidance/belmont.html

Vallgarda, S. (2012). Nudge: A new and better way to improve health? *Health Policy*, *104*(2), 200–203. doi:10.1016/j.healthpol.2011.10.013

PART TWO

FUNDAMENTALS OF HEALTH PROMOTION RESEARCH

CHAPTER 4

OBSERVATIONAL RESEARCH DESIGNS

Laura F. Salazar
Richard A. Crosby
Ralph J. DiClemente

The research design of a study is the *strategy* the investigator chooses for answering the research question. The research question directs the type of design chosen. If the nature of the research question involves making observations rather than making causal inferences, then it would be considered observational research. There are a variety of observational research designs from which to choose, each with its own strengths and weaknesses. Ultimately, the design chosen should be tied to the research question; however, other factors—such as ethical issues, cost, feasibility, and access to the study population—may play a significant role as well. It is critical for the investigator to choose the most appropriate design, as this will affect the success of the research project and will determine the conclusions that may be drawn from the research.

In general, scientific inquiry can be conceptualized as an interlocking chain, with each link being a precursor of the next. The first link in the chain represents exploratory research, and the subsequent links represent varying levels of conclusive research. The model shown in Figure 4.1 can be applied to health promotion research, and, as shown, exploratory research is often conducted when the health issue has not been clearly defined, or a scientific basis for inquiry has not yet been established. In other words, little is known about the topic. In this early stage, observations are needed to provide investigators with data to define health issues, to begin to understand

LEARNING OBJECTIVES

- Differentiate the two stages of research in the context of health promotion research.

- Understand the difference between qualitative and quantitative research and data.

- Learn the different observational research designs used in health promotion research.

- Distinguish the strengths and weaknesses of each observational research design.

- Develop a basic understanding of data analytic approaches for each research design.

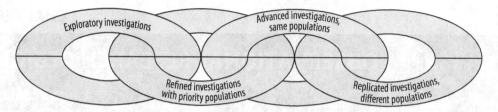

Exploratory investigations generate (rather than test) specific research questions. Refined studies initially test a given set of research questions, and priority populations are defined through surveillance and epidemiological studies. Advanced investigations are built on findings from previous tests of research questions. After the research questions have been adequately addressed in a priority population, investigations should be replicated with a second priority population.

Figure 4.1 The Chain of Research in Health Promotion

etiology
the cause of a health condition

the **etiology** of those health issues, to generate insight into a problem, to formulate theories, to reveal relevant factors, and to identify potential relationships.

The research conducted in the exploratory stage is regarded as preliminary and serves as the basis for future conclusive research efforts. Some examples of exploratory research questions follow, and, as these examples indicate, the research question involves investigations that will describe the issue. Depending on the outcomes, this type of research is usually viewed as a springboard for further inquiry.

- Are college students being harassed online?

- What does "using condoms" mean for Latino immigrants?

- Do family-level factors contribute to obesity among toddlers in the United States?

- What barriers exist, if any, to getting vaccinated for the human papillomavirus among young men?

- Does the built environment contribute to respiratory disorders in global megacities such as Mumbai, Mexico City, Jakarta, Tokyo, or Karachi?

- Does intimate partner violence affect HIV risk for men who have sex with men?

- Is intimate partner violence related to women's health-seeking behaviors?

Conclusive research, on the other hand and as the term suggests, provides information that is useful for reaching conclusions or in making decisions. Research in this phase generally has five overarching purposes: (1) to document the scope of the issue (see Box 4.1 for common public health indicators of scope), (2) to test causal or etiological theories, (3) to identify the sequelae of disease or health conditions, (4) to evaluate measurement instruments, and (5) to evaluate treatments or interventions. Take the issue of HIV/AIDS, previously mentioned in Chapter One. At the onset of the epidemic in the early 1980s, the research conducted was exploratory in nature, as little was known about the condition at the time. Now that we are in the third decade of research and much knowledge has been generated, most of this research is conclusive. To glean a better idea of what types of research purposes would be considered as conclusive research, a sample of questions pertaining to HIV/AIDS research from each of these five research purposes is provided. As these examples illustrate, conclusive research is marked by clearly defined research questions. In comparison with exploratory research, the process is more formal and structured. Findings inform hypothesis testing and decision making.

- How many new cases of HIV infection occurred among men who have sex with men (MSM)?

- How many new cases of AIDS were diagnosed among injection drug users in the Northeastern United States?

- What are the risk factors for HIV infection among African-American women?

- What are the psychological and psychosocial effects of HIV diagnosis among adolescents?

- Does social support protect against negative effects of HIV diagnosis among homeless women?

- How well does a sexual risk-reduction program reduce unsafe HIV-related behaviors as compared with an abstinence program?

- What are the long-term side effects of highly active antiretroviral therapy?

- What are the side effects of an HIV vaccine among African-American men?

BOX 4.1. PREVALENCE VERSUS INCIDENCE

Prevalence and *incidence*, two very important concepts in health promotion research, are also two very different ways of measuring a disease's occurrence. *Prevalence* of a condition refers to the total number of people who currently have the condition, whereas *incidence* refers to the number of people diagnosed with the condition annually. A chronic incurable disease such as AIDS can have a low incidence but high prevalence. A short-duration curable condition such as a bacterial sexually transmitted disease (STD) can have a high incidence but low prevalence because many people get an STD each year, but few people actually have a bacterial STD at any given time.

The two stages in the research process, exploratory and conclusive, can be further subdivided into two overarching categories of research purpose: descriptive and causal research. Figure 4.2 provides a graphic depiction of health promotion research in terms of stages, purpose, and designs. Descriptive research provides data describing the "who, what, where, when, and how" of a health issue versus what caused it. Therefore studies that reveal which individuals either are at risk or have a particular health issue or condition; that document incidence, prevalence, or both; that examine risk factors; that look at the effects of having the health issue; and that assess scale properties designed to measure a construct related to a health issue would be categorized as descriptive research. The main limitation with descriptive research is that it cannot assess what caused the health issue. This is where causal research steps in. Determining a cause-and-effect relationship is imperative in situations in which the investigator must reveal the true cause(s) of a particular disease or when evaluating whether or not a program caused the observed changes. In some instances, however, it may not be ethical to use an experimental design to reveal the true cause and effect. For example, it would be unethical to randomize pregnant women to drink alcohol or not drink alcohol to determine the effects of alcohol on the fetus

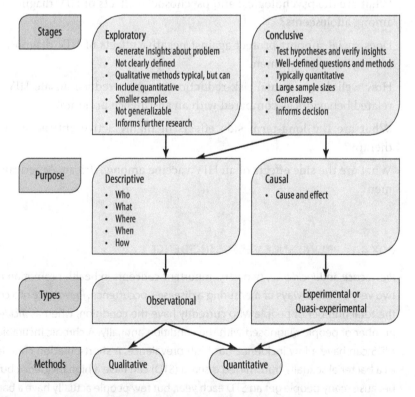

Figure 4.2 Health Promotion Research Stages, Purpose, Types, and Methods

IN A NUTSHELL

Descriptive research provides data describing the "who, what, where, when, and how" of a health issue, versus what caused it.

in utero. In this scenario, an observational study would be the only option. In this chapter, we provide an overview of the observational research designs used for conducting descriptive research in health promotion. Subsequently, in Chapter Five, we provide an overview of experimental and quasi-experimental designs used for conducting causal research in health promotion.

Observational Research

Qualitative versus quantitative. As shown in Figure 4.2, descriptive research, whether in the exploratory or the conclusive stage, utilizes observational research to achieve its objectives. Observational research or nonexperimental research refers to research in which phenomena are observed either in the real world or in a laboratory setting—yet no *manipulation* of the participants and their decision making occurs. Observational research can take many forms and varies depending on the extent to which the investigator intrudes on or attempts to control the environment. Furthermore, observational research can vary depending on the nature of the data collection methods involved, such as using either **qualitative** or **quantitative** methods. In simple terms, qualitative methods involve making observations or collecting data that typically cannot be expressed numerically. Observational research that uses qualitative methods aligns with the exploratory stage. Qualitative research typically does not entail the use of specific research designs per se; rather, depending on the research question, different strategies are used (Morse, 1994). A few qualitative strategies are naturalistic observation, phenomenology, ethnography, and grounded theory. For example, naturalistic observation—also known as nonparticipant observation—involves studying behaviors or other phenomena that occur naturally as opposed to occurring within the artificial environment of a controlled laboratory setting. The investigator either covertly or overtly observes certain behaviors of the people he or she is studying. Conducting a naturalistic observation study allows the investigator to observe and measure what behavior is *really* like because it is done in real-life settings. Because of this advantage, naturalistic observation is especially conducive for generating insight into a problem so that further inquiries can be made on a larger scale.

qualitative
making observations or collecting data that typically cannot be expressed numerically

quantitative
observations or data that can take on numerical values.

Collins et al. (2012) conducted a naturalistic observation study at a service organization that implemented a program for homeless persons with significant alcohol use. Investigators observed verbal exchanges between staff and residents, made observations during staff rounds, and audio-recorded staff focus groups and resident interview sessions in order to better understand the role of alcohol use in the lives of homeless individuals enrolled in the housing program. The qualitative data collected thus included field notes and audio recordings. They found that a harm reduction approach, that is, a focus on prevention of harm associated with alcohol or drug use rather than prevention of alcohol) was more desirable to program residents than a traditional abstinence approach and that programs for the homeless must consider the residents' motivations for using alcohol. Thus these results could be used to strengthen similar programs and evaluate them on a larger scale. One of the advantages of using naturalistic observation is that it has high **ecological validity**, meaning it can be generalized to real-life circumstances. It allows the investigator to *observe* what people do rather than *asking* them what they do. The main weaknesses of naturalistic observation are (1) conclusions cannot be drawn as to the exact causes of the behaviors under investigation, and (2) the presence of the investigator may exert some influence on the behavior being observed, resulting in bias.

ecological validity
results of study that can be generalized to real-life circumstances

Other types of qualitative methods are more intrusive than naturalistic observation and can involve actual interaction with people, such as conducting interviews. The data collected in interviews consist of verbal responses to either structured or semistructured questions. These responses may be audio-recorded and then transcribed. The investigator would then perform an analysis by reviewing the transcriptions and identifying **themes** that emerged. In general, themes are abstract constructs, which the investigators may identify before, during, or after data collection. A review of transcripts would entail inducing themes from the text. All results are conveyed through description. An example of a qualitative study that involved face-to-face interviews, which were audio-recorded, transcribed, and analyzed for themes, was conducted by Hailemariam, Kassie, and Sisay (2012). The purpose of the study was to explore the experiences of HIV-discordant couples living in Addis Ababa, Ethiopia, regarding their sexual life and fertility desire. Discordant, or serodiscordant, in this context indicates that one member of the couple is HIV-positive and the other is HIV-negative. They conducted interviews with twenty-eight participants who were living in an HIV serodiscordant long-term relationship. Interviews were audiotaped and field notes taken. The overarching theme was "struggling to maintain the relationship," which was conceptualized as a process whereby couples passed through a series of phases such as "entering

themes
abstract constructs that investigators identify before, during, or after data collection

a transition," "dealing with the discordancy," "shared life," and "ups and downs" (Hailemariam, Kassie, and Sisay, 2012, p. 5). Hence the results of the interviews were used to conceptualize a theoretical model involving these themes as interrelated constructs that could be tested with future research using quantitative methods. We have provided only a brief introduction to some types of qualitative research here; however, you will find additional qualitative methods and strategies described in much greater depth in Chapter Eight.

In contrast to qualitative methods, quantitative methods involve observations or data that can take on numerical values. Quantitative data might include frequency of responses or occurrences, or it might entail a process whereby participants' verbal or written responses are quantified by transforming them into numerical values. Analyses of quantitative methods require the use of statistical procedures. Observational research that uses quantitative methods would entail the use of cross-sectional designs, successive independent samples designs, longitudinal or cohort designs, cohort-sequential designs, case-control designs, and case-crossover designs. We describe these designs in greater detail in the following sections.

Cross-Sectional Design

One of the most commonly used research designs in health promotion is the cross-sectional design. The hallmark of this design is that time is fixed. The collection of data at one point in time can be thought of as taking a "snapshot" of health conditions at that moment/month/year (see Figure 4.3). Because this data collection occurs at only one time, the cross-sectional design can measure only *differences* between or among a variety of people, subjects, or phenomena rather than any type of *change*. Thus cross-sectional designs focus on studying and drawing inferences from existing differences among people, subjects, or phenomena. Differences could be in race or ethnicity, gender, age, or socioeconomic level or in exposure to a certain health risk; phenomena could include prevalence of various health-related conditions, treatments, services, or other outcomes and the factors associated with such outcomes. To make valid inferences using a cross-sectional design, it is extremely important that the results generalize to the larger population; Therefore the sample selected should be a random sample if possible and of sufficient size (see Chapter Six for more on sampling).

Most survey-research designs are cross-sectional; however, other types of research besides survey research may use cross-sectional designs. Survey research constitutes a field of scientific inquiry in its own right and

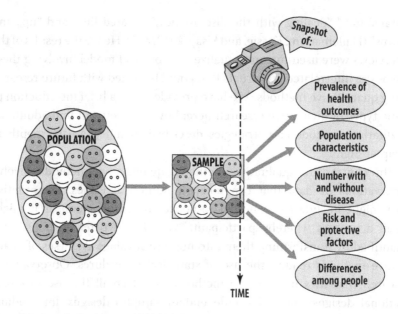

Figure 4.3 Cross-Sectional Design with Multiple Purposes

we have dedicated Chapter Thirteen to describing this type of research. For now, we provide some basic highlights of survey research. It is best defined as a scientific method to help understand the characteristics of a population. By characteristics, we mean people's thoughts, opinions, feelings, and behaviors. Surveys are conducted for myriad reasons and are used not only by public health professionals but also by political scientists, psychologists, sociologists, and marketing researchers. Surveys vary according to their mode of administration. They can be conducted over the telephone or in person. They can be self-administered using paper and pencil in a classroom or using a computer. Some surveys are administered via mail, others via the Internet. Regardless of the mode of administration, data analysis for cross-sectional surveys typically involves descriptive statistics in which frequencies or percentages are calculated and are of interest.

As an example of survey research, consider a study examining exposure to, frequency of, and perceived seriousness of cyberbullying. Self-administered questionnaires were mailed to a representative sample of 12- to 18-year-olds in Finland in 2009 (Lindfors, Kaltiala-Heino, and Rimpela, 2012). The respondents could either answer via the mailed paper questionnaire or the Internet. Respondents were asked questions about four dimensions of cyberbullying: being a cyber victim, being a cyberbully, being both a cyber victim and cyberbully, and witnessing the cyberbullying of friends. The results showed that the proportion of adolescents indicating exposure to at least one of the measured dimensions was 23 percent. The proportion was higher among girls than boys. The proportion was lowest among 18-year-olds and highest among 14-year-olds of both sexes.

In another example, a study conducted by Holt et al. (2013) examined counseling and provision practices for female condoms in sub-Saharan Africa with a nationally representative sample of 1,444 nurses and physicians. Holt and colleagues conducted surveys and in-depth interviews, in which they asked questions regarding female and male condoms counseling and provision practices as well as demographic and professional practice characteristics. A total of 614 providers from South Africa and 830 providers from Zimbabwe completed the survey, with an overall response rate of 73.2 percent. In South Africa, the response rate did not differ between hospitals (61 percent) and clinics (60 percent), although results showed that nurses were more likely to respond than physicians (66 percent versus 39 percent). In Zimbabwe, providers in hospitals were more likely to respond than in clinics (92 percent versus 81 percent), and physicians were more likely to respond than nurses (100 percent versus 87 percent).

Although there is only one criterion to a cross-sectional design (that is, measurement is conducted at one point in time), research that uses a cross-sectional design can have more than one purpose. Cross-sectional designs can be used to document the prevalence of a specific health issue. Studies with this purpose are sometimes referred to as surveillance or prevalence studies. Data analysis for prevalence studies is similar to survey research in that it is mostly descriptive, meaning that frequencies of responses, means, and percentages are calculated for the specific health issue or disease for the overall sample or possibly for specific subgroups of the sample. For example, Yu et al. (2013) conducted serologic surveillance for H5 and H9 influenza subtypes among poultry workers in Beijing, China, from 2009 to 2010. In addition, the researchers used surveys to test poultry workers' knowledge, attitudes, and beliefs regarding avian flu infection. Serum specimens were collected from 305 workers who were in close contact with poultry. The serum specimens were subtyped using microneutralization assay to identify the presence of either H5 or H9 influenza antibodies.

Other types of surveillance studies can be used to document the prevalence of health-related *behavior*. For example, the Centers for Disease Control and Prevention (CDC) is interested in knowing how many adolescents engage in certain health-risk behaviors. The Youth Risk Behavior Surveillance System (YRBSS) monitors six categories of priority health-risk behaviors among youths and young adults—behaviors that contribute to unintentional injuries and violence; tobacco use; alcohol and other drug use; sexual behaviors that contribute to unintended pregnancy and STDs, including human immunodeficiency virus (HIV) infection; unhealthy dietary behaviors; and physical inactivity plus being overweight. Some results from the 2013 national Youth Risk Behavior Survey (YRBS) demonstrated that among the high school students surveyed:

- 7.6 percent had never or rarely worn a seatbelt in the preceding 30 days;

- 21.9 percent had ridden one or more times with a driver who had been drinking alcohol;

- 10.0 percent had driven a car one or more times after they had been drinking alcohol;

- 41.4 percent had texted or emailed while driving on at least one day in the last 30 days;

- 15.7 percent had smoked cigarettes on at least one day in the preceding 30 days;

- 17.7 percent had carried a weapon (gun, knife or club) on at least one day in the last 30 days;

- 19.6 percent had been bullied at least once on school property while 14.8 percent had been electronically bullied in the preceding 12 months;

- 10.5 percent of females had been physically forced to have sexual intercourse;

- 34.9 percent had at least one drink of alcohol on at least one day in the preceding 30 days; and

- 46.8 percent had ever had sexual intercourse. [Kann et al., 2014, pp. 6-24]

In addition to assessing prevalence of disease or health-related behaviors, cross-sectional designs can also be used to estimate levels of knowledge and health-related attitudes, beliefs, and opinions. For studies with this purpose, descriptive analyses would again be applied and would include frequencies of responses, percentages, and means for continuous scale measures. For example, Ahmed and el-Guindy (2011) conducted a survey among baccalaureate nursing students in Cairo, Egypt, to measure their breastfeeding knowledge and attitudes. Results showed that the mean breastfeeding knowledge score was 12.41 points out of a possible 24.0 and the attitudes mean score was 3.13 out of a possible 5.0. Thus the results revealed weak breastfeeding knowledge and neutral breastfeeding attitudes.

Another function addressed by cross-sectional designs is the ability to assess the relationships among variables for a given population. In health promotion research, this may involve determining the risk or protective factors for a given health-related outcome or determining the significant theoretical factors related to a given health-related outcome. Data analysis for these types of studies would involve calculating correlation coefficients, prevalence ratios and odds ratios, or chi-square test for independence. When investigating relationships among variables, the research is often referred to as correlational; however, there is a distinction between the statistical technique and the design. Using a cross-sectional design to investigate the correlation between two variables by applying statistical techniques (for instance, the Pearson product moment correlation coefficient) precludes the ability to infer causal relationships. In a correlational relationship, changes in one variable accompany changes in another; however, it cannot be said that one variable influenced or caused changes in another when the two variables were measured at the same point in time and observational methods were employed.

For example, in a cross-sectional study that found a significant and positive relationship between knowledge of HIV and consistent condom use, we could not infer that high levels of knowledge caused a high degree of condom use. An exception would be made, however, if the data were collected using experimental methods. For example, if we measured knowledge of HIV and consistent condom use among a group of people (baseline), randomized them to either an HIV educational curriculum group or a control group, and compared groups following the intervention, then in this scenario a positive correlation between the same two variables in the treatment group as compared to the control may imply a causal relationship. This is an important distinction that needs to be made: it is the manner in which the data are collected and not the statistical technique that allows one to make causal inferences. A classic example to support this assertion is that crime rates and ice cream consumption tend to be correlated. Yet you would not conclude that eating more ice cream causes crime rates to increase unless you conducted a controlled experiment and randomized people to an "ice cream eating" condition or to a placebo control condition. If people in the ice cream eating condition exhibited more aggression than people in the control condition, then you could possibly conclude that ice cream causes an increase in crime. Logic and reasoning applied to this example suggest that more likely, the ice cream and crime rate correlation is due to a **third-variable problem**, in which there is another unmeasured variable affecting both of the measured variables and causing the two variables to appear correlated with each other (for example, hotter temperatures in the summer affect people's

third-variable problem
another unmeasured variable affecting both of the measured variables and causing the two variables to appear correlated with each other

IN A NUTSHELL

It is the manner in which you collect the data and not the statistical technique that allows one to make causal inferences.

moods and levels of aggression and also influence people to eat more ice cream). Unless this potential third variable is measured in the study, one would only be able to guess as to what the real explanation is.

Voisin, Salazar, Crosby, and DiClemente (2013) conducted a study that demonstrated the potential for the third-variable problem. In their study, they examined ethnic identity and its correlation with chlamydia and gonorrhea infection among female detained adolescents. Findings indicated that participants who indicated high ethnic identity were 4.3 times more likely to test positive for either of these infections compared to those scoring low on the measure of ethnic identity. Clearly, ethnic identity cannot *cause* a sexually transmitted disease (STD)—a bacterial pathogen transmitted by an infected partner is the culprit (the third variable). In this study, the authors did not purport a cause-effect relationship between ethnic identity and STD, but rather they wanted to identify potential risk factors for acquiring an infection so that subgroups of the population who are at heightened risk could be identified for possible intervention. However, in other studies, in which investigators are attempting to establish correlations as a basis for further conclusive research, the omission of a key variable could potentially undermine the results.

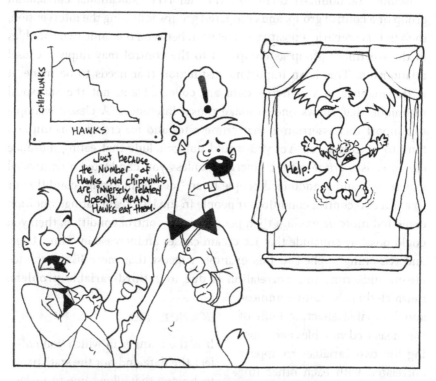

Mincus Iterates That Correlation Does Not Mean Causation
Copyright 2005 by Justin Wagner; reprinted with permission.

Table 4.1 Strengths and Weaknesses of Cross-Sectional Research Designs

Design	Strengths	Weaknesses
Cross-sectional	Quick and relatively inexpensive because data are collected once	Not good for documenting rare health outcomes or ones that are of short duration
	Low or no attrition	May need an extremely large sample size to power the study
	Participation rate usually high due to low commitment	Results may be affected by selection bias due to accessibility to targeted population members
	Burden of risk factors in relation to illness can be determined	No evidence for the temporal relationship between exposure and outcome
	Can formulate hypotheses regarding causal and preventive factors	Cannot determine cause and effect
	Able to measure prevalence	Unable to measure incidence
		Omission of significant variable can undermine results (third variable)
		Cohort effects (such as different ages) may bias results

Although cross-sectional designs are used frequently in correlational research, the design has several weaknesses (see Table 4.1). The design is limited in inferring causation—only an experimental design is capable of establishing cause and effect. Furthermore, it is important to note that in a cause-and-effect relationship, there is a temporal order to the relationship of cause and effect. Establishing this temporal order is a necessary condition for determining which is the cause and which the effect, but a cross-sectional design is unable to establish this temporal order, or directionality. Consider the significant inverse correlation (as one variable increases, the other variable decreases) between depression and self-esteem found frequently in the available literature. It is unclear whether depression leads to low self-esteem or whether low self-esteem leads to depression. In reality, both propositions are equally plausible; therefore, a cross-sectional design is incapable of distinguishing cause from effect. In an example from published research, Shen, Pickard, and Johnson (2013) conducted a study on the effects of volunteering on depression in African-American female caregivers.

IN A NUTSHELL

Although cross-sectional designs are used frequently in correlational research, the design is limited in inferring causation. The design is also unable to establish directionality.

Shen and colleagues were able to demonstrate that volunteerism was inversely related to depressive symptoms, but the authors also suggested that self-esteem may be a third variable. Volunteerism may increase self-esteem, which in turn may decrease depressive symptoms. However, based on the cross-sectional study design it is impossible to determine with a high degree of certainty the temporal order or directionality of these relationships.

Another weakness is that cross-sectional designs do not control for **cohort effects**. Traditionally, the term cohort refers to the part of the population born during a particular period (for instance, in the United States, there are cohorts with names such as the baby boomers, Gen X, and millennials); however, in research, a cohort can refer to any group who shares a common characteristic or experience within a defined period—for example, "men who were exposed to Agent Orange while fighting in Vietnam" or "factory workers exposed to asbestos." Thus in a cross-sectional study, which does not typically recruit a specific cohort, results could be attributed to the life experiences of the cohort rather than developmental age. For example, if a study wanted to ascertain internet addiction among U.S. adults with an internet connection at home, and results showed that people age 60 and older tended to not access the Internet as often as people who were younger, it may be incorrect to conclude that internet usage decreases with age. Rather, the results could be explained by a cohort effect—people in the age 60 and older group may use the Internet less often because while growing up they had less experience with computers compared to younger people.

Even with these shortcomings, we nonetheless continue to conduct observational research using cross-sectional designs as it provides the necessary foundation for more elaborate studies that can improve on the limitations of a cross-sectional design. Also, there are many instances in which it is not feasible or ethical to conduct an experimental research study because manipulation of the variable is impossible, or it is unethical to do so (for instance, you cannot assign a person to any condition that entails risk). Furthermore, cross-sectional correlational studies in health promotion research can be very useful in identifying significant correlates of health-related behaviors and disease outcomes, though not necessarily variables that have a cause-and-effect relationship.

Successive Independent Samples Design

An improvement over the cross-sectional design is the successive independent samples design, also known as a trend study. This design incorporates a series of cross-sectional studies conducted over a period of time. Each cross-sectional survey is conducted with an independent sample, which means that a new sample is drawn for each of the successive cross-sectional surveys and the same questions are asked of each successive sample.

cohort effects
the effects of the study that could be due to a group who shares a common characteristic or experience within a defined period

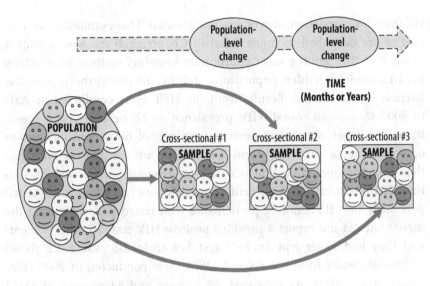

Figure 4.4 Successive Independent Samples Design

This design is used to assess change in a population characteristic (for example, tobacco use, condom use, pregnancy rates) over time; hence the name "trend" study. This design is depicted in Figure 4.4.

As an example, we may want to document the change in certain health-risk behaviors or the prevalence of disease for a given population over a period of time. This would be very important information to have and could inform programs and policy. In fact, this type of design is used quite often in **epidemiology**—the discipline of studying the incidence, distribution, and control of disease in a population. Data analyses for successive independent samples design would be similar to cross-sectional designs but would expand to include a comparison of study outcomes by year or month or other defined periods of time.

The CDC conducts and sponsors many studies using the successive independent samples design. One example is the CDC's National HIV Behavioral Surveillance (NHBS) system, which is used to monitor the prevalence of HIV-related risk behaviors, HIV testing behaviors, access, and use of preventive services as well as to provide context for its HIV surveillance results (Lansky, Sullivan, Gallagher, and Fleming, 2007). NHBS uses the successive independent samples design to study three different high-risk populations (men who have sex with men [MSM]; injection drug users [IDUs]; and heterosexuals at increased risk [HETs]) in rotating annual cycles. Since 2003, NHBS has recruited three successive cross-sectional samples from each of the three populations. For the MSM cycle, venue-based sampling is used to recruit, whereas for the IDUs and the

epidemiology
the discipline of studying the incidence, distribution, and control of disease in a population

HETs cycles, respondent-driven sampling is used. These sampling methodologies are described in more detail in Chapter Six; for now, suffice it to say that they are the most appropriate sampling method for reaching hard-to-reach or hidden populations and for enhancing the representativeness of the sample. Results from the HET cycle conducted in 2006 to 2007 showed an overall HIV prevalence of 2.0 percent and a prevalence of 2.3 percent among persons with annual household incomes at or below the poverty level, and 2.8 percent among persons with less than a high school education (Centers for Disease Control and Prevention, 2013). Overall, 25.8 percent of participants had never been tested previously for HIV. Among participants who tested positive during the survey but did not report a previous positive HIV test, 36 (43.9 percent) said they had never had an HIV test before NHBS. Table 4.2 shows additional results from the second MSM cycle conducted in 2008 (Finlayson et al., 2011). As indicated, 49 percent and 44 percent of MSM reported engaging in unprotected, receptive anal sex with their main and a casual partner, respectively—a high-risk sexual behavior that spreads STDs, including HIV.

At this juncture, we hope you have gleaned that these NHBS results pertain to *only one time point*—in other words, these findings are for *only one* of the cross-sectional studies rather than looking at several of the cross-sections to assess changes over time. You are therefore probably wondering: where are the results for the trend analyses? To answer the ultimate research question associated with using a successive independent samples design, investigators at the CDC have recently (as of this writing) been able to report trends for the time period of 1994 to 2011. They examined cross-sectional HIV prevalence and past twelve-month HIV testing behavior among young MSM using data from five cities across multiple cross-sectional surveys. Overall, trend analyses showed an increase in HIV prevalence among MSM ages 23 to 29, driven by an increase in the city of Baltimore. There was no change in HIV prevalence among MSM ages 18 to 22 overall, although prevalence increased in Baltimore. HIV testing behaviors increased significantly for both age groups (Oster et al., 2014).

Although an improvement over the cross-sectional design, successive independent samples design also suffers from limitations (see Table 4.3). It is very useful for measuring changes over time for a characteristic such as disease or infection; however, for other characteristics, such as behavior, attitudes, or opinions, the researcher cannot determine with certainty the extent to which the population truly changed because the results are based on different samples of people. To attribute documented changes to the time factor, the same group of people must be followed and surveyed over time.

Table 4.2   Number[a] and Percentage of Participants Who Reported Having Had Anal Sex during Their Most Recent Sexual Encounter with a Male Partner, by Type and HIV Status of Partner, Location of Encounter, and Substance Use during Encounter

Characteristic	Insertive anal sex[b] Total[d] No.	(%)	Unprotected[e] No.	(%)	Receptive anal sex[c] Total[d] No.	(%)	Unprotected[e] No.	(%)	Total
Partner type									
Main[f]	2,905	(78)	1,368	(47)	2,267	(61)	1,117	(49)	3,742
Casual[g]	2,886	(65)	1,202	(42)	2,128	(48)	928	(44)	4,427
Partner's HIV status									
Not infected	2,639	(55)	1,190	(45)	2,031	(42)	975	(48)	4,794
Infected	181	(53)	87	(48)	126	(37)	58	(46)	339
Unknown	1,388	(46)	557	(40)	1,026	(34)	417	(41)	3,042
Location where participant met partner of most recent sexual encounter[h]									
Bar or club	1,444	(54)	587	(41)	1,023	(38)	440	(43)	2,699
Internet or chat line	663	(48)	268	(40)	582	(42)	247	(42)	1,392
Cruising area or adult bookstore	218	(45)	88	(40)	139	(29)	55	(40)	483
Bathhouse, sex club, or sex resort	83	(51)	24	(29)	46	(28)	14	(30)	164
Circuit party, rave, or private sex party	67	(50)	22	(33)	69	(52)	26	(38)	133
Other	1,048	(53)	439	(42)	799	(40)	362	(45)	1,984
Substance use during most recent sexual encounter									
None	2,316	(50)	992	(43)	1,864	(40)	842	(45)	4,649
Alcohol only	1,256	(52)	519	(41)	861	(36)	371	(43)	2,400
Drugs only	214	(60)	101	(47)	150	(42)	75	(50)	354
Alcohol and drugs	421	(56)	221	(52)	305	(40)	160	(52)	755
Total	4,208	(51)	1,834	(44)	3,183	(39)	1,450	(46)	8,175

[a] Numbers might not add to total because of missing or unknown data.

[b] The participant placed his penis in the anus of his sex partner.

[c] The participant's sex partner placed his penis in the participant's anus.

[d] Insertive and receptive sex categories were not mutually exclusive. Men might have engaged in both insertive and receptive sex with their partner.

[e] Neither the participant nor his partner used a condom. Proportion reported is that of all participants who engaged in that type of anal sex with that type of partner.

[f] A man with whom the participant had sex and to whom he felt most committed (e.g., boyfriend, spouse, significant other, or life partner).

[g] A man with whom the participant had sex but to whom he did not feel committed, whom he did not know very well, or with whom the participant had sex in exchange for something such as money or drugs.

[h] Among those who reported a relationship duration of ≤3 years with the most recent partner (n = 6,855).

Source: National HIV Behavioral Surveillance System: Men Who Have Sex with Men, 21 U.S. Cities, 2008.

Longitudinal Designs

A longitudinal design is one in which the same participants are followed over a period of time and interviewed more than once during the time period (see Figure 4.5). Longitudinal designs are therefore capable of

Table 4.3   Strengths and Weaknesses of Successive Independent Samples Research Designs

Design	Strengths	Weaknesses
Successive Independent Samples	Can document trends or patterns over time	Samples must be drawn from same population and be equally as representative
	Low attrition and refusal rates	Cannot identify *causes* of any documented change
	Internal validity higher than cross-sectional	

Source: Finlayson et al. (2011), 1–34.

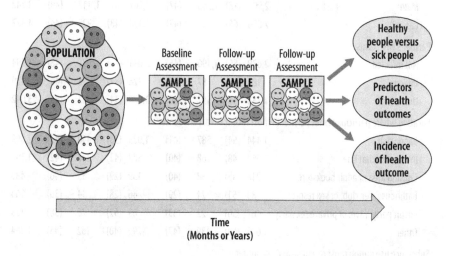

Figure 4.5 Longitudinal/Cohort Design with End Purposes

determining *changes* in health-related outcomes, behavior, attitudes, and opinions over time. Thus longitudinal designs can capture new cases of disease or incidence in a population, unlike cross-sectional designs. Moreover, longitudinal designs can establish a temporal order of exposure to risk and health-related outcomes. The time period of a longitudinal study could range from months to years. Such a study—sometimes referred to as a cohort study, prospective study, trend study, or panel study—begins with a baseline assessment and then proceeds with subsequent follow-up assessments to determine rates of disease, behavior, or other variables of interest in the cohort during a defined period of observation. Within this context, the term cohort study describes an investigation of any designated group of persons who are followed over a period of time.

risk ratios
frequencies calculated by comparing those who were exposed to a possible risk factor to those who had no exposure

Achieving the purpose of longitudinal studies typically involves (1) documenting exposure to risk factors and other confounding variables to determine associations with health outcomes over time (such as **risk ratios**), (2) determining the predictive ability of certain risk and protective factors as they relate to health-related outcomes over time (such as regression coefficients), or (3) estimating rates of disease or behavior changes during the observation period (such as incidence). In the first scenario, frequencies of disease or behavioral outcomes are tested between persons who had exposure to the possible risk factor and persons with no exposure (that is, comparing healthy people to sick people). Thus with a longitudinal design you can ascertain the likelihood that the risk factors are the underlying cause of the health-related outcome. In these types of studies, risk ratios or relative risk would be calculated by comparing those who had developed the health outcome and had been "exposed" to those who developed the health outcome and had not been exposed.

In studies that examine associations between risk and protective factors on the one hand and health-related outcomes on the other hand (the second scenario), with a longitudinal design you can have more confidence that observed correlations may have a causal relationship if they are present over time periods. General estimating equations (GEEs) are an appropriate statistical technique for these types of studies as GEEs accommodate correlated data stemming from multiple time points with the same individuals and can be used to calculate unbiased estimation of population-averaged regression coefficients. Voisin, Tan, and DiClemente (2013) conducted a longitudinal study that examined sexual risk behaviors. Specifically, they determined the correlational relationship between higher sexual sensation seeking (SSS) and condom use. SSS is a trait that is characterized by frequently seeking novel and unusual sexual experiences. A sample of 751 females attending an STD clinic was given a baseline survey with follow-up surveys at 6 and 12 months. GEE regression models were used to evaluate the influence of SSS on STD-related risk factors over the 6-month and 12-month follow-up periods. Using GEE allows researchers to control for repeated within-subject measurements over the longitudinal course of the study. Outcomes included condom use in the last 14 and 60 days, consistency of condom use, number of lifetime sexual partners, partner sexual communication, self-efficacy to refuse sex, and fear of condom negotiation. Results showed that higher SSS predicted lower percent of condom use in the last 14 and 60 days, lower consistent condom use, and a higher number of lifetime sexual partners. Additionally, higher SSS predicted lower partner sexual communication, diminished self-efficacy to refuse sex, and a higher fear of condom negotiation.

In the third scenario, newly diagnosed cases (incidence) of a disease for a cohort could be calculated for the observation period so that both the **density incidence** (DI) and **cumulative incidence** (CI) could be determined. Calculating incidence cannot be done in cross-sectional studies, but incidence is extremely useful to know so that an evaluation of trends

regression coefficients
the predictive ability of certain risk and protective factors as they relate to health-related outcomes over time

density incidence
the ratio of incident cases to the population at risk during a particular time period

cumulative incidence
the ratio of incident cases to the at-risk population at the beginning of the observation period

can be documented (for example, how many people are contracting HIV each year?) and a determination of the effectiveness of prevention efforts can be made. DI is defined as the ratio of incident cases to the population at risk during the course of a time period. The ratio of the numerator to the denominator thus acts as a measure of the *concentration* of observed events (density) by individual and time period and serves as a measure of risk of developing the disease or outcome. In this instance, individual and time period refers to the years (or days/months) of observation time each person contributes (in other words, **person-years**). So for each individual you would have to calculate the time they were in the study in order to calculate their person-year. Thus if you have a cohort of 2,000 people, all of whom are followed for a period of 30 years, 200 of whom develop the disease, then the DI would be the ratio of newly diagnosed cases (200) to a denominator equal to 2000 × 30 years = 60,000. The DI ratio would equal .00333 cases per person-year. Typically the DI is expressed in terms of 100,000 person-years and in this example would be 333 cases per 100,000 person-years.

person-years
the amount of observation time each person contributes

CI is simply defined as the ratio of incident cases to the at-risk population at the beginning of the observation period. The denominator of CI is neither time nor any sum of contributed time periods; rather, it is the number of individuals at risk. Therefore CI provides the best estimate of how many people will eventually get the disease. CI would be calculated as the number of newly diagnosed cases divided by the number of people in the cohort at the beginning of the study. In a cohort of 2000 people, if 200 of them develop the disease over two years, then the CI would be 200/2000 × 100 = 10 percent. In another study that used longitudinal design, Norwegian researchers Brumpton, Camargo, Romundstad, Langhammer, Chen, and Mai (2013) conducted a prospective cohort using 23,191 participants who were asthma-free at baseline. Obesity is both a risk factor for asthma and a major component of metabolic syndrome; thus the researchers aimed to explore the association between metabolic syndrome and its mechanisms related to the incidence of asthma in adults. Results showed that metabolic syndrome was associated with an increased risk of incident asthma (AOR=1.57; CI 1.31–1.87).

Longitudinal designs greatly improve on some of the limitations of cross-sectional designs and of the successive independent samples design (see Table 4.4). For instance, by following the same cohort over a long period of time you can establish the temporal order of occurrences, and you may therefore be able to attribute change to the time factor. Additionally, you may be able to ascertain the effects of naturally occurring events. For example, if within the time frame of your longitudinal study an event such as a natural disaster, a divorce, or a heart attack

Table 4.4 Strengths and Weaknesses of Longitudinal Research Designs

Design	Strengths	Weaknesses
Longitudinal (Cohort/Panel)	No cohort or generation effects	Time-consuming and expensive
	Can study the natural development of multiple health outcomes or disease	Generally require large samples
	Can assess the stability and continuity of several attributes	Attrition and missing data
	Can document trends or patterns over time	Individuals measured multiple times may result in "testing" effects
	Can establish a temporal order	Dependency of data must be accounted for
	Can assess reasons for change or outcome	Not very useful for rare outcomes
	Sampling error minimized	

occurs, you could investigate whether or not there were any differences between those in the cohort who experienced the event and those who did not. If significant differences were found, then you could reasonably attribute them to the event. Of course, one major problem with longitudinal studies is **attrition**. Also referred to as **mortality**, attrition can bias the results. Severe attrition can be dealt with statistically by comparing those who returned for follow-up interviews (or completed follow-up questionnaires) with those who did not, identifying critical differences between the two groups, and determining whether any bias has occurred. For example, in sex research, if those lost to attrition had baseline indicators of more frequent risky sexual activity than those who remained in the study, the loss to follow-up could bias the study conclusions.

attrition
also referred to as mortality, the loss of participants from the research study

mortality
also referred to as attrition, the loss of participants from the research study

IN A NUTSHELL

Longitudinal designs greatly improve on some of the limitations of cross-sectional designs and of the successive independent samples design.

The Cohort-Sequential Design

The cohort-sequential design is essentially a hybrid of cross-sectional and longitudinal designs that corrects for cohort effects. Starting with an initial cohort and following it over a period of time, another cohort or cohorts are then added at varying intervals within that time period. Researchers can assess changes over time for the first cohort while also being able to make cross-sectional comparisons among the different cohorts at specific time points. This design is depicted in Figure 4.6.

In health promotion research, this design clearly has distinct advantages over the cross-sectional and the longitudinal designs, as it encompasses

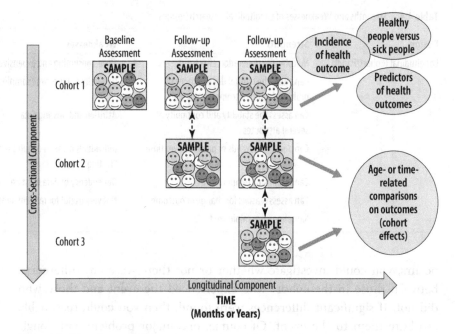

Figure 4.6 Cohort-Sequential Design

both. The longitudinal component of the cohort-sequential design would help to track trajectories of disease, risk factors, and health-related outcomes and incidence over time at the individual level (rather than the population level, as would be the case for a strictly cross-sectional design) by following the cohort. These purposes are essentially the same as a strictly longitudinal design and therefore can be deemed as a trend study; however, in addition, because this design adds in additional cohorts at later time points, it allows for comparisons between or among all cohorts on the relevant study outcomes at a single point in time. Thus this design helps to better our understanding of any potential cohort effects that may influence or explain the results found for the longitudinal component. Data analyses for a cohort-sequential design would employ similar procedures, previously described, for examining the separate components (that is, the longitudinal and the cross-sectional), but would also include latent growth curve methodology for analyzing the longitudinal data and combining information from the different overlapping cohorts to form a single developmental trajectory. An example of cohort-sequential design was conducted by Duncan, Duncan, and Strycker (2006). In their study, they assessed changes in alcohol use among children ages 9–16. Participants were recruited from 1999 to 2003 from a large metropolitan area in the Northwest United States via telephone, using a computer-assisted telephone interviewing system. The sample comprised 139 9-year-olds, 138 11-year-olds, and

128 13-year-olds. In addition to the target participant, all family members over the age of eight were invited to participate. Annual surveys were completed in the participants' homes to ascertain adolescent alcohol use, parent/guardian alcohol use, family alcohol problems, family cohesion, parent supervision, adolescent peer alcohol use, peer encouragement of alcohol use, alcohol use norms among school peers, and peer deviance. The study employed latent growth modeling (LGM), which offers a "flexible and efficient means of modeling longitudinal behavioral outcome variables, such as alcohol use, and of handling non-normal distributions" (Duncan, Duncan, and Strycker, 2006, p. 15). Results showed that proportions of adolescents using alcohol increased steadily from the ages of 9 to 16. In addition, being female and having higher levels of parental alcohol use were both associated with higher initial rates of alcohol use. Interestingly, greater encouragement of alcohol use by friends was related to lower *initial* rates of alcohol use. In contrast, more peer deviance and friends' encouragement of alcohol use was related to an increase in alcohol use rates from ages 9 to 16 years, as was being White and from a single-parent family.

When each of the individual components is viewed in isolation—that is, the longitudinal and cross-sectional components are viewed separately—the cohort-sequential design has the same strengths and weaknesses previously attributed to those designs. However, when viewing the design as a whole, it provides the additional strength of examining cohort effects (see Table 4.5). As previously mentioned, cohort effects are a product of aging or of the passage of time, so it would be appropriate only for research questions for which age and time are main factors in studying the development of health-related phenomena such as alcohol use, drug use, or sexual risk behavior.

The Case-Control Design

The case-control study is another observational research design that has its roots in epidemiology. John Snow, a British physician aptly referred to as the father of modern epidemiology, investigated a cholera epidemic in 1854 in Soho, London, by mapping where victims lived, then marking the sites of public water pumps on the map to test his hypothesis that water

Table 4.5 Strengths and Weaknesses of Cohort-Sequential Designs

Design	Strengths	Weaknesses
Cohort-Sequential Design	Same as cross-sectional and longitudinal	Same as cross-sectional and longitudinal
	Controls for cohort or generation effects	Does not control for history effects
	Can also examine contribution of cohort effects	

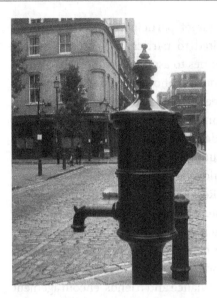

Figure 4.7   John Snow Memorial and Pub,
Broadwick Street (formerly Broad Street), London
Source: "John Snow Memorial and Pub" by justinc is licensed
under CC BY 2.0.

contaminated by fecal material was the source of infection. Snow determined, through interviews with people who had cholera and those who did not, that one particular water pump (the Broad Street pump) lay at the center of a cluster of cholera cases; in fact, all of the local cholera patients had consumed water from this one pump (see Figure 4.7). Other pumps on his map were shown to be used much less frequently. Accordingly, Snow concluded that this pump (that is, the water flowing from it) was the source of the infection and persuaded health officials to remove the pump handle so that its use would be discontinued. Removal of the handle prevented additional cholera deaths. Since Snow's study, the case-control design has been used extensively. A more recent example (in the 1950s) of major import was the case-control study that found an association between cigarettes and lung cancer.

cases
participants in a study selected because they have the disease or health-related outcome

controls
participants in a study who are matched on key characteristics to cases and who do not have the disease or health-related outcome

The logic of the case-control design is that participants are selected on the basis of whether they have or do not have the disease or other health-related outcome of interest. Those who have the disease or outcome are termed **cases**; those who do not are termed **controls**. Although assessment occurs once, as is the case in a cross-sectional design, exposure to putative risk factors is assessed retrospectively for both cases and controls. Then comparisons are made to determine the likelihood of the contribution of different risk factors deemed "exposures" to the outcome. For instance, people who have lung cancer (cases) could be compared to people without lung cancer (controls) in terms of their smoking behaviors (exposure) to determine whether more cases were smokers than controls. Thus the central feature of the case-control is the comparison of the cases' and controls' exposure *histories*. This differs from the longitudinal/cohort study design in which the key comparison is made of disease incidence between the exposed and unexposed groups, so the disease or health-related outcome occurs naturally and *prospectively*. The case-control design is depicted in Figure 4.8.

In health promotion research, the case-control design is used to determine the relative importance of a predictor variable or a set of

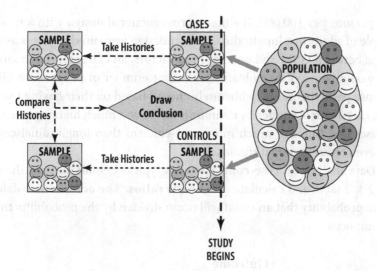

Figure 4.8 The Case-Control Design

predictor variables (such as smoking, lack of exercise, diet, lead exposure, asbestos exposure, or other environmental exposures) in relation to the presence or absence of the disease. Ideally, cases may be selected at random from all cases of interest in the source population (such as vital data or registry data). Typically, cases are selected from available cases at some type of medical care clinic or facility. Controls should mirror characteristics of the cases as close as possible, including the hypothesized risk factors, but of course controls must be free of the disease. If cases are a random sample of all cases in the population, then controls should be a random sample of all non-cases in the population. The key to choosing controls is that comparability is more important than representativeness.

In terms of risk factors or exposures, health promotion researchers may consider many possible determinants to explain patterns of illness or disease, which can range from physical, biological, social, cultural, and behavioral factors. This assessment of multiple etiologic factors is accomplished through interviews or surveys with the cases and controls or preexisting sources from medical, pharmacy, registry, employment, insurance, birth, death, and environmental records, and biological specimens. Because of this ability to assess multiple types of exposures, case-control designs are considered cost-efficient, especially when the disease or outcome is rare (usually defined as a frequency of less than 20 percent in the population). In fact, where the outcome is very rare, case-control studies may be the only feasible approach. For example, take the disease glioblastoma multiforme (GBM). Although GBM is the most common and deadliest of malignant primary brain tumors in adults, the incidence is 2 to 3 persons per 100,000. If either a cross-sectional design with a random sample of adults or a longitudinal/cohort design were used to assess associations between GBM and potential risk factors, an extremely large sample size would be needed to obtain a sufficient number of people with GBM. Because participants are deliberately chosen based on their having the disease, case-control studies by definition will have a much higher percentage of cases and thus are much more cost-efficient than longitudinal/cohort and even cross-sectional studies.

odds ratios
the probability that an event will occur divided by the probability that it will not occur

Data analysis for case-control studies typically entails putting the data in a 2 × 2 table and calculating the **odds ratios**. The odds ratio is defined as the probability that an event will occur divided by the probability that it will not occur.

	Outcome	
Case		**Control**
Yes	a	b
Exposure		
No	c	d

For a case-control study, you would calculate the odds of being a case among the exposed (a/b) compared to the odds of being a case among the nonexposed (c/d). The odds ratio for the case-control is deemed an approximation of risk because the controls are a sample of the population that produced the cases. In this instance, the sampling fraction is not known; thus an estimate of the total population, which is needed to obtain the rates and risks of disease, cannot be determined. An example of case-control design was conducted by Sanderson et al. (2013). This study aimed to assess whether perinatal factors were associated with breast cancer among Hispanics. Participants were recruited through clinics in the Lower Rio Grande Valley between 2003 and 2008. The sample comprised 188 participants who were breast cancer incident cases (identified through surgeons and oncologists) and 974 controls. All participants completed interviews. Results showed that there appeared to be no association with breast cancer among women whose child's birth weight was 4000 g or more relative to women whose child's birth weight was 2500 to 3999 g, as suggested by an adjusted odds ratio of .76 (CI .47–1.21). Women who delivered preterm were not at risk of breast cancer relative to women who delivered at term (AOR = .32; CI = .08–1.40).

The case-control design provides several additional strengths over cross-sectional and longitudinal/cohort designs (see Table 4.6). The main advantage is that case-control studies are efficient—when little is known

Table 4.6   Strengths and Weaknesses of Case-Control Research Designs

Design	Strengths	Weaknesses
Case-Control Design	Quick and relatively inexpensive	Cannot account for rare exposures
	Well-suited for diseases with long latency periods	Restricted to only one outcome
	Well-suited for rare diseases	Recall bias
	Can examine multiple etiologic risk factors	Sample bias in creating groups and if controls are not properly matched to cases
	Useful for outbreak investigations or new diseases	Cannot determine incidence

about a disease or health-related outcome, multiple risk factors can be assessed even when the disease or outcome is rare. The main weaknesses related to the case-control are sample bias and recall bias stemming from the retrospective assessment of the risk factors.

Case-Crossover Design

The case-crossover design, not to be confused with a crossover study or crossover trial (see Chapter Five), is our final observational study design and is a relatively new (less than 20 years old) variant of the case-control design (Lombardi, 2010; Maclure, 1991). The case-crossover design is considered a hybrid design and is novel in that it involves sampling only cases. No controls are sampled; rather, cases serve as their own controls. The case-crossover design was conceptualized to examine the influence of risk factors or exposures that are transient and difficult to measure on outcomes with an acute onset. Recall that in the case-control design, cases and controls must have comparability of their risk factors to ensure that similar levels of exposure are used to match cases with controls. For many types of risk factors, comparability on exposure levels is not difficult; such is the case when assessing how often and how many cigarettes a person smokes or how often and how many drinks of alcohol are consumed, for example. In contrast, consider a risk factor that may be more of a challenge to compare and match, such as heavy physical exertion. Heavy physical exertion is considered a physical trigger or risk factor for myocardial infarction (MI) and would be considered a transient behavior (Mittleman, Maclure, and Robins, 1995). If a case-control study was conducted to determine the association of heavy physical exertion with MI, it would be a challenge to find controls, who experienced similar periods and levels of physical exertion, to match with a sample of hospital-based cases (who experienced a MI). The case-crossover design eliminates this issue by having the cases serve as their own controls.

In health promotion research, a case-crossover study would be used to examine whether the risk of a health-related outcome increased

hazard period
the period in which a person is at risk of exposure

case-exposure window
the time period immediately preceding the onset of the health outcome

pair-matched interval approach
comparing the risk exposure during the case window statistically to risk exposure during the control window

usual frequency approach
using an expected frequency of exposure based on a subject's reported usual frequency over a specified time period before the health-related outcome occurred as the control window

immediately following the exposure period. Thus a basic requirement is that subjects must have crossed at least once from lower to higher levels of exposure. For instance, the case-crossover design would be an appropriate design to test whether texting while driving (a transient risk exposure) among 16-year-olds was related to an increased risk of accidents (acute onset of an outcome). The risk exposure period is called the **hazard period** or the **case-exposure window** and refers to the time period immediately preceding the onset, so the person is deemed a case during this time period. In this example, the day of the accident would be the case-exposure window, and the amount of text messages sent or whether texting occurred would be examined as the risk exposure. The "control" window refers to an earlier time period; Therefore it is the period of time associated with not being a case. In this example, we could use the day prior to the accident as the control window and examine the amount of text messages sent or whether texting occurred. The risk exposure during the case window is then compared statistically to risk exposure during the control window. This two-window approach is called the **pair-matched interval approach** (Lombardi, 2010). In addition to this comparison, it may be relevant in some studies to conduct a second comparison in which risk exposure during the case exposure window is compared to the frequency of exposure that is *expected*. Expected frequency of exposure is based on a subject's reported usual frequency over a specified time period before the health-related outcome occurred. In other words, a more in-depth understanding of the typical levels of exposure over a longer time period leading up to onset are compared to the case window. In the texting while driving example, this would be the texting behavior of the teen over the course of the previous month or 6 months leading up to the accident so that a better picture of the subject's typical texting behavior is determined. This second approach is called the **usual frequency approach** (Lombardi, 2010). Because of the transient nature of the risk factor, using two or more control windows strengthens the conclusions that can be drawn when making comparisons to the case exposure window. The case-crossover design using both these approaches is depicted in Figure 4.9.

Data analysis for the case-crossover design is dependent on the approach. For the matched-pair interval analysis, similar analyses for matched case-control data would be used, such as the odds ratio.

In our hypothetical example of teens and texting while driving, suppose we recruited 200 teens who had been involved in a car crash to be in our case-crossover study. Their cell phone billing records could be used to determine their texting behaviors (risk exposure) for both the case window and control window. Crude numbers could be assessed and put into a 2 × 2 table as shown. Among the 200 teens in our study, 40 had

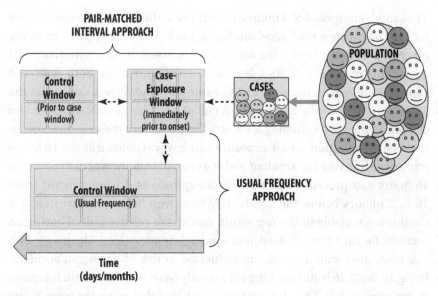

Figure 4.9 The Case-Crossover Design

text-messaged right before the crash (case) and during the same period on the day before the crash (control), 60 had texted during the case period but not during the control period, 20 had not texted during the case period but had during the control period, and 80 had not texted during either periods. The estimated odds ratio (relative risk) in this table is the ratio of the discordant pairs (N in row 1 – column 2 divided by N in row 2 – column 1), yielding a ratio of 3 (60/20). So in this hypothetical example it appears that there is a positive association between texting and the occurrence of a car accident.

	Control	
	Yes	**No**
Case Yes	40	60
No	20	80

For the usual frequency analysis, the relative risks would be determined and would be calculated as the ratio of the observed frequency of exposure to each transient risk factor at the time of the onset to the expected frequency of exposure in the previous time period (control window), using the Mantel-Haenszel estimator for person-time data. An example of a case-crossover design was conducted by Lombardi (2010). The purpose of the study was to measure the association of acute sleep deprivation, prolonged wakefulness, and long working hours and road traffic accidents.

The sample comprised 574 injured drivers presenting to an emergency room for care following a road accident. Sleep, work, and driving patterns in the preceding 48 hours before the accident were assessed via a semistructured questionnaire. The authors adopted two definitions for both case and control windows. In the first, a case exposure window was defined as the 24 hours immediately before the accident and the control window was defined as the corresponding 24 hours the day before the case window. In the second definition, a case exposure window was defined as the 16 hours immediately before the accident and the control window was defined as the 16 hours that preceded the most recent episode of driving, ranging from 16 to 23 hours before the accident. When sleep hours were treated as a continuous variable in the regression model, the relative risk of having an accident for each hour of sleep hour was slightly attenuated. Sleeping ≥ 11 h was associated with a significant reduction in risk of having an accident; being awake ≥ 16 h and working > 12 h daily were associated with increases in the relative risk. Thus the authors concluded that extended work hours and prolonged wakefulness increased the risk of road accidents.

Because cases serve as their own controls, the case-crossover design has several advantages over the case-control design, including the elimination of confounding by time invariant characteristics such as gender and race and the elimination of a type of bias that results from selecting unrepresentative controls (see Table 4.7). In addition, because variability is reduced, this design requires fewer subjects than the traditional case-control study. The main weakness with this design is that determining the appropriate control window(s) with enough variability can be a challenge; Therefore different control window periods should be examined and tested.

Summary

Choosing an appropriate research design is a critical part of the overall research process and depends to a large degree on the nature of the research question. Observational research designs, although considered less rigorous

Table 4.7   Strengths and Weaknesses of the Case-Crossover Design

Design	Strengths	Weaknesses
Case-Crossover	Efficient—self-matching, so requires fewer subjects	Information bias—inaccurate recall of exposures during control window(s)
	Eliminates between-person confounding	Requires careful selection of the time period during which the control window occurs
	Can use multiple control windows for one case	Requires careful selection of the length and timing of the windows

than experimental designs, are nonetheless critical to answering important health promotion research questions that can further our understanding of a range of health-related outcomes and risk factors. The selection of one observational design over another depends on the research question and other factors, such as how much is known about the health outcome and the underlying risk factors, the prevalence of the health outcome, resources available, time frame, access to the study population, and the feasibility of a control group. Although most students find that their initial research project can effectively use a cross-sectional design, you are obligated to always ask, "Is there a better observational research design that would give my findings greater rigor?" When contemplating these alternatives, simply match your research question to the best design. If your question looks for trends in a population, then you will need the successive independent samples design. If your question requires that you establish a temporal relationship between variables, then you will need a longitudinal design. The cohort-sequential design is unlikely to be one of the first designs you apply in your career; however, it is highly versatile, and you would do well to keep this one in mind as your career progresses—especially if you have an interest in adolescents and their developmental trajectories related to health outcomes. If your interest and your research question lie within the identification of behavioral or environmental risk factors, you will certainly want to use the case-control study. Finally, if you have a need to conduct the definitive study of risk factors on outcomes, you should consider whether the case-crossover design is a fair match for your research question.

KEY TERMS

Attrition	Mortality
Case-exposure window	Odds ratios
Cases	Pair-matched interval approach
Cohort effects	Person-years
Controls	Qualitative
Cumulative incidence	Quantitative
Density incidence	Regression coefficients
Ecological validity	Risk ratios
Epidemiology	Themes
Etiology	Third-variable problem
Hazard period	Usual frequency approach

For Practice and Discussion

1. Some public health issues are complicated in terms of the myriad causal influences underlying the health behavior or the disease outcome. For example, obesity results from poor diet and sedentary lifestyle, but it is important to identify the specific factors that contribute to those behaviors , so that preventive interventions can be developed. Design a study that would first document the prevalence of childhood obesity and then design a study that would allow you to identify a range of contributing factors to childhood obesity. What design(s) would you use? Provide a rationale for each design, and identify the strengths and weaknesses of your approaches.

2. Pre-exposure prophylaxis or PrEP is the use of the antiretroviral medication that is typically used to treat people who have HIV, by people who are HIV-negative, as a form of HIV prevention. PrEP has been shown to be effective in clinical trials if taken regularly. One critique of PrEP is that it may contribute to abandoning the regular use of condoms (referred to as "condom migration"), thereby resulting in acquiring other STDs. Discuss how you would design a study that would answer whether or not PrEP contributes to condom migration among a high-risk population such as MSM and whether this condom migration has resulted in more STDs. What design would you choose and why? What would be the limitations?

3. In the United States, the Family Smoking Prevention and Tobacco Control Act (FSPTCA), also known as the Tobacco Control Act, became law on June 22, 2009. It gives the U.S. Food and Drug Administration (FDA) the authority to regulate the manufacture, distribution, and marketing of tobacco products to protect public health. Tobacco regulatory science is needed to inform new policies to help prevent youth from initiating both tobacco use and use of novel tobacco products such as e-cigarettes. E-cigarettes are electronic cigarettes and are currently not regulated. There is much controversy surrounding their safety and use, especially among youth. Discuss how you would design a study that would determine adolescents' use of e-cigarettes, their risk perceptions of e-cigarette use, and whether use of e-cigarettes contributes to use of regular cigarettes. Describe the design you would use (for example, cross-sectional, case-control, case-crossover, longitudinal) and provide the rationale for your choice. List the limitations of your design.

4. Read a journal article that describes an empirical observational research study. Discuss the design that was used in terms of its appropriateness

in answering the research question(s). Is there another design that would have been stronger and that you would have chosen instead? What were the limitations of the design? Did the investigators draw appropriate conclusions based on the design or did they overstep their data?

References

Ahmed, A., and el-Guindy, S. R. (2011). Breastfeeding knowledge and attitudes among Egyptian baccalaureate students. *International Nursing Review, 58*(3), 372–378. doi:10.1111/j.1466–7657.2011.00885.x

Brumpton, B. M., Camargo, C. A., Jr., Romundstad, P. R., Langhammer, A., Chen, Y., and Mai, X. M. (2013). Metabolic syndrome and incidence of asthma in adults: The HUNT study. *European Respiratory Journal.* doi:10.1183 /09031936.00046013

Centers for Disease Control and Prevention. (2013). HIV infection among heterosexuals at increased risk—United States, 2010. *Morbidity and Mortality Weekly Report, 62*(10), 183–188.

Collins, S. E., Malone, D. K., Clifasefi, S. L., Ginzler, J. A., Garner, M. D., Burlingham, B., . . . and Larimer, M. E. (2012). Project-based housing first for chronically homeless individuals with alcohol problems: Within-subjects analyses of 2-year alcohol trajectories. *American Journal Of Public Health, 102*(3), 511–519. doi:10.2105/AJPH.2011.300403

Duncan, S. C., Duncan, T. E., and Strycker, L. A. (2006). Alcohol use from ages 9 to 16: A cohort-sequential latent growth model. *Drug and Alcohol Dependence, 81*(1), 71–81. doi:10.1016/j.drugalcdep.2005.06.001

Finlayson, T. J., Le, B., Smith, A., Bowles, K., Cribbin, M., Miles, I., . . . Dinenno, E. (2011). HIV risk, prevention, and testing behaviors among men who have sex with men—National HIV Behavioral Surveillance System, 21 U.S. cities, United States, 2008. *Morbidity and Mortality Weekly Report. Surveillance Summaries, 60*(14), 1–34.

Hailemariam, T. G., Kassie, G. M., and Sisay, M. M. (2012). Sexual life and fertility desire in long-term HIV serodiscordant couples in Addis Ababa, Ethiopia: A grounded theory study. *BMC Public Health, 12*, 900. doi:10.1186 /1471–2458–12–900

Holt, K., Blanchard, K., Chipato, T., Nhemachena, T., Blum, M., Stratton, L., . . . Harper, C. C. (2013). A nationally representative survey of healthcare provider counseling and provision of the female condom in South Africa and Zimbabwe. *BMJ Open, 3*(3). doi:10.1136/bmjopen-2012–002208

Kann, L., Kinchen, S., Shanklin, S. L., Flint, K. H., Hawkins, J., Harris, W. A., . . . Zaza, S. (2014). Youth risk behavior surveillance—United States, 2013. *Morbidity and Mortality Weekly Report, 63*(4), 1–168.

Lansky, A., Sullivan, P. S., Gallagher, K. M., and Fleming, P. L. (2007). HIV behavioral surveillance in the U.S.: A conceptual framework. *Public Health Reports, 122* Suppl 1, 16–23.

Lindfors, P. L., Kaltiala-Heino, R., and Rimpela, A. H. (2012). Cyberbullying among Finnish adolescents—A population-based study. *BMC Public Health, 12*, 1027. doi:10.1186/1471-2458-12-1027

Lombardi, D. A. (2010). The case-crossover study: A novel design in evaluating transient fatigue as a risk factor for road traffic accidents. *Sleep, 33*(3), 283–284.

Maclure, M. (1991). The case-crossover design: A method for studying transient effects on the risk of acute events. *American Journal of Epidemiology, 133*, 144–53.

Mittleman, M. A., Maclure, M., and Robins, J. M. (1995). Control sampling strategies for case-crossover studies: An assessment of relative efficiency. *American Journal of Epidemiology, 142*(1), 91–98.

Morse, J. (1994). Designing funded qualitative research. In N. K. Denzin and J. S. Lincoln (Eds.), *Handbook of qualitative research* (pp. 220–235). Thousand Oaks, CA: Sage.

Oster, A. M., Johnson, C. H., Le, B. C., Balaji, A. B., Finlayson, T. J., Lansky, A., . . . Paz-Bailey, G. for the Young Men's Survey (YMS) and National HIV Behavioral Surveillance System (NHBS) Study Groups. (2014). Trends in HIV prevalence and HIV testing among young MSM—Five United States cities, 1994–2011. *AIDS & Behavior, Suppl 3*, S237-47.

Sanderson, M., Perez, A., Weriwoh, M. L., Alexander, L. R., Peltz, G., Agboto, V., . . . Khoder, W. (2013). Perinatal factors and breast cancer risk among Hispanics. *Journal of Epidemiology and Global Health, 3*(2), 89–94. doi:10.1016/j.jegh.2013.02.004

Shen, H. W., Pickard, J. G., and Johnson, S. D. (2013). Self-esteem mediates the relationship between volunteering and depression for African American caregivers. *Journal of Gerontological Social Work, 56*(5), 438–451. doi:10.1080/01634372.2013.791907

Voisin, D. R., Salazar, L. F., Crosby, R., and DiClemente, R. J. (2013). The relationship between ethnic identity and chlamydia and gonorrhea infections among low-income detained African American adolescent females. *Psychology, Health & Medicine, 18*(3), 355–362. doi:10.1080/13548506.2012.726361

Voisin, D. R., Tan, K., and Diclemente, R. J. (2013). A longitudinal examination of the relationship between sexual sensation seeking and STI-related risk factors among African American females. *AIDS Education and Prevention, 25*(2), 124–134. doi:10.1521/aeap.2013.25.2.124

Yu, Q., Liu, L., Pu, J., Zhao, J., Sun, Y., Shen, G., . . . Liu, J. (2013). Risk perceptions for avian influenza virus infection among poultry workers, China. *Emerging Infectious Diseases, 19*(2), 313–316. doi:10.3201/eid1902.120251

CHAPTER 5

EXPERIMENTAL RESEARCH DESIGNS

Laura F. Salazar
Richard A. Crosby
Ralph J. DiClemente

Causal research in health promotion entails two overarching objectives: isolating etiological causes of health behavior and associated disease outcomes as well as determining whether health promotion interventions are effective in achieving their intended outcomes. These two objectives can be accomplished by implementing experiments. Experiments can be classified according to whether there is a control group, the level of control instituted, and whether there is randomization. This chapter describes the different types of experimental designs that are used for causal research in health promotion along with the respective threats to their internal validity and strengths.

In Chapter Four we outlined and described two stages in the research process—exploratory and conclusive—which we further subdivided into two overarching categories, *descriptive* and *causal*. The focus of this chapter is on causal research. To help clarify, we refer you back to Figure 4.2, which provides a graphic depiction of health promotion research in terms of stages, purpose, and designs. Compared with descriptive research, causal research transcends the natural order of things through manipulation and enables researchers to make cause-effect statements. Causal research employs *experimental designs* and in some instances *quasi-experimental designs* so that causal inference can be made with a high degree of certainty. In basic terms, experimental designs entail the manipulation of a variable to test the effects of the

LEARNING OBJECTIVES

- Understand the role of causal research in the context of health promotion research and practice.

- Identify the necessary conditions for causation and the two hallmarks of experimental designs.

- Describe the threats to internal validity.

- Distinguish between true experiments and quasi-experiments.

- Learn the various types of experimental designs used in health promotion research.

- Learn the quasi-experimental designs used in health promotion research.

Table 5.1   Three Necessary Conditions for Causation

To conclude that changes in variable A cause changes in variable B:	
Condition 1: **The relationship condition**	Variable A and variable B must be related.
Condition 2: **The temporal antecedence condition**	Proper time order must be established.
Condition 3: **The lack of an alternative explanation condition**	The relationship between variable A and variable B must not be due to a confounding extraneous "third" variable.

manipulation on some outcome. Quasi-experimental designs approximate experimental designs but do not use randomization. Additionally, causal research entails three main conditions that are always required when making claims that changes in one variable cause changes in another variable. These three conditions, considered necessary for causality, are summarized in Table 5.1.

In the context of health promotion research, causal research allows us not only to understand and predict health behavior but also to *change* health behavior. Health promotion research is at the forefront of first understanding the underlying individual and environmental factors that influence health behavior and health outcomes. Understanding and predicting behavior could entail using some of the observational designs described in Chapter Four, but this type of research would not allow for causal inferences and would be categorized as descriptive. Only when experimental designs are used can causal inferences be made.

Why should we care so much about making cause-effect statements? Making cause-effect statements provides both theoretical and practical benefits. For example, many of the theories we use in health promotion guide our research and our programs by providing us with a framework to better understand behavior. By testing these theories in terms of specific health behaviors, we can begin to identify determinants and isolate causes of a condition, disease, or behavior. Then we may begin devising a treatment or developing a health promotion program. Although observational designs are useful and can be used to meet necessary condition 1, and to some degree necessary condition 2, experimental designs meet all three necessary conditions. In other words, by using an experimental design, we can ensure that A is related to B, we can definitively establish a temporal order of A and B, and we can rule out alternative explanations so that the true etiological causes can be isolated.

Once research has been conducted to identify significant determinants or causes, then interventions can be designed to modify those factors that are modifiable. Ultimately, the crux of health promotion is improving public health by changing health-related behavior and thereby positively affecting health-related outcomes. Changing health-related outcomes entails the implementation of health promotion and disease prevention interventions that are culturally appropriate, promote the adoption of healthy lifestyles, improve behaviors and social conditions, improve environmental conditions related to disease, change poor diet and use of tobacco, alcohol, and other recreational drugs, and ameliorate mental illness, HIV infection, and unintentional or intentional injury. Once implemented, causal research is critical to determining whether a particular program is helpful in solving the problem. If the treatment or program is *efficacious*—meaning it can produce the desired effect—then it can be implemented on a wider scale.

Health promotion practice is at the forefront of designing and implementing interventions. To be effective, it is generally agreed that health promotion interventions should be multidimensional, which means they target not only individuals but also schools, communities, or political structures (such as public policy). This multilevel approach, shown in Figure 5.1, has been deemed an ecological approach. As the figure indicates, health promotion interventions that involve educational and skill-building programs happen at the individual level, whereas interventions that target relational factors such as social support networks are at the interpersonal level. Evaluating the effectiveness of these types of health promotion interventions equates with causal research and would entail implementing experimental or quasi-experimental designs, depending on the ecological level. Generally speaking, the level at which you intervene will ultimately determine the design you choose: higher levels equate with quasi-experimental designs, whereas lower levels are more conducive to true experimental designs.

IN A NUTSHELL

The level at which you intervene will ultimately determine the design you choose: higher levels equate with quasi-experimental designs, whereas lower levels are more conducive to true experimental designs.

In the following sections, we provide an overview of the related concepts and terminology associated with causal research and the various experimental and quasi-experimental research designs that make up causal research. We illustrate these concepts with examples drawn from the scientific literature. Because the focus of this book is on the research methods used in health promotion and practice, we describe designs and methods related to health promotion. For example, research concepts

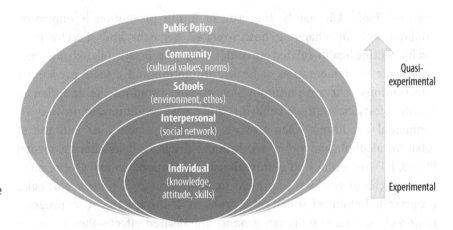

Figure 5.1 Ecological Model with Associated Experimental Design by Levels

independent variable

the variable chosen by the investigator to modify or administer to determine its effect on the dependent variable

extraneous variables

variables outside of the investigator's purview that could influence the outcome of the study

dependent variable

the primary outcome or the main variable of interest in an experiment that is hypothesized to be affected by the independent variable

factor

the independent variable in an experiment

single-factor design

a research design in which the investigator is manipulating only one factor

factorial design

a research design in which the investigator is manipulating more than one factor

or methods used in the study of pathogen isolation (such as Koch's postulates; Falkow, 2004), though important, are outside the scope of this text and will not be covered.

Manipulation and Control

The two defining characteristics of experimental research designs are (1) manipulation of an **independent variable** (IV) and (2) control over **extraneous variables**. The independent variable is the variable chosen by the investigator to determine its effect on the **dependent variable** (DV) and is manipulated or controlled by the investigator. In this context, manipulation in an experiment does not involve unfair or insidious actions in order to influence an outcome; rather, it means to change or implement something that serves a purpose, which should directly relate to the research question. Although the degree of manipulation of conditions in experiments theoretically can go too far (see "Mincus Participates in a Nutrition Experiment"), in general, manipulation in health promotion research entails implementing a health promotion program that involves minimal risk. If the investigator is manipulating only one **factor**, then the design is a **single-factor design**; if there is more than one factor, it is called a **factorial design**. The number of different IVs equates with the number of factors in the design. For instance, a study that tests the effects of a physical activity health promotion program on teens' physical activity levels and ultimately their body mass index (BMI) would be a single-factor design even when a comparison condition is used, because only one IV—treatment—is being manipulated. Although the investigator in this example is using only one IV, the single factor is manipulated at two levels (the physical activity health promotion program and the comparison program).

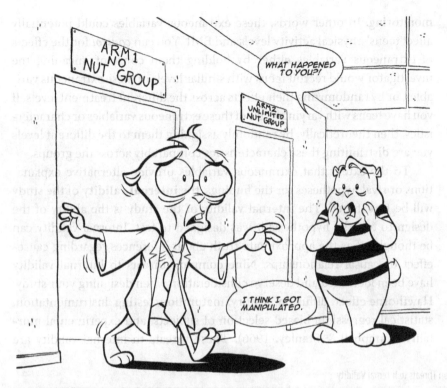

Mincus Participates in a Nutrition Experiment

Copyright 2014 by Justin Wagner; reprinted with permission.

It is important to distinguish between factors and levels. A factor is what the investigator is manipulating, whereas the level refers to variations in the factor. If this same study were to add another IV, it would have to be qualitatively different from the first IV to be considered another factor. In this example, another IV could be age, and it could have two levels (13–14 years old and 15–18 years old). The DV is the outcome variable of interest and is measured by the investigator. In this example, the DVs are physical activity level and body mass index (BMI).

IN A NUTSHELL

Extraneous variables are not directly related to the hypothesis being tested, but may nevertheless have an effect on the dependent variable.

The second defining characteristic is control over those pesky extraneous variables. Extraneous variables are considered pesky because they are not directly related to the hypothesis being tested but may nevertheless have an effect on the DV. Potential extraneous variables in this example could be family structure, family socioeconomic status, or parental monitoring. In other words, these extraneous variables could potentially affect teens' physical activity levels and BMI. You can *control* for the effects of extraneous variables either by holding them constant, meaning the investigator would recruit teens with similar levels of these extraneous variables, or by randomizing their effects across the different treatment levels. If you have teens with varying levels of these extraneous variables or characteristics, then theoretically, by randomly assigning them to the different levels you are distributing these characteristics comparably across the groups.

internal validity
the ability of the design to test the hypothesis it was designed to test

To the extent that extraneous variables provide alternative explanations or rival hypotheses for the findings, the **internal validity** of the study will be threatened. The internal validity of the study is the ability of the design to test the hypothesis it was designed to test. Internal validity can be thought of as the approximate truth about inferences regarding cause-effect or causal relationships. Nine common threats to internal validity have been identified and deserve consideration when designing your study: Hawthorne effect, diffusion, history, maturation, testing, instrumentation, statistical regression, biased selection of subjects, and experimental mortality (Campbell & Stanley, 1966). These threats to internal validity are

Table 5.2   Nine Common Threats to Internal Validity

Threat	How Caused	Research Design Affected
Hawthorne effect	Results might be due to the time and attention paid to participants.	One-group design and two-group design without placebo-attention group
Diffusion	Results might be due to contamination of control group.	Two-group or multigroup design
History	Results might be due to an event that occurred between observations.	One-group design
Maturation	Results might be due to participants growing older, wiser, stronger, or more experienced between observations.	One-group design
Testing	Results might be due to the number of times responses were measured.	One-group design
Instrumentation	Results might be due to a change in the measuring instrument between observations.	One-group design
Statistical regression	Results might be due to the selection of participants based on extreme scores, and when measured again, scores might move back to an average level.	One-group design
Differential selection	Results might be due to differences that existed between participants in groups before treatment occurred.	Two-group or multigroup design
Differential attrition (mortality)	Results might be due to the differential loss of participants from each group.	Two-group or multigroup design

defined in Table 5.2. Before conducting your study, you must address common threats that may seriously threaten internal validity so you can rule out alternative hypotheses.

When thinking about these threats in more detail, it may be helpful to know two very simple and basic experimental designs. The first is a one-group experimental design sometimes referred to as a "pre"-experimental design due to the lack of a control group. As the name implies, a one-group design involves only one treatment group—no comparison or control group is involved, hence the qualifier "pre." Observed effects on the DV would involve the difference in the pretest (O_1) and posttest scores (O_2). This design is depicted as follows:

$$O_1 \qquad X_{treatment} \qquad O_2$$

The second design essentially involves two groups, with the second group being a comparison or control group. Observed effects on the DV would involve the difference between groups in posttest scores (O_2). This design is depicted as follows:

$$X_{treatment} \qquad O_2$$
$$X_{control} \qquad O_2$$

- *Hawthorne effect.* The Hawthorne effect (also referred to as the observer effect) refers to a phenomenon whereby participants improve or modify an aspect of their behavior in response to the fact of some change in their environment (such as researchers paying attention to them), rather than in response to the nature of the change itself. The "Hawthorne effect" study suggested that the novelty of having research conducted and the increased attention could lead to temporary increases in productivity. For example, a Hawthorne effect could result from the added attention and time given to hospital staff (for example, RNs, LPNs, and nurses' aides) by the research staff in an experimental study designed to increase adherence to hand washing protocols through an educational intervention. The Hawthorne effect is similar to the placebo effect sometimes seen in medical or drug trials, but stems from the social interaction between the participant and the researcher. The Hawthorne effect is a threat for the one-group experimental design and can be for two-group or multigroup designs unless the control group also receives what is called an **placebo-attention comparison** intervention: this mimics the treatment intervention in terms of time and attention, but should not have an effect on the primary outcome. In the hand washing experiment, an placebo-attention comparison intervention could be a nutritional educational program or a

placebo-attention comparison characterizing an intervention that mimics the treatment intervention in terms of time and attention but should not have an effect on the primary outcome

smoking cessation program. If both groups are paid equal amounts of attention and receive similar instructional sessions in terms of duration, then observed effects can more likely be attributed to the treatment intervention.

- *Diffusion.* Diffusion is another threat to internal validity and can only occur in two-group or multigroup designs when treatment effects spread from the treatment group to a control group. This "contamination" of the control group could occur if, for example, participants are recruited from small, contained locations where participants may know each other outside the context of the research study, such as in clinics, small towns, or schools. The no-treatment control group becomes aware of what is being done in the treatment group and their behavior is affected. Therefore diffusion results in no observed differences between groups and essentially eliminates having a true control group. In situations where diffusion may occur, the researcher may have to switch to a quasi-experimental design.

- *History.* As Table 5.2 shows, this threat refers to any external event that occurs during the course of the study that may be responsible for the effects observed on the DV rather than the manipulation of the IV. A history effect would preclude meeting necessary condition 3. If both a treatment and a history effect occur during the course of the study, then you will not know for certain whether observed differences between the pretest and the posttest are due to the treatment or the history effect. In short, these two events are confounded. For example, a history effect could occur if a famous celebrity was diagnosed with breast cancer during a community-level intervention designed to promote mammograms among high-risk populations. The history effect is a threat for the one-group experimental design but not for the multigroup design. All or part of the difference in a one-group design could be due to a history effect; therefore, you don't know whether the change in scores is due to the treatment (X) or the history effect. They are confounded. The basic history effect, however, is not a threat to the two-group or multigroup design, as you are comparing groups, and any history effect would theoretically occur for both groups. Therefore any observed difference between groups would not be attributable to a history effect.

- *Maturation.* Maturation is present when some type of physical or mental change occurs naturally over the course of the study and affects participants' performance on the DV. Typically, maturation is more of a threat for research studies involving children or youth, as they are undergoing dramatic developmental changes. For example, there could be a maturation effect in a study that is evaluating whether a new sexual health curriculum is effective in delaying or reducing sexual activity among ninth or tenth grade students as they mature. Increased sexual activity would probably be due to their natural maturation rather than an ineffective curriculum. Maturation is a threat in a one-group design but not a threat in the two-group design because as long as both groups mature at the same rate, the difference between groups will not be due to maturation.

- *Testing.* As Table 5.2 shows, testing (also called "reactivity to testing") refers to observed changes that result from having previously taken the test or survey. Something about taking the test the first time leads to a change in responses the second time. Being sensitive to the nature of the questions, learning the answers, or learning how the skip patterns are set up are some of the explanations suggested to account for this change. For example, a testing effect could occur in a study that measures drug use behaviors among injection drug users enrolled in a drug treatment program. Testing in this example would be a threat with a one-group design, as you cannot know for certain, if the injection drug users showed improvement from pretest to posttest, whether it was due to the treatment or a testing effect. Testing is not a threat in the two-group design because as long as participants in both groups are affected equally by the pretest, any observed differences between groups would not be due to a testing effect.

- *Instrumentation.* Instrumentation is a common threat to internal validity; it occurs when observed changes or differences are due to a change in the measuring instrument for the DV. Instrumentation differs from testing in that instrumentation is attributed to the measurement instrument itself rather than to participants' behavior as a result of taking the test. Instrumentation is most commonly found with observational measures, in which observers or interviewers are the "measuring instrument." For example, instrumentation could occur if some preschool children are being observed on certain behaviors to evaluate a behavior modification program and several types of good behaviors are missed initially but are counted in another assessment. The positive "gain" would be attributed to an instrumentation effect rather than an effect from the behavior modification program. In the one-group design, instrumentation would be a threat, whereas in the two-group design it would not, because as long as both groups are affected equally by the instrumentation, any differences between groups could be attributed to the treatment rather than to instrumentation.

- *Statistical regression.* This common threat occurs when very high pretest scores become lower on subsequent tests or when very low pretest scores become higher on post testing. This is more likely to occur when the selection of participants is based on extreme scores (either high or low) and, when they are measured again, their scores move back to an average level. For example, statistical regression could occur in a study in which an investigator wants to affect negative attitudes (such as homophobia) and selects people who have extremely high scores on a homophobia scale to be in the study. Some of these scores may be artificially high due to other factors (such as the instrumentation or the measurement scale having low reliability) rather than the participants' truly having a high level of homophobia. Therefore, if scores on the homophobia scale go down from pretest to posttest, some or all of the change may be due to a regression effect. In the one-group design, statistical regression could be a threat, as you cannot say for certain that any improvement from pretest to posttest is due to your treatment. Statistical regression is not a threat in the two-group design, as people in both groups are affected equally by the statistical regression effect.

- *Differential selection bias.* Another common threat is called differential selection bias and occurs typically when there is a lack of randomization to groups; it is a threat only for two-group or multigroup designs when there are differences between groups prior to any treatment. Participants could differ by age, gender, skill level, race or ethnicity, or socioeconomic status, to name just a few examples. The main point is that groups should be similar to avoid any confounding with the outcome of the study. For instance, assume that you have selected two high school classes for a study on improving physical activity levels; each class would constitute a "group." One group will receive the health promotion intervention ("treatment") and the other will act as a control. The problem is that these two groups may differ in variables other than the treatment variable, and any differences found at the posttest may be due to these "selection" differences rather than your treatment. Selection bias is an internal validity problem only for the two-group or multigroup design but not for the one-group design.

- *Differential attrition.* Attrition (also known as experimental mortality) is the loss of participants during the course of a study. When there is a *differential* loss of participants from the experimental group and the control group, the study is threatened by differential attrition. A differential loss is when one group—say, the treatment group—experiences more attrition than the control group, and this attrition relates to the outcome. For example, in our physical activity study, results would be compromised if teens in the health promotion group were more likely to drop out because those teens had the most weight to lose compared to teens in the control group; then, in this instance, any differences observed at posttest could now be the result of differential attrition. Differential attrition is an internal validity problem for two-group or multigroup designs but not for the single-group design.

Before we discuss the different types of experimental designs in greater detail, we need to understand an important and related concept: conducting experiments in a controlled laboratory environment is markedly different from conducting experiments with people. Although controlling for extraneous variables is critical to the integrity of an experiment so that necessary condition 3 is met, the level of control may vary widely when the experiment takes place in a real-world setting (such as a classroom or community) as opposed to a laboratory or other controlled setting (for instance, an isolated room), and when the subjects compose a heterogeneous group. Having a lower level of control over human subjects and environmental factors threatens internal validity and may introduce **error variance**. (*Error variance* refers to the variability in the dependent variable that *cannot* be attributed to the independent variable, but rather is attributed to extraneous variables or to variability among human subjects.) Reducing or controlling error variance is an important matter to consider, as error variance may affect the ability to attribute observable effects to the manipulation of the IV. Furthermore, different types of designs handle error variance differently and this should be a consideration when choosing an appropriate design.

error variance
the variability in the dependent variable that cannot be attributed to the independent variable, but is attributed to extraneous variables or variability among the subjects

To illustrate the two main experimental concepts of manipulation and control, consider the research question, What are the side effects of a hepatitis vaccine on African-American men? The IV in this instance would be the administration of the hepatitis vaccine. There must be at least two levels to an IV or it is not a variable. In this instance, manipulation of the IV could mean using two vaccines that are qualitatively different, such as a surface antigen vaccine as one and a different type of hepatitis vaccine as the second, or even a *placebo* (an inactive substance that may look like medicine but contains no medicine—a "sugar pill" with no treatment value). If all three of these were used, the IV would have three levels. Moreover, different levels of the IV could be quantitatively different—for example, when the same vaccine type is used, but in different dosages. The latter scenario is referred to as a dose-ranging study, in which two or more doses (starting at a lower dose and proceeding to higher doses) of a vaccine are tested against each other to determine which dose works best and has acceptable side effects. The DV in this hypothetical study is the side effects and could include measures of fatigue, quality of life, and nausea.

In terms of control, there are two main issues to consider: first, control related to subject selection and assignment, and second, control related to the type of experimental design chosen. Control over extraneous variables through the use of experimental designs increases the confidence that observed outcomes are the result of a given program, treatment, drug, or innovation instead of a function of extraneous variables or events, so it greatly enhances internal validity. Given these two important issues, referring back to our hepatitis vaccine study, the first issue to consider would be the method in which potential participants will be selected from the population of African-American men. A *random sampling* procedure, such as the use of a random numbers table, would ensure a high degree of control in that each potential participant would have an equal chance of being selected. This procedure helps to control variables that could be introduced into the sampling process and that could cause low **generalizability**. Generalizability is the degree to which the research findings can be applied to the population under study (for example, African-American men). Using random sampling techniques helps to reduce **sampling bias** and increase the representativeness of the sample, thereby enhancing generalizability (see Chapter Six). If random selection is used, then sampling bias should not be an issue unless the response rate or the rate at which participants agreed to be in the study is extremely low. Furthermore, if random selection is not possible, then a nonrandom sampling technique, such as *convenience sampling* (using individuals who are convenient to access) or *snowball sampling* (using recruited participants to identify others) would have to be used and would not reduce sampling bias. Accordingly, if participants differ in ways that affect the DV (side effects of the HIV vaccine), then the results might be attributed to these differences rather than to the vaccine. Chapter Six provides detailed information about sampling techniques.

Once the sample is recruited, the next factor to consider is how to assign participants to two groups. Other sources of error variance—such as socioeconomic status, age, and education level, to name a few—must be controlled. One method that would control (in this instance, by "control" we mean hold the effects of these variables constant) these sources of error variance would be to use **random assignment a.k.a. randomization** as the method to assign participants to respective groups. Randomization entails assigning participants by chance to one of two or more groups. There are different methods, such as using a random numbers table, using a software program, or even flipping a coin. Randomization minimizes any differences between or among groups by equally distributing subjects with particular characteristics between or

generalizability
the degree to which the research findings can be applied to the population under study

sampling bias
a type of bias that is attributed to nonrandom sampling methods used to generate a sample that results in the sample not being representative of the population under study

random assignment a.k.a. randomization
assigning participants by some technique involving chance to one of two or more groups

IN A NUTSHELL

Randomization minimizes any differences between or among groups by equally distributing subjects with particular characteristics between or among all the trial arms.

among all the trial arms. Randomization is clearly a powerful control technique and rules out many threats to internal validity—but not all of them.

The second and probably the most important issue of control is the choice of specific experimental design; however, keep in mind there are usually different ways in which research questions can be answered. The various designs that are used to conduct causal research vary in the quality of evidence they provide for making causal inference and in the level of control. Moreover, there are distinctions between pre-experimental designs, "true" experimental designs, and quasi-experimental designs that further influence the level of control and the ability to attribute changes in the DV to the manipulation of the IV. The following sections describe various types of experimental designs in detail and explore the strengths and weaknesses of each in terms of causal inference and level of control.

True Experimental Research Designs

In health promotion research, as previously stated, experimental designs are often used to answer specific health questions under the umbrella of causal research. By definition, experimental designs employ both a control group and a means to measure the change that occurs in both groups. Thus there is a high level of control for many confounding variables, and causal inferences can be made. It is important to also note that a distinction is made between a "true" experimental design and an experimental design. According to Campbell and Stanley (1966), a true experimental design, in addition to having a control group and common measured outcome(s), must also include random assignment. True experimental designs used in health promotion could involve determining the effects of disease or the etiological causes of certain diseases; however, for the most part, they typically involve testing the efficacy of prevention programs for reducing health risk behaviors and ultimately disease.

Posttest Control Group Design

The **posttest control group design** is considered the weakest of the true experimental designs. This design is deemed a between-subjects design in that there are at least two groups or **arms** between which to assess differences on the DV following the manipulation of the IV. Each group or arm is formed by random assignment and then presented with either the treatment or some type of control. No pretest is administered, but posttests are given to identify any difference between or among groups or arms. This design may be used if treatment started before the researcher

posttest control group design
experimental design involving more than one group but lacking a pretest

arms
groups involved in an experiment

was consulted, if testing would be considered a major threat to the internal validity of the study, or if the researchers were confident that the sample was homogenous (that is, similar in relevant characteristics including the DV). Although this is a true experimental design, the posttest control group design's major weakness is its lack of a pretest measure. Without a pretest, it is difficult to determine definitively if any differences observed at the end of the study are due to an actual change stemming from the treatment. Its major strength lies in having a control group, which controls for most common threats to internal validity except for differential selection and attrition. Randomization should theoretically control for differential selection; however, without a pretest, we cannot be assured that randomization worked and truly created an equivalency between groups. A posttest control group design is depicted in Figure 5.2.

An example of a three-group posttest-only control group design was implemented by Silverman (2011) in a study to examine the effects of a single session "rockumentary" music therapy intervention on patients in a detoxification unit. Silverman randomized 141 patients to either the "rockumentary" music therapy group, a standard music therapy group, or a verbal therapy group. Silverman utilized the posttest-only design, indicating that it would be inappropriate in a short-term situation (that is, one-session therapeutic intervention) to implement a pretest prior to randomization. Posttests were administered to patients after they received therapy to measure readiness to change and cravings. Posttest results showed that there was a significant difference in readiness to change between the verbal therapy group and the two music therapy groups. Patients in the two music therapy groups had lower cravings

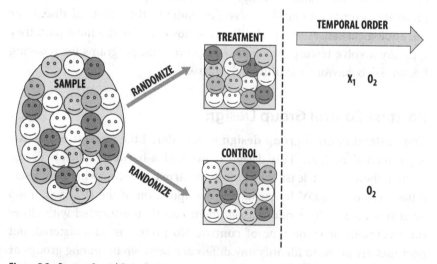

Figure 5.2 Posttest Control Group Design

than the verbal therapy group. However, there was no difference in readiness to change between the standard and "rockumentary" music therapies.

Pretest-Posttest Control Group Design

A common and more rigorous experimental design employed in health promotion is the **pretest-posttest control group design**. This design represents a significant improvement over the posttest control group design in that it adds a pretest that can be used to assess differences between groups prior to the implementation of the treatment. It is also considered a between-subjects design, as differences between groups are made on the DV and it involves exposing the *arms* or treatment groups to different levels of the IV. Furthermore, because you randomly assign subjects to the different arms, it is also referred to as a **randomized controlled trial** (RCT), which is considered one type of true experimental designs and is viewed as the "gold standard" of experimental designs. We provide specific details on how to conduct an RCT in health promotion in Chapter Ten as well as how to analyze RCTs in Chapter Fifteen; for now, suffice it to say that most health promotion researchers concur that the RCT is the most effective and most rigorous design for testing the efficacy of a program or treatment because it allows for causal inference and has the highest level of control possible in a real-world setting. Indeed, this design controls for most common threats to internal validity except for attrition. The strengths of this design are numerous; weaknesses may include **low external validity**, being time intensive, and being expensive to conduct. It is important to emphasize that a primary criticism of the RCT, in health promotion practice, is that the high level of internal validity precludes a high level of external validity. (Overreliance on the RCT in health promotion may indeed be a detriment to the development of programs given their cost and time intensity for implementation and evaluation).

The number of levels of the IV dictates the number of arms to be employed in an RCT. For example, if you were examining the efficacy of an HIV-preventive intervention relative to a general health promotion intervention, then you would require two groups (two levels); if you

pretest-posttest control group design
a between-subjects design consisting of a pretest that can be used to assess differences between groups prior to the implementation of the treatment in addition to a posttest

randomized controlled trial
a subset of true experimental designs that involves randomization to two or more arms, one of which is a control group, and allows for causal inference and controls for common threats to internal validity

low external validity
the ability to generalize results outside the setting of the RCT

IN A NUTSHELL

The RCT is the most effective and most rigorous design for testing the efficacy of a program or treatment because it allows for causal inference and has the highest level of control possible in a real-world setting.

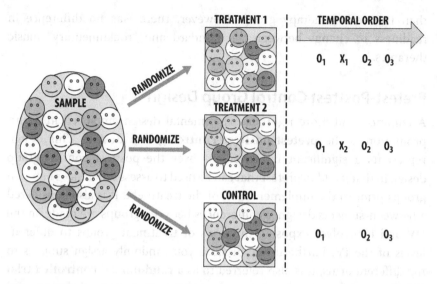

Figure 5.3 Three-Arm Randomized Controlled Design

were examining the efficacy of an HIV-preventive intervention and an HIV-preventive intervention with booster sessions relative to the general health promotion intervention, then you would need three groups or arms (three levels). A three-arm RCT design is depicted in Figure 5.3.

As the figure demonstrates, the RCT is considered a mixed design when subjects are randomized to groups and assessed at multiple time periods, and comparisons are made between groups and over time; it is called a mixed design because it incorporates a between-subjects factor (groups) and a within-subjects factor (movement of time changes in the DV observed across the waves of follow-up assessment). In simplest terms, implementation of an RCT as shown would involve (1) assessing subjects at baseline, (2) randomizing subjects into groups, (3) exposing subjects to the respective treatment, (4) assessing subjects after completion of the treatment (this could be immediately following or at a follow-up period), and (5) assessing them again at a subsequent follow-up period(s). Analysis goals for this design could include determining overall differences between groups (main effect for group), overall differences within groups (main effect for time), and whether subjects in the treatment group changed differentially over time as compared with subjects in the control group (an interaction of group and time).

Ditekemena and colleagues (2011) applied a mixed design RCT to test whether male participation rates in HIV voluntary counseling and testing (VCT) services could be enhanced by varying the venue in which VCT services were offered. The sample for the study was 591 male partners of pregnant women attending a maternity unit of a hospital located in

Kinshasah, the Democratic Republic of Congo. Men were randomized to obtain VCT services at either (1) a neighborhood health center, (2) a bar, or (3) a church, so this randomized controlled trial study had three arms. Participation in VCT was measured. Male participation was more likely to occur at the bar venue (OR=1.61; 95% CI=1.28–2.01) compared to the neighborhood health center venue. Male participation was higher at the church than at the health center, but the difference was not significant (OR=1.18; 95% CI=.93–1.48).

Matched Pairs Group Design

Another type of between-subjects design that is useful in health promotion research is the **matched pairs group design**. This design is employed when the researcher is aware of a particular subject characteristic or attribute that is strongly associated with the DV. Even when randomization is used, the characteristic may not get equally distributed between or among groups and could result in a significant amount of error variance. To ensure that the characteristic is distributed equally, subjects or even communities can be matched on the characteristic prior to random assignment. Depending on the number of groups in the experiment, subjects or communities are matched with other subjects or communities as closely as possible to form pairs (two groups), triplets (three groups), or even quadruplets (four groups). Then, taking each set, subjects are assigned at random into groups. The main advantage of this design is a significant reduction in the potential confounding effect of the matched characteristic on the DV. One example would be matching adolescents on alcohol and drug use who are enrolled in a two-arm sexual-risk-reduction intervention prior to randomization into groups. In this instance, prior to randomization, subjects would be measured on their alcohol and drug use. Subjects who reported similar alcohol and drug use behaviors (matching variable) would be paired together. Next, each subject, within each pair, would be randomly assigned to one of the two conditions.

Matched pairs group design allows for the control of differential selection that results from groups differing significantly on characteristics that would otherwise affect the DV. In essence, it creates balance between groups relative to key variables. The weaknesses of matched pairs design are that it is a time-consuming method to employ and it may not be possible to truly match all participants

matched pairs group design
a between-subjects design that matches subjects on a key characteristic and then randomizes each to a different condition or arm

IN A NUTSHELL

Matched pairs group design allows for the control of differential selection that results from groups differing significantly on characteristics that would otherwise affect the DV.

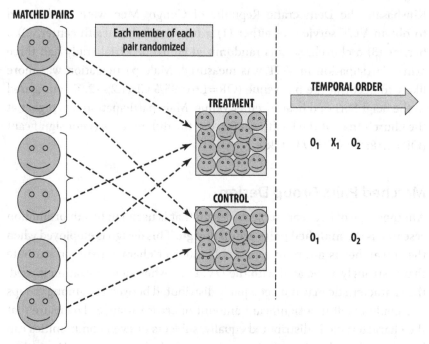

Figure 5.4 Matched Pairs Control Design

in one group with a suitable partner in the other group. A matched pairs group design is shown in Figure 5.4.

In health promotion research, often the use of this design could also involve the site rather than individual subjects as the unit of assignment. Examples of sites are places like schools, communities, workplaces, and even entire states. For example, Le Roux and colleagues (2013) evaluated the effect of community health workers' home visits on maternal and infant well-being for women living with HIV in South Africa. Maternal and infant well-being was assessed for the first six months of life. The study employed a randomized matched pairs design in which neighborhood was the unit of assignment. Women were assigned to either standard comprehensive healthcare at a clinic or home visits by community health workers in addition to standard care. Women were assessed during pregnancy and at one week and six weeks post-birth. Results showed that women participating in the arm involving home visits by community health workers arm were more likely to complete tasks to prevent vertical transmission of HIV, avoid birth-related medical complications, breast-feed exclusively for six months, have infants with healthy height-for-age measurements, and use condoms consistently than women in the standard healthcare arm.

Within-Subjects or Repeated-Measures Design

The **within-subjects design**, also referred to as the *repeated-measures design*, is another experimental design that is effective in reducing error variance due to human subject differences. In this design, only one arm is used, so between-group differences are not considered. The one-arm design uses subjects as their own controls, by exposing the same people to the different levels of the IV. For example, if there are two levels of the IV, condition one is formed when subjects are exposed to the first level; condition two is formed when subjects are exposed to the second level. Although matching in a between-groups design reduces error variance due to individual differences to a large degree, the within-subjects design is more effective because the same subjects are exposed to the different treatments, thereby significantly reducing or eliminating error variance due to subject differences. Again, this is true because subjects are their own controls—the goal is to detect within-subject change. With this level of reduction in error variance, the ability to detect the effects of the IV is greater than in other designs. Although the within-subjects design is classified as an experimental design because of manipulation and control, it is important to note that because this design does not have random assignment, it cannot be considered a true experimental design.

In health promotion research that involves a behavioral intervention, the within-subjects design is rarely used mainly because of **carryover effects**, which occur when exposure to the first treatment (in this instance, it could be an educational intervention) affects the subjects' performance during subsequent treatments. This is the main weakness of the within-subjects design. Depending on the carryover effect, performance can be enhanced or reduced. For example, subjects may learn a skill in the first treatment that may enhance the observed outcomes after subsequent treatments; however, the observed change in outcome may be from the first treatment and not the second. This effect is called **learning**. Other types of carryover effects include **fatigue** (deterioration in performance due to being tired from the first treatment), **habituation** (repeated exposure to stimulus leading to reduced responsiveness), **sensitization** (stronger responses to stimuli stemming from initial exposure to a different stimulus), and **adaptation** (adaptive changes to a stimulus leading to a change in outcome). The within-subjects design is presented in Figure 5.5.

An applied example of a repeated-measures design study was conducted by Reed and colleagues (2013) in the United Kingdom. The purpose of the study was to examine whether exercising in a green natural space affected enjoyment and perceived exertion in 75 children. The participants ran 1.5 miles in an urban setting and one week later ran 1.5 miles in a

within-subjects design
an experimental design that uses subjects as their own controls by exposing the same people to different levels of the independent variable

carryover effects
effects that occur when exposure to the first treatment affects the subjects' performance during subsequent treatment

learning
type of carryover effect in which what is learned in the first treatment enhances observed outcomes after subsequent treatments

fatigue
type of carryover effect in which deterioration in a subject's performance results from being tired from the first treatment

habituation
type of carryover effect in which a subject's repeated exposure to stimulus leads to reduced responsiveness

sensitization
type of carryover effect in which subjects respond stronger to stimuli stemming from initial exposure to a different stimulus

adaptation
type of carryover effect in which a subject's adaptive changes to a stimulus lead to a change in outcome

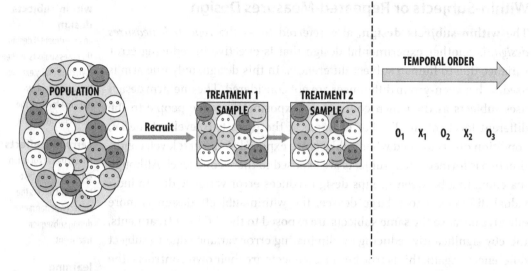

Figure 5.5 Repeated-Measures or Within-Subjects Design

nearby park. Immediately following each exercise, the participants provided retrospective levels of enjoyment and exertion during exercise. Results showed that there was no significant difference in levels of enjoyment and level of perceived exertion between the two conditions. However, it is important to note that the exercise in the park was more physically demanding because running on rough terrain requires greater energy than running on artificial surfaces.

Crossover Trial

crossover trial

an experimental design in which subjects act as their own controls; it involves randomizing subjects to receive the different levels of the independent variable in a particular order so that they receive all possible levels

A specific form of the within-subjects design used in some health promotion research, in particular in drug efficacy trials, is called a **crossover trial**. With a crossover trial, it is possible to reduce the negative impact of carryover effects by counterbalancing, which means varying the order in which participants take part (for example, group 1 does treatment 1 followed by treatment 2; group 2 does the reverse), which means that any carryover effects are equally balanced for both conditions of the IV. In this type of design, the same group of subjects is exposed to all levels of the IV, but the order in which groups of subjects are exposed is varied. Thus for every possible order combination a group is formed. For example, if researchers wanted to examine the efficacy of a drug on reducing pain, then using a crossover trial, they could randomly assign half the subjects to receive the drug first and then the placebo, while the other half receives the placebo first and then the drug. When each group of subjects switches from the first treatment condition to the next, this is the point at which they "cross over." By random assignment into the groups in this way, the more simple within-subjects design can be classified as a true experiment.

Crossover studies are not the most appropriate design in certain instances. They are appropriate in studies where the effects of the treatment(s) are short-lived and reversible (such as in drug efficacy trials) or in trials related to symptomatic but chronic conditions or diseases. It is generally agreed that the crossover design should not be used when the condition of interest is unstable (such as influenza) and may change regardless of interventions. A significant strength of this design is that error variance due to human subjects' differences or between-subject variability is eliminated, as each subject acts as his or her own control, allowing for within-group comparisons, but the design also permits between-group comparisons. Weaknesses are similar to other experimental designs; these may include attrition, whereby some subjects drop out before undergoing the other condition. Because it is a within-subjects repeated measure design, carryover effects may also be a threat, depending on the nature of the treatment. The crossover trial design is shown in Figure. 5.6.

IN A NUTSHELL

A significant strength of this design is that error variance due to human subjects' differences or between-subject variability is eliminated, as each subject acts as his or her own control, allowing for within-group comparisons, but the design also permits between-group comparisons.

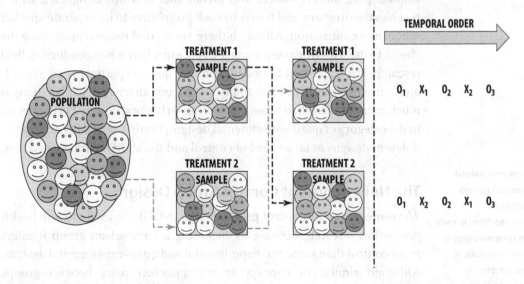

Figure 5.6 Randomized Crossover Trial Design

A randomized crossover trial design was used in a sexual health promotion study conducted among women attending an urban reproductive health clinic in the southeastern United States to assess their acceptance and use of male and female condoms (Kulczycki, Kim, Duerr, Jamieson, & Macaluso, 2004). The sample of women was randomly assigned to one of two groups: the first group used ten male condoms first followed by a crossover to using ten female condoms; the second group was the reverse order. An intervention, consisting of a nurse providing instruction in correct condom usage, was given to all women. Overall, the results indicated that regardless of order, women preferred male condoms to female condoms and judged them to be superior.

Quasi-Experimental Designs

The word *quasi* means "as if" or "almost"; thus a quasi-experiment approximates a true experiment. Quasi-experiments are similar to true experiments in that there is a treatment of some kind to examine and there are outcome measures; the main difference is that quasi-experiments do not use random assignment to create the groups necessary for comparison on the outcome measures. Often, conducting health promotion research precludes using random assignment into groups or conditions because it may not be feasible, possible, ethical, or legal. For example, withholding a drug treatment or critical health program from vulnerable populations such as prisoners or pregnant women would be unethical or illegal in some instances, when one group benefits and one group is deprived. For school-based health educational programs, resources may dictate that only one designated school receives the program, and it may be cost-prohibitive to incorporate another school as a comparison. Although there are myriad reasons underlying the choice to use a quasi-experimental design, especially when conducting field research, it is important to understand that quasi-experiments are considered causal research, but the ability to rule out alternative explanations is much more limited than when using an experimental design. Furthermore, in the category of quasi-experimental designs, there is variability among the different designs as far as level of control and the ability to infer causation.

nonequivalent control group design
a research design in which the comparison group is matched as closely as possible to the experimental group

The Nonequivalent Control Group Design

The **nonequivalent control group design** (NCGD) is used often in health promotion research, because by including a comparison group it offers more control than some pre-experimental and quasi-experimental designs. Although similar in concept to the matched pairs between-groups design, the nonequivalent control group design deviates from the matched-subjects design in that there is no randomization of the matched subjects, sites, workplaces, or communities into respective groups. Because the investigator does not control the assignment to groups through randomization, this design is deemed to have "nonequivalent groups." In the NCGD, a group is matched as closely as possible to the experimental group and is used as a comparison group; however, the groups may be different prior to the study. Because of this nonequivalence of groups at the start, the NCGD is especially susceptible to the threat of differential selection, which means that prior differences between the groups may affect the outcome of the study. Under the worst circumstances, this can lead us to conclude that our health promotion program did not have an effect, when in fact it did—or that the program did have an effect, when in fact it did not.

IN A NUTSHELL

Because of this nonequivalence of groups at the start, the NCGD is especially susceptible to the differential selection threat to internal validity.

The Nonequivalent Group, Posttest-Only

The **nonequivalent group, posttest-only design** is one of two main types of designs that fall under the general category of NCGD. The nonequivalent group, posttest-only design consists of administering an outcome measure to two groups—such as a program-treatment group and a comparison group, or possibly two program groups—each receiving a different version of the program. This design might be used when you are not able to do a pretest (for various reasons) but you can get a comparison or control group. For example, one group of students at a high school received an abstinence-only program while students at another school received a comprehensive sexual-risk-reduction program, and the school superintendent decided an evaluation was necessary even though no pretest had been administered. After twelve weeks, a test measuring sexual debut and risky sexual behaviors was administered to see which program was more effective. A major problem with this design is that, as stated previously, the two groups (in this instance schools) might not necessarily be the same before the program takes place and may differ in important ways that may influence the outcomes. Differential selection is therefore a threat to internal validity. For instance, if it is found that the students in the abstinence-only program reported a delay in sexual debut and less engagement in sexual risk behavior compared to students in the sexual-risk-reduction group, there is no way of determining if they were less likely to engage in those behaviors before

nonequivalent group, posttest-only design
a type of nonequivalent control group design which consists of administering an outcome measure to two groups that receive a different version of the program

the program or whether other factors existed. For example, students at the school that received the abstinence-only program may come from households that are of a higher socioeconomic status and contain a higher percentage of two-parent households as compared to the other school. Accordingly, the students from the former school may differ in their levels of parental monitoring or parental communication about sex, and these differences may have influenced their sexual behavior. For this reason, this design cannot definitively show whether observed changes are due to the treatment or to existing differences between the groups prior to the treatment.

In addition to differential selection, the nonequivalent group, posttest-only design has other weaknesses such as differential attrition as well as additive and interactive effects, meaning that threats to internal validity can be layered with such factors as selection history, which occurs when history affects one group but not the other. For example, in the school example, imagine that a major event occurs at one school (for example, a rape or shooting) but not at the other, and this event affects the outcome of the study. The design is depicted in Figure 5.7.

Shepherd, McBride, Welch, Dirks, and Hill (2011) conducted a study employing the nonequivalent group, posttest-only design, which compared the health-related quality of life of individuals residing near wind farms to individuals not residing near wind farms. Samples were drawn from two geographically matched areas in New Zealand. This study was conducted after the wind turbines were installed; thus a pretest survey was not an option. In other words, households in both areas were given questionnaires to assess their health-related quality of life at posttest. Results showed that individuals living near wind farms reported a lower mean score on physical health than those not living near wind farms.

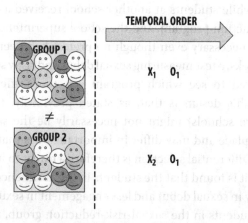

Figure 5.7 Nonequivalent Groups, Posttest-Only Design

The Nonequivalent Group, Pretest-Posttest

The **nonequivalent group, pretest-posttest design** improves on a major limitation of the nonequivalent group, posttest-only design by allowing the researcher to empirically assess differences in the two groups prior to implementation of the program. If the researcher finds that one group performs better than the other on the posttest, then initial differences (if the groups were in fact similar on the pretest) can be ruled out as explanations for the differences. Furthermore, if in fact the groups did differ on the pretest measure, then the researcher could potentially control for these differences statistically. This design is depicted in Figure 5.8.

Thato and Penrose (2013) used a nonequivalent control group, pretest-posttest design to evaluate the effects of a brief, theory-based HIV intervention among college students in Bangkok, Thailand. Undergraduate students taking a sexual health class were asked to participate as peer leaders. The peer leaders first went through a training that included activities such as interviewing HIV/AIDS patients in a hospital temple, learning negotiation skills, and learning how to properly use a condom. The peer leaders used convenience sampling to recruit n=435 students for both the intervention group (the sexual health program led by the peer leaders), and the control group (information about 2009 flu prevention). Unfortunately, the researchers do not provide a rationale for their lack of randomization in this study. It may have been a matter of convenience in how students were recruited and where they were recruited; however, details on this issue were not provided. Sexual behavior and AIDS prevention knowledge was assessed via questionnaire at baseline and after the intervention for both the intervention and the control group. A total of 226 students participated in the intervention, and 209 students served as the control group. Results showed that at post-intervention and 2 months later,

nonequivalent group, pretest-posttest design
a type of nonequivalent control group design in which the researcher assesses differences in the two groups prior to implementing the program

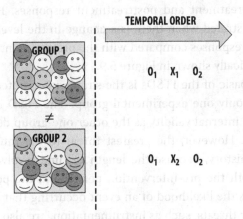

Figure 5.8 Nonequivalent Groups, Pretest-Posttest Design

students in the intervention group reported statistically significantly higher knowledge of AIDS prevention behaviors than those in the control group. However, the intervention did not improve AIDS preventive behaviors among sexually active Thai college students.

The Interrupted Time Series Design

interrupted time series design
a research design that involves collecting data at multiple instances over time before and then after implementation of a treatment or intervention

The **interrupted time series design** (ITSD) is the strongest quasi-experimental approach for evaluating the longitudinal effects of interventions. It involves collecting data at multiple instances over time before and after a treatment of some kind. The treatment can be a health promotion program, implementation of a new health policy, or a naturally occurring event. Data used in a time series design can range from individual behavior to cumulative incidence of diseases such as myocardial infarction, cancer, and diabetes. It does require knowledge about the specific time in which the program or intervention occurred in the time series. An advantage of collecting a series of observations both before and after the treatment is that a reliable picture regarding the outcome of interest can be gleaned. Thus the time series design is sensitive to trends in performance.

maturational trend
observations involving human subjects who are changing their behavior as they age

seasonal trend
phenomenon in which observations are influenced by the season in which data are collected

The aim of the ITSD is to determine whether or not the intervention had an effect over and above any trend present in the data. For example, the data collected prior to the treatment may reveal several trends in the data such as a **maturational trend** (in which observations involve human subjects who are changing their behavior as they age) or a **seasonal trend** (in which observations are influenced by the season in which data are collected). These trends can be identified and assessed, and treatment effects ascertained. A treatment effect is demonstrated only if the pattern of posttreatment responses differs significantly from the pattern of pretreatment responses. That is, the treatment effect is demonstrated by a discontinuity in the pattern of pretreatment and posttreatment responses. For example, an effect is demonstrated when there is a change in the level or slope of the posttreatment responses compared with the pretreatment responses. This effect is dramatically shown in Figure 5.9.

The most basic of the ITSDs is the simple interrupted time series, in which there is only one experimental group. The ITSD is subject to the same threats to internal validity as the other one-group designs described in this chapter. However, the greatest threat to the internal validity of this design is history, because the length of time involved in collecting the data for both the pre-intervention period and the post-intervention period increases the likelihood of an event occurring that might affect the outcome. Other threats, such as instrumentation, are also likely if the way in which the data are collected changes over time. Maturation may also be

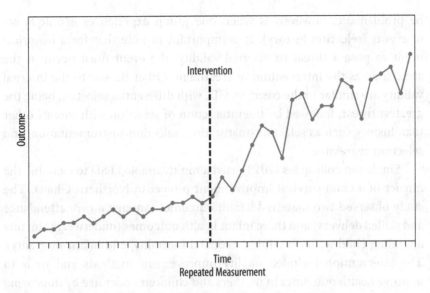

Figure 5.9 Interrupted Time Series Intervention Effect

an issue if the data points represent assessments with human subjects or other outcomes that normally would change over time. Testing could pose another threat if not using archival data; however, testing would most likely become evident in the pre-intervention phase. This design is diagrammed in Table 5.3.

Adding a nonequivalent control group to the simple interrupted time series will significantly improve on some of the limitations mentioned. This design, called an interrupted time series with a nonequivalent control group, is also diagrammed in Table 5.3. As shown, a series of observations is collected both prior to and following the administration of the treatment for the experimental group; during this same time period, a series of observations is also collected for a comparison group. This design allows the researcher to control for history effects, as a historical event would most likely affect both treatment and control groups equally. What may

Table 5.3 Interrupted Time Series Designs

Design								Threats
Simple Interrupted Time Series								
O_1	O_2	O_3	O_4	X_1	O_5	O_6	O_7	O_8 Hawthorne effect, History, Instrumentation, Maturation, Testing, Statistical Regression
Interrupted Time Series with Nonequivalent Control Group								
O_1	O_2	O_3	O_4	X_1	O_5	O_6	O_7	O_8 Diffusion, Differential Selection, Selection-maturation,
O_1	O_2	O_3	O_4	O_5	O_6	O_7	O_8	Selection-instrumentation, Selection-regression

be problematic, however, is when one group experiences a unique set of events (selection history). It is important to note that for a historical event to pose a threat to internal validity, the event must occur at the same time as the intervention or treatment. Other threats to the internal validity are similar to the basic NCGD, with differential selection being the greatest threat, followed by the interaction of selection with threats other than history such as selection-maturation, selection-instrumentation, and selection-regression.

Singh and colleagues (2013) used a multivariable ITSD to examine the impact of a child survival improvement project in Northern Ghana. The study observed two maternal health outcomes (antenatal care attendance and skilled delivery) and three infant health outcomes (underweight infants attending child wellness clinics, neonatal mortality, and infant mortality). The intervention included quality improvement methods and tools to improve health outcomes in mothers and children under five by improving the coverage, quality, reliability, and patient-centeredness of a national program implemented in all public and faith-based health facilities in Ghana. Comparisons of the study outcomes were made on a monthly basis, to detect whether the intervention was associated with a change in an

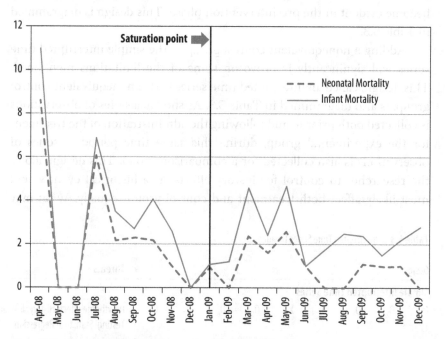

Figure 5.10 Means of the Mortality Outcomes Over Time (per 1000)
Source: Singh et al. (2013).

underlying trend for an outcome variable. The timeframe for the evaluation periods was from April 2008 to December 2009; the project did not reach full implementation until January 2009; thus the pre-intervention data period was 9 months. Results showed that neonatal mortality decreased from a mean of 2.5/1000 to 0.9/1000 and infant mortality decreased from a mean of 3.5/1000 to 2.3/1000 from the pre-intervention to post-intervention periods. Furthermore, the mean for skilled delivery increased from 55.9 to 64.7%. These time series results are presented in Figure 5.10.

Summary

Causal research identifies etiological causes of health-related outcomes and evaluates whether health promotion programs are effective. Typically, in health promotion we focus mainly on evaluation of programs. This chapter focused on describing the designs frequently used in conducting causal research in health promotion. Perhaps the most important decision to make when embarking on any study—but especially causal research studies due to the resources involved—is the selection of a research design. The experimental and quasi-experimental designs described in this chapter all have their associated strengths, limitations, and varying levels of rigor. Some designs control for most internal threats to validity, whereas others control for far fewer. The important thing is to know the strengths and limitations of each research design, and how these may affect the internal validity and, in turn, the study results and interpretation of those results. To make the process easier, this seemingly complicated decision about which design to choose can be broken down into three smaller decisions: (1) Is randomization an option? (2) Is having a control group feasible? and (3) Can a pretest be administered? All of these decisions should be examined carefully by every member of the research team, with the pros and cons of each option weighed with great attention to rigor. In addition, it is critical to consider what resources are available to the project, so that the selected study design is not only functional but also feasible. Although implicit in this chapter, it is important to remain vigilant regarding your obligation to design studies that are ethical and that do not violate the rights or well-being of the participants. Considering all of these factors, at a basic level you want your research design to optimize the ability to provide a rigorous and valid test of the research question(s), because your work may have great potential to shape health promotion practice and policy and contribute another link in the chain of research.

KEY TERMS

Adaptation

Arms

Placebo-attention comparison

Carryover effects

Crossover trial

Dependent variable

Error variance

External validity

Extraneous variables

Factor

Factorial design

Fatigue

Generalizability

Habituation

Independent variable

Internal validity

Interrupted time series design

Learning

Levels

Low external validity

Matched pairs group design

Maturational trend

Nonequivalent control group design

Nonequivalent group, posttest-only design

Nonequivalent group, pretest-posttest design

Posttest control group design

Pretest-posttest control group design

Random assignment

Randomization

Randomized controlled trial

Repeated-measures design

Sampling bias

Seasonal trend

Selection bias

Sensitization

Within-subjects design

For Practice and Discussion

1. For each research goal listed here, please select the best research design that could be applied to most effectively address the goal. Be prepared to justify your answers. Identify the threats to internal validity that each design does and does not control for.

   a. To determine the efficacy of a brief, clinic-based health promotion program that is designed to promote correct and consistent condom use among high-risk young women and also incorporates a social media component to affect the social networks of the young women enrolled.

b. To determine the efficacy of a community-based health promotion intervention designed to promote physical activity among high-risk youth in the Southeastern United States.

c. To assess whether a media campaign can reduce initiation of e-cigarette use among teens in the Pacific Northwestern United States.

d. To test the hypothesis that low perceived risk of cancer causes adolescents to start smoking and using novel tobacco products.

e. To test the effectiveness of a prescription drug abuse awareness program (note: you have a strong suspicion that the assessment instrument used for measuring prescription drug abuse is also likely to foster awareness—you would like to test this suspicion as well).

2. Read a journal article that describes a randomized controlled trial (the gold standard) in the field of health promotion. Discuss how randomization was implemented. Did it work (that is, were groups equivalent at baseline?)? How many arms did it have? What was the DV? What was the IV? What were the extraneous variables that were controlled for? Were there any noticeable threats to internal validity? Did the authors describe the limitations fully?

3. List potential research questions that would be appropriate for a within-subjects design. Why would this design be more appropriate than a between-subjects design?

4. What are the ethical considerations involved when using an experimental design with a placebo-control group for testing a health promotion intervention among HIV-positive patients to enhance their adherence to high-active anti-retroviral therapy?

References

Campbell, D. T., and Stanley, J. C. (1963, 1966). *Experimental and quasi-experimental designs for research.* Chicago: Rand McNally.

Ditekemena, J., Matendo, R., Koole, O., . . . and Ryder, R. (2011). Male partner voluntary counseling and testing associated with the antenatal services in Kinshasa, Democratic Republic of Congo: A randomized controlled trial. *International Journal of STD & AIDS, 22*(3), 165–170.

Falkow, S. (2004). Molecular Koch's postulates applied to bacterial pathogenicity—A personal recollection 15 years later. *Nature Reviews Microbiology, 2*(1), 67–72.

Kulczycki, A., Kim, D., Duerr, A., Jamieson, D., and Macaluso, M. (2004). The acceptability of the female and male condom: a randomized crossover trial. *Perspectives on Sexual & Reproductive Health, 36*(3), 114–119.

Le Roux, I. M., Tomlinson, M., Harwood, J. M., . . . and Rotheram-Borus, M. J. (2013). Outcomes of home visits for pregnant township mothers and their infants in South Africa: A cluster randomized trial. *AIDS, 27*(9):1461–1471.

Reed, K., Wood, C., Barton, J., Pretty, J. N., Cohen, D., et al. (2013). A repeated measures experiment of green exercise to improve self-esteem in UK school children. *PLoS ONE, 8*(7), e69176.

Shepherd, D., McBride, D., Welch, D., Dirks, K., and Hill, E. (2011). Evaluating the impact of wind turbine noise on health-related quality of life. *Noise & Health, 13*(54): 333–339.

Silverman, M. J. (2011). Effects of music therapy on change readiness and craving in patients on a detoxification unit. *Journal of Music Therapy, 48*(4), 509–531.

Singh, K., Speizer, I., Handa, S., . . . and Twum-Danso, N. (2013). Impact evaluation of a quality improvement intervention on maternal and child health outcomes in northern Ghana: Early assessment of a national scale up project. *International Journal for Quality in Health Care, 25*(5), 477–487.

Thato, R., and Penrose, J. (2013). A brief, peer-led HIV prevention program for college students in Bangkok, Thailand. *Journal of Pediatric and Adolescent Gynecology, 26*(1), 58–65.

CHAPTER 6

PRINCIPLES OF SAMPLING

Richard A. Crosby
Laura F. Salazar
Ralph J. DiClemente

One of the most important decisions you will make about any research study involves the very basic question of whether the sample fairly represents the **population** (the defined segment of people being targeted by your study) you have chosen to study. The answer is a matter of degree rather than an absolute "yes" or "no." When designing a study, your job is to ensure that the degree of representativeness is as high as possible. This chapter will provide you with the tools needed to achieve this goal. It will also give you an important skill set for accessing samples, tracking your success, and calculating sample size requirements.

Deciding how research participants will be selected is a turning point in the research process. The "how" in this case is known as sampling, and successfully choosing the correct method of sampling is as critical as using that method correctly. As with most endeavors, the key aspect of successful sampling is a great deal of attention to planning. Planning is, in a sense, the "art" of sampling; it requires creativity and cautious optimism regarding possibilities. At the foundation of this planning, the researcher is formulating an operationally defined goal. To formulate this goal, three vital decisions are needed: (1) What is the sampling element? (2) Is a sampling frame accessible? and (3) What type of sampling technique should be employed? Ultimately, the utility of a research project is a function of its generalizability. In turn, generalizability is a function of how well the sample represents the selected priority population. Sampling is a science unto itself—one that is

LEARNING OBJECTIVES

- Distinguish between probability and nonprobability samples.

- Understand when probability sampling can be used appropriately.

- Describe the concept of a sampling frame.

- Identify multiple techniques of sampling and determine the advantages and limitations of each.

- Enumerate issues pertaining to accessing a sample and estimating how many sampling elements are required.

population
the defined segment of people being targeted by a study

used to predict winners of political elections before the polls even close, and one that may someday be used in place of a "head by head" count for the U.S. census.

In health promotion research, sampling methods can be divided into two main categories: (1) methods that are admittedly weak in generalizability (nonprobability methods) and (2) methods that yield high generalizability (probability methods). Despite its limitations, the former category is often very useful in the early stages of the research chain or when the nature of the selected population precludes the application of probability methods. The latter category, although far more rigorous, is often problematic to apply, as it depends on the existence of a sampling frame. In this chapter you will learn about sampling techniques, sampling frames, and a host of issues related to sampling in health promotion research. As you read this chapter, bear in mind that nearly all research is vulnerable to challenges as to whether the sample fairly represents the population, but the degree of this vulnerability varies tremendously from one study to the next.

Once you have determined the most appropriate sampling technique for your research question, your next challenges will involve accessing the sample, tracking your success rates in the sampling process, and determining the final sample size required for analytic purposes. Thus this chapter will also prepare you to learn the fundamental concepts that apply to these challenges. As you learn this material, you will begin to see that the rigor of health promotion research is partly a product of the sampling techniques you select, your diligent use of those techniques, and your skillful navigation of the aforementioned challenges. Indeed, the work of health promotion research serves as an apt reminder of the complexity and the exciting challenges inherent in the pursuit of scientific rigor.

Sampling Elements

The goal of any sampling technique is to maximize the *generalizability* of the sample to the population. In this sense, the term *population* refers to all possible *elements* of a defined group. An **element** (the basic unit that defines the study population) can, in turn, be people (as is usually the case) or well-defined units (also called clusters) that have importance in public health (such as emergency care centers, schools, and homeless shelters). When people are the sampling element, the research questions are centered on the person; for example, Do outpatients from cardiac care centers consume a healthy diet? Conversely, when well-defined units are the sampling element, the research questions will involve "behavior" of an entire system, such as, How effectively do cardiac care centers teach outpatients to consume

element
the basic unit that defines the study population

healthy diets? Therefore an initial step in defining the sampling goal is to determine whether the research questions necessitate investigation of behavior at the individual level or the collective behavior of an organized system. Making this distinction is vital. Table 6.1 presents several examples of health promotion research questions shown by this essential division in purpose.

IN A NUTSHELL

An initial step in defining the sampling goal is to determine whether the research questions necessitate investigation of behavior at the individual level or the collective behavior of an organized system.

Sampling Frame Accessibility

Once the type of element has been identified, the next question that presents itself is whether a *sampling frame* exists (or can be created). A **sampling frame** is a formal list (often an exhaustive list) of units or elements that constitutes the population. The word *exhaustive* is critical here because the list must represent every possible element in the population. For example, imagine that the research question is, Are unemployed men residing in rural counties more likely to be heavy smokers than unemployed men residing in urban counties? At first, the existence of a sampling frame seems intuitive—unemployed men are "listed" by offices that provide government assistance (that is, unemployment benefits). Ignoring for a moment whether such lists would even be made available, the researcher needs to ask the question, Is this frame exhaustive of the population?

sampling frame
a formal list (often an exhaustive list) of units or elements that constitute the population

Table 6.1   Examples of Research Questions Displayed by Level of Analysis

Person-Level Research Questions	System-Level Research Questions
How does condom availability influence teens' use of condoms?	What factors influence school systems to adopt condom distribution programs?
Is religiosity associated with lower rates of domestic violence?	Do churches actively teach couples and families conflict-resolution skills?
Are first-time parents able to properly install infant car seats?	Do hospitals offer first-time parents training in the installation of car seats?
Do women residing in low-income nursing homes consume diets adequate in fiber?	Do low-income nursing homes provide women with diets that are adequate in fiber?
Is affiliation with social organizations associated with decreased substance abuse?	To what extent do urban social organizations provide teens with alternatives to substance abuse?
Do people with adult-onset diabetes practice the consistent and correct use of insulin?	What is the extent of postdiagnostic education provided to adults newly diagnosed with diabetes in state-funded health clinics?

An unfortunate reality of sampling is that very few sampling frames are truly exhaustive of the population. For example, do all unemployed men collect government assistance? The answer is no, and thus you can quickly imagine that this sampling frame would not be exhaustive. Even seemingly clear-cut cases of an effective sampling frame can be problematic. A classic example is the use of telephone directories as a sampling frame. The directory is not exhaustive because it will not include people who use mobile phones exclusively, people who cannot afford phone service, people who pay extra for an unlisted number, or people who have recently moved into the listing area. So the question, "Is this frame exhaustive of the population?" is answered by degree rather than by a simple "yes" or "no" (otherwise "no" would almost always be the answer). Table 6.2 displays examples of sampling frames that adequately represent the population (providing a higher degree of generalizability) and those less likely to represent the population (providing a lower degree of generalizability).

Careful scrutiny of Table 6.2 will reveal two important points. First, note that none of the examples involves units as the sampling element. In each example, including the one about pediatricians, the research question is about behavior of people rather than organizations. Table 6.2 does not provide examples for elements defined by units rather than people because, with some exceptions, units typically have a sampling frame that will offer a high degree of exhaustion. As a principle, exhaustion is generally far more likely when the sampling element is defined by a unit rather than by people. The difference is that social structures and law often protect individual identities, whereas group identities (for units) are often made public by intention. For example, churches, voluntary health agencies, schools, and neighborhood organizations are units that, by design, can be easily identified. Hospitals, soup kitchens, youth organizations, and drug treatment centers are just a few other examples of potential elements that are amenable to sampling for research questions at the system level.

Second, deeper scrutiny of the left-hand column in Table 6.2 raises an essential question: Can these sampling frames be accessed? Access to lists of pediatricians with hospital privileges may be possible; however, one can easily imagine "lists" that could not be obtained (for example, people receiving psychotherapy, convicted felons, persons living with tuberculosis, people who have survived cancer, or persons living with HIV/AIDS). This key concern leads to compromise between two competing conditions: (1) the need for the sample to be generalizable to the target population and (2) the practical reality of obtaining sampling frames that list people.

This compromise is often inevitable, and it may shape the research question. For example, looking again at Table 6.2, imagine that the initial research question is to investigate the relationship of parental monitoring

Table 6.2   Sampling Frames with High and Low Degrees of Generalizability

Higher Generalizability	Lower Generalizability
Research Question:	Research Question:
Is parental monitoring associated with health risk behavior among boys thirteen to sixteen years of age from low-income homes?	Are cancer patients who remain optimistic likely to survive longer than those who lose hope?
Sampling Frame:	Sampling Frame:
Boys enrolled in reduced-cost lunch programs at public schools	People diagnosed with cancer at publicly funded medical offices.
Note: Findings could be generalized to low-income boys attending public schools, but not to those who have dropped out or been placed in an alternative setting (including juvenile detention)	Note: Publicly funded medical offices may represent only a very small portion of the locations where cancer is diagnosed—thus generalizability is quite low.
Research Question:	Research Question:
Are women who receive WIC benefits at risk of rapid repeat pregnancy?	What behavioral factors predict iron-deficiency anemia among pregnant women?
Sampling Frame:	Sampling Frame:
Women enrolled in WIC programs	Women receiving prenatal care
Note: In this scenario, the sampling frame and the research question line up perfectly! Thus generalizability would be optimal.	Note: The key question to consider is what portion of pregnant women do not receive prenatal care. To the extent that pregnant women in any given setting may not receive this care, generalizability decreases.
Research Question:	Research Question:
To what extent do hospital-based pediatricians meet guidelines for children's vaccination schedules?	Are low-income elderly women less likely than their male counterparts to exercise on a regular basis?
Sampling Frame:	Sampling Frame:
Hospital registry of pediatricians with privileges	Women and men receiving Medicare benefits
Note: Again, the sampling frame and the research question appear to line up quite nicely, so potential for generalizability is high.	Note: Here it is important to realize that all low-income elderly people may not receive Medicare benefits. Further, not all people receiving Medicare benefits are likely to be low-income, and many may not perceive themselves to be "elderly." Thus generalizability is likely to be quite low.

to health risk behavior among boys in low-income households attending public schools. That the sampling frame exists is not in question, but whether this list will be provided to a researcher is another question entirely. A compromise is achieved by altering the research question to accommodate the sampling frame that *is* accessible. For example, the question could become, What is the relationship of parental monitoring to health risk behavior among boys attending public schools? Note that the slightly altered research question no longer includes the term *"low-income."* Because of privacy regulations, disclosing a comprehensive list of boys who qualify for a reduced or free lunch is problematic, whereas disclosing a comprehensive list of *all* boys may be acceptable. Moreover, the advantage of this inclusive sampling frame is that the original research question could still be evaluated. For example, the study questionnaire could ask all boys, Do you qualify for a free or reduced-price lunch at school? Then the analysis could compare boys in low-income households (defined by the "lunch" criterion) to remaining boys. In fact, such a comparison could lead to a more elaborate version of the initial research question: What is the relationship of parental monitoring to health risk behavior among low-income boys attending public schools compared with boys not classified as low-income? Therefore, when sampling is being considered, the art of planning research requires that you understand the reciprocal relationship between framing the research question and accessing a sampling frame. In this regard it is appropriate to think of steps 2 and 6 from the nine-step model (Chapter One) as being necessarily linked to one another. That is, defining the research goal and specifying the exact research question, on the one hand, and selecting the sampling procedure, on the other, should happen correspondingly.

Sampling Techniques

Effective sampling from the sampling frame, referred to as the selection process, is predicated on a thorough understanding of techniques. The overarching goal of this selection process is to maximize the representativeness of the sample with respect to the sampling frame and ultimately the population that is represented by the sampling frame. This ostensibly simple goal is illustrated in Figure 6.1.

The extent to which the sample, denoted by the small circle shown in Figure 6.1, mirrors the exact composition of the population, depicted by the larger circle, will increase the degree of representativeness. Stated differently, the sample must be a mirror image (only smaller) of the

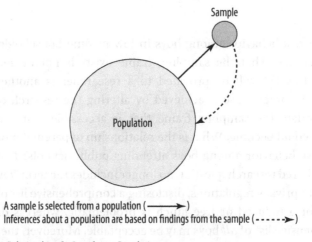

A sample is selected from a population (———▶)
Inferences about a population are based on findings from the sample (- - - - -▶)

Figure 6.1   The Relationship of a Sample to a Population

population. Because gauging the representativeness (namely, is it truly a mirror image?) of the sample relies on determining the extent to which the sample mirrors the population, an important consideration is, how do you determine the exact composition of the population? It must be stated that it is not possible to know with certainty the infinite parameters of any given population. The best we can do in science is to use rigorous sampling techniques that enhance the likelihood that the sample represents the population. Learning of each of these techniques is requisite to success as a researcher.

The lack of correspondence between the sample and the population *not* attributed to chance represents the **sampling bias** (the difference between the sample and the population that is missed by imperfect sampling) in a research study. Because the element of chance cannot be controlled, it is critically important to eliminate other factors that may introduce sampling bias. As with other forms of bias in research, sampling bias may yield inaccurate results that are not generalizable. Choosing the most rigorous and appropriate sampling technique will ensure that sampling bias is reduced to as close to "zero" as possible. Reducing sampling bias enables researchers to *extrapolate* the findings to the population. **Extrapolation** (the process of using a sample to make inferences about an entire population) implies making an inference based on the quality of the sampling technique. These inferences are an accepted and expected product of the research process. Indeed, health promotion research is very much about achieving large-scale change, and it is therefore necessary to think far beyond the relatively small numbers of people who make up the sample.

sampling bias
the difference between the sample and the population that is missed by imperfect sampling

extrapolation
the process of using a sample to make inferences about an entire population

Common Probability Sampling Techniques

In the behavioral and social sciences, probability sampling techniques represent the most rigorous category of sampling because they employ a *random selection* technique (a technique that ensures that each element has an equal probability of being selected), which greatly reduces the probability of sampling bias. **Random selection** (allowing chance to operate in the selection of units from a sampling frame) is the key procedure to

random selection
allowing chance to operate in the selection of units from a sampling frame

minimizing sample bias and therefore enhancing generalizability of the findings. A word of caution: random selection should not be confused with random assignment! (See Chapter Ten for a description of random assignment.) The following section describes the different types of probability sampling techniques.

Simple Random Sampling

The guiding principle behind this technique is that each element must have an equal and nonzero chance of being selected (see Figure 6.2). This can be achieved by applying a table of random numbers to a numbered sampling frame. An approach that could be used for a small sample involves drawing numbers from a container. The product of this technique is a sample determined entirely by chance. It should be noted, however, that chance is "lumpy" (Abelson, 1995), meaning that random selection does not always produce a sample representative of the population. Imagine, for example, a sampling frame comprising 10,000 people. Furthermore, consider that race is a critical variable, and that the composition of the sampling frame is as follows: 1,500 are African American; 7,500 are White, and 1,000 are Asian. You are going to select a sample of 500 people from this sampling frame, using a simple random sampling technique. Unfortunately, the simple random selection process may or may not yield a sample that has racial proportions equivalent to the sampling frame. Due to chance, disproportionate numbers of each racial category may be selected. This failure to perfectly mirror the population is especially likely when sample

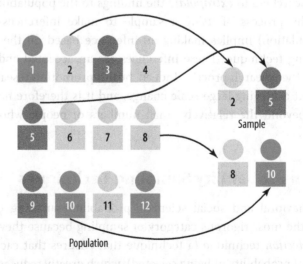

Figure 6.2 Simple Random Sampling Illustration

Source: "Simple Random Sampling Illustration" by Dan Kernler from http://faculty.elgin.edu/dkernler/statistics/ is licensed under CC by BY-NC-SA 1.0.

sizes are small (fewer than 1,000 elements). Although simple random sampling has an intuitive appeal, it is less than ideal for most studies.

Systematic Random Sampling

In contrast to simple random sampling, systematic random sampling does not ensure that every element has an equal and nonzero probability of being selected. The systematic random sampling technique begins with selecting one element at random in the sampling frame as the starting point; however, from this point onward, the rest of the sample is selected systematically by applying a predetermined sampling **interval** (the predefined distance between elements in a sampling frame) (see Figure 6.3). An interval is a defined number of elements that separate the selected elements in a sampling frame. In this sampling technique, after the initial element is selected at random, every "Nth" element will be selected (Nth refers to the size of the interval—such as the twentieth element in the sampling frame), and that element becomes eligible for inclusion in the study. The "Nth" element is selected over and over again until reaching the end of the sampling frame and then from the beginning of the sampling frame until a complete cycle is made back to the starting point (that is, the place where the initial random selection was made). Note that all of the selections become predetermined as soon as the first selection is made. So, for example, if element 29 is the initial selection (and the interval equals 20), elements 30 through 48 have a zero chance of being selected.

interval
the pre-defined distance between elements in a sampling frame

IN A NUTSHELL

As opposed to simple random sampling, systematic random sampling does not ensure that every element has an equal and nonzero probability of being selected.

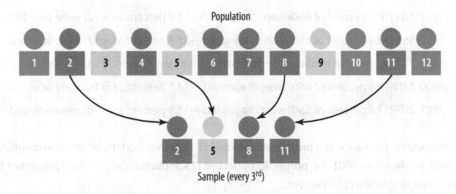

Figure 6.3 Systematic Random Sampling Illustration

One important question is, when is systematic random sampling more appropriate than simple random sampling? The answer involves the term *periodicity*. **Periodicity** refers to the inherent ordering of a particular characteristic within the sampling frame (for example, periodicity exists if the list is ordered by date of birth). Sampling frames that are arranged in any meaningful fashion may possess periodicity. For example, a sampling frame of women receiving abnormal Pap test results may be arranged by date of the test (that is, women with abnormal Pap results in 2007 might be listed first, followed by those having abnormal Pap results in 2008, and so on). This inherent ordering of elements has the potential to greatly enhance the representativeness of the sample. Systematic sampling from this sampling frame of abnormal Pap test results would ensure that each year of diagnosis is proportionately represented in the selected sample. Box 6.1 provides a comparison of simple random sampling and systematic random sampling with respect to this example. Note that because of the periodicity of the sampling frame, in this instance systematic random sampling has an advantage in comparison with simple random sampling.

periodicity
inherent ordering of elements in a sampling frame

BOX 6.1.   A COMPARISON OF TWO TECHNIQUES TO SAMPLE WOMEN WITH ABNORMAL PAP TEST RESULTS IN THE PAST FIVE YEARS

Technique 1 (Simple Random Sampling)

Given a sampling frame of 650 women and a desired sample size of 100, the corresponding quantity of random numbers were drawn. This yielded 12 women diagnosed in 1997, 37 diagnosed in 1998, 7 diagnosed in 1999, 16 diagnosed in 2000, and 28 diagnosed in 2001. The proportions of women selected, by year, in comparison to those diagnosed were as follows:

1997: 105 (16.1 percent of 650) were diagnosed—11.4 percent ($n = 12$) were selected

1998: 155 (23.8 percent of 650) were diagnosed—23.8 percent ($n = 37$) were selected

1999: 73 (11.2 percent of 650) were diagnosed—9.6 percent ($n = 7$) were selected

2000: 110 (16.9 percent of 650) were diagnosed—14.5 percent ($n = 16$) were selected

2001: 207 (31.8 percent of 650) were diagnosed—13.5 percent ($n = 28$) were selected

Comment: By chance, the proportion selected in 1998 matched the proportion diagnosed in 1998. However, in 2001 the proportion selected (13.5) dramatically underrepresented the proportion diagnosed (31.8 percent).

Technique 2 (Systematic Random Sample)

Given a sampling frame of 650 women and a desired sample size of 100, a sampling interval of 6.5 was used. The first woman selected was selected at random (#456). The next woman selected was #462 (rounding down from 6.5 to 6.0) and the next woman was #469 (rounding up from 6.5 to 7.0). The sampling procedure continued until 100 women were selected (which brought the sequence back to the starting point of #456). The proportions of women selected, by year, in comparison to those diagnosed were as follows:

1997: 105 (16.1 percent of 650) were diagnosed—16.0 percent ($n = 16$) were selected

1998: 155 (23.8 percent of 650) were diagnosed—24.0 percent ($n = 24$) were selected

1999: 73 (11.2 percent of 650) were diagnosed—11.0 percent ($n = 11$) were selected

2000: 110 (16.9 percent of 650) were diagnosed—17.0 percent ($n = 17$) were selected

2001: 207 (31.8 percent of 650) were diagnosed—32.0 percent ($n = 32$) were selected

Comment: By design, the proportion selected in each of the five years matched the proportion diagnosed in each corresponding year. The periodicity of the sampling frame was used to ensure proportional representation for women in each of the five diagnostic years.

Stratified Random Sampling

Stratified random sampling begins with the identification of some variable, which may be related indirectly to the research question and could act as a **confounding variable** (a variable that has an undue influence on the analytic outcome of a study—such as geography, age, income, race or ethnicity, or gender—is known as a confounding variable). This variable is then used to divide the sampling frame into mutually exclusive *strata* (also known as subgroups). Once the sampling frame is arranged by strata, the sample is selected from each stratum using random sampling or systematic sampling techniques (see Figure 6.4). This stratification achieves the goal of ensuring that the critical variable of race, for example, is mirrored perfectly between the sample and the population. This means that sample bias for at least one aspect of representativeness (race) is reduced to zero (a very good thing indeed). Imagine, for example, the following research goal: *Identify key nutritional risk factors among adults living in New York State.* Through conversations with people in the State Health Department, you have learned that people in the southeastern part of the state (New York City and surrounding areas) are likely to be quite different from those in the northeastern part of the state and, furthermore, that people in the

confounding variable
a variable that has an undue influence on the analytic outcome of a study

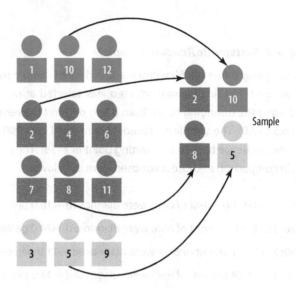

Figure 6.4 Stratified Random Sampling Illustration

Source: "Stratified Random Sampling Illustration" by Dan Kernler from http://faculty.elgin.edu/dkernler/statistics/ is licensed under CC by BY-NC-SA 1.0.

remaining part of the state (central and western New York) will be different from people in the east. Thus a sample that does not fairly represent each of these three regions will have sampling error. This error can be averted by dividing the sampling frame into three strata (southeastern, northeastern, and the remainder of the state). Each stratum then becomes its own independent sampling frame, and a simple random sample or a systematic random sample is taken from each frame. It is important that the sample selected within each stratum reflects proportionately the population proportions; thus, you can employ **proportionate** *stratified sampling* (proportionate sampling means that the number of elements selected is a function of the larger makeup of the sampling frame). In this case, for instance, if 40 percent of the adults reside in the southeastern stratum, then 40 percent of the total sample should be selected from this stratum.

proportionate

as applied to sampling, meaning that the number of elements selected is a function of the larger makeup of the sampling frame

Cluster Sampling

Cluster sampling is a technique used when the research question is about organizational behavior or policy rather than the health behavior or disease status of individuals. As you have learned already in this chapter, this means that sampling elements are units rather than persons. Application of the technique is simple. First, a sampling frame of clusters is developed or obtained. Then a random sample of clusters is selected (simple random

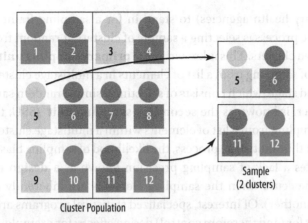

Figure 6.5 Cluster Sampling Illustration

Source: "Cluster Sampling Illustration" by Dan Kernler from http://faculty.elgin.edu/dkernler/statistics/ is licensed under CC by BY-NC-SA 1.0.

sampling or systematic random sampling could be used to achieve this goal). The cluster itself is the intended unit of analysis for the research being conducted (see Figure 6.5). Examples include research goals such as the following:

* To assess the established exercise programs in nursing homes

* To determine whether worksite health promotion programs provide financial incentives to employees for wellness indicators

* To assess the proportion of Nevada counties that treat their municipal water supplies with fluoride

* To identify the presence or absence of counseling protocols designed to promote proper infant hydration practices for women being discharged from maternity wards

In each case, data from individuals would not be appropriate. Instead, the unit of analysis (that is, the source of data) is the cluster. This type of research is especially applicable to health services research and to formulating policy related to health promotion.

Multistage Cluster Sampling

Multistage cluster sampling is used when an appropriate sampling frame does not exist or cannot be obtained. Rather than revert to a nonprobability sampling technique, multistage cluster sampling combines cluster sampling with simple random sampling. First, multistage cluster sampling uses a collection of preexisting units or clusters (such as health districts, counties,

primary sampling unit

the first level of sampling from a list of elements in a multistage cluster sample

secondary sampling unit

the second level of sampling from a list of elements within a multistage cluster sample

design effect

the effect that occurs when the sampling elements are inherently correlated with one another

or voluntary health agencies) to stand in for a sampling frame. The first stage in the process is selecting a sample of clusters at random from the list of all known clusters. This is known as the **primary sampling unit** (PSU, the first level of sampling from a list of elements in a multistage cluster sample). The second stage, which consists of selecting a simple random sample from each cluster, is known as the **secondary sampling unit** (SSU, the second level of sampling from a list of elements within a multistage cluster sample). Because of this multistage process, the likelihood of sampling bias increases. This creates a lack of sampling precision known as a **design effect** (the effect that occurs when the sampling elements are inherently correlated with one another). Of interest, specialized statistical programs are available to account for (and therefore control) design effects; for example, SUDAAN (Shah, Barnwell, and Beiler, 1997).

An inflated design effect (see Henry, 1990, p. 108, for a computational formula) can be avoided by selecting a larger number of clusters or PSUs. Clusters are likely to be homogenous (meaning that people within the clusters are relatively similar to one another, and homogeneity reduces sampling error. Given that sample size is always limited by the researcher's financial or practical constraints, the question at hand is whether to select more clusters or to select more people within a smaller number of clusters. By sampling more clusters (as opposed to more people within clusters), the likelihood of sampling error can be reduced and the design effect can be minimized.

Two relatively common terms must be understood when reading or reporting research that uses a multistage cluster sampling technique. The PSU is the first set of clusters used in the process of obtaining a sample. For example, counties may be the PSU in a study designed to assess the prevalence of farm accidents in the state of Montana. However, a second set of clusters could also be employed. For example, after randomly selecting a group of counties (that is, the PSU) from a list of all rural counties, the research team could then select zip code areas to be the second set of clusters. In this case, zip code areas would be the SSU. The final sampling unit might be Montana farmers; these individuals would be selected at random from the zip code areas. By convention, all steps in the sampling process that follow the PSU are labeled SSUs. Thus the step of randomly selecting farmers from zip code areas would also be an SSU. The final sampling unit becomes the intended unit of analysis. At each stage, selection of sampling units (whether PSU or SSU) is made at random.

Stratified Multistage Cluster Sampling

A simple extension of multistage cluster sampling is stratified multistage cluster sampling. Contrary to its rather complicated-sounding name, this technique is nearly identical to multistage cluster sampling. The only difference is that the clusters may be divided into strata before random selection occurs. As previously noted, stratification reduces sampling error to "zero" for variables that may otherwise introduce sampling bias into a study.

An important note: probability sampling does not need to be overwhelming! To the contrary, the techniques used are simply variants of three basic tools. Box 6.2 illustrates the logic of probability sampling by showing that basic techniques (see step 1) can be applied in numerous ways to create a sample that best fits the needs of the research question.

BOX 6.2. PROBABILITY SAMPLING MADE EASY

Step 1. Consider three basic options:

A. Simple random sampling

B. Systematic sampling

C. Cluster sampling

Use any of these options (*alone*) to meet the needs of your research question.

Step 2 (if needed). For some research questions, you may need to begin by dividing the sampling frame into strata. This creates three possibilities based on the options in step 1:

Stratified random sample = stratification + a

Stratified systematic sample = stratification + b

Stratified multistage cluster sample = stratified c + a or b

Step 3 (if needed). In some cases you may need to *combine* the options listed in step 1:

Multistage cluster sample = c + a or c + b

Common Nonprobability Sampling Techniques

Although the benefits of probability sampling are tremendous, it is nonetheless important to note that whenever the population being studied is narrowly defined or hard to reach, it may be difficult to employ these techniques. The term "narrowly defined" signifies that certain distinguishing parameters are used to delineate a target population, such as those highlighted in the following research objectives:

•   To examine associations of perceived parental monitoring with biologically confirmed tobacco cessation among adolescents with severe mental illness

- To identify factors that may preclude people in high-risk populations (gay men, injection drug users, and low-income African-American men) from accepting an AIDS vaccine when one is approved for use

- To compare HIV-associated sexual health history, risk perceptions, and sexual risk behaviors of unmarried rural and nonrural African-American women

As indicated, the population is narrowly defined in each of the three research goals. Because the existence of sampling frames for each of these three narrowly defined populations is unlikely, using a probability sampling technique is not feasible. In these instances, although a probability technique would be more rigorous, a nonprobability sampling technique may be more realistic.

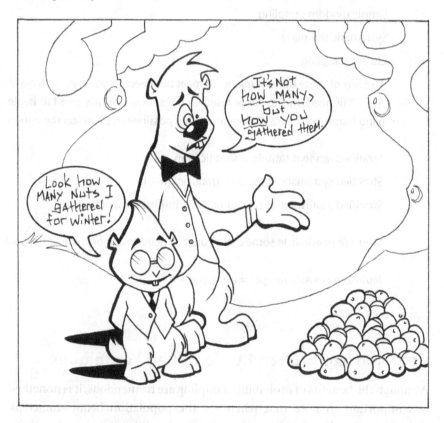

Dincus Worries About Their "Sample" of Nuts for the Winter

Source: Copyright 2005 by Justin Wagner; reprinted with permission.

Convenience Sampling

Convenience sampling, perhaps the most widely used technique in health promotion research, is deemed as such because it provides convenient access to a population by using preexisting groups such as a classroom of students, a support group for people with cancer, people in a waiting room of a public health clinic, people celebrating gay pride at a public event, or employees at a workplace to facilitate recruitment of the sample. People in these groups may be approached and asked to volunteer for the study. Of course, the simplicity of this technique is attractive, but it comes with a high risk of yielding sampling bias because it does not implement any type of systematic procedure to ensure a representative sample. For example, imagine that the research question is, What are the correlates of breastfeeding among women in third-world countries? Using a convenience sample of women recruited from family health clinics, for example, may provide a skewed view of the population in that the women who go to health clinics may have quite different attitudes about breastfeeding from those who do not.

When using a convenience sample, the key issue to consider is how well the preexisting group represents the population. Substantial and identifiable differences between the preexisting group and the population may result in study findings may not adequately represent the population. Box 6.3 provides several examples of this problem. In each example, it is important to note that the conclusion (despite intuitive appeal) is quite broad in scope—reaching far beyond the limitations imposed by a convenience sample.

BOX 6.3. EXAMPLES OF CONVENIENCE SAMPLES WITH "LARGE CONCLUSIONS"

Sample	Conclusion
952 low-income women in San Francisco	The involvement of male partners in decision making about condoms ensures greater protection against HIV infection.
789 adults recruited from a comprehensive service center in a Southeastern city	Clinicians working with adolescents should explore risk taking and prevention measures with their clients.
1,000 adolescents receiving prenatal care at one clinic	The experience of family violence is correlated with rapid repeat pregnancy among U.S. adolescents.
569 men recruited from one university	Prevention-intervention programs in high school and college reduce risk behaviors for chronic disease.

Venue-Based-Time Sampling

As indicated previously, accessing hard-to-reach populations through traditional probability sampling techniques is typically not feasible. Although convenience sampling may be used in some instances, for some populations finding a convenience sample still poses challenges because the population is numerically small, stigmatized, or engages in illegal activity, rendering the formation of a viable preexisting "group" from which to recruit nearly impossible. Commercial sex workers or injection drug users are two populations for which a convenience sample is likely not feasible. An alternative approach for these hard-to-reach populations is called venue-based-time sampling; it can be viewed as a quasi-probability sampling method. Venue-based-time sampling is a two-stage sampling design that allows the researcher to generate a sample with known properties from hard-to-reach populations; it improves on convenience sampling because it interjects systematic procedures so that inferences relating to the venue-visiting population can be made. However, it involves several steps before recruitment can begin; thus it is much more involved than traditional convenience sampling. First, in-depth ethnographic research must be conducted that helps identify a list or "universe" of all potential venues the targeted population might visit. In this context, a venue is not narrowly defined; rather, it is any place where the population might gather. For example, a retail establishment, a street corner, a park, a bar or restaurant, a church, a bath house or sex club, special events (such as a gay pride parade), a formal establishment, or a shooting gallery are all potential venues for certain hard-to-reach populations. Because the goal is to gain access to the population, these venues should be broad in scope and include a range of potential places, so the ethnography must be thorough.

Once a venue universe has been developed, enumeration of specific days and times that will yield the most potential participants must be conducted. Typically, time periods of 4 hours are used (such as 10 P.M. to 2 A.M. or 8 P.M. to 12 A.M.) and should not be limited by Monday through Friday, 9 to 5; rather, the days and times enumerated should correspond to a high volume so that recruitment events will be successful. Enumeration at this point essentially entails counting the number of people who visit the venue and who most likely represent the targeted population during these days and times so that the best days and times for that venue can be determined. Other considerations—such as safety of the research team at the venue; permission from proprietors, if applicable; and whether the venue allows for survey research to be conducted with adequate protection of human subjects—must all be addressed as well. The third step is to create a final sampling frame that represents all potential venue-day-times, from which a random sample is drawn. This is the first stage of the sampling process— a random sample is drawn, which in turn becomes the recruitment calendar for the current month, outlining each venue that will be visited on a specific day and during a specific time. No matter the number of venue-day-times in the sampling frame, the random sample drawn

Sunday	Monday	Tuesday	Wednesday	Thursday	Friday	Saturday
	1	2	3 Power Fitness 1800-2200	4	5	6 Piedmont Park 1400-1800
7	8	9	10	11	12 West End Video 2000-0000	13
14	15	16 Blake's 1800-2200	17	18	19	20
21	22	23	24	25	26	27
28 Gay Pride 1100-1500	29	30	31			

Figure 6.6 Sample Venue-Day-Time Recruitment Calendar

should correspond to the number of recruitment events that need to be scheduled for that month. A sample recruitment calendar is presented in Figure 6.6.

The second stage of this two-stage design involves the actual recruitment at the venue and also involves a systematic approach. Depending on the venue, an imaginary line, area, or swath is predetermined so that only potential participants who cross into the area or the line are approached, screened for eligibility, and, if eligible, asked to participate. During the screening process, it is important to ask if the potential participant has previously participated in the study. This application of systematic selection at the venue reduces the selection bias that occurs from convenience sampling, although those who agree to participate may still differ from those who do not participate. Venue-based-time sampling can be viewed as an improvement over traditional convenience sampling, as it expands the reach to many more venues than one or two and selects the venues for recruitment events at random, thereby reducing some of the sampling bias associated with convenience sampling. Although we acknowledge that some members of the targeted population may not visit any of the venues during the specified days and times or may rarely visit them, it does allow for generalizations to the targeted population of "venue visitors."

Purposive Sampling

Purposive sampling is a technique that is targeted and specifies pre-established criteria for recruiting the sample. The need for purposive sampling is dependent on the research question. For example, consider this research purpose statement: "The purpose of the study is to determine the correlates of condom use among men who test positive for an STD."

This is a research question that necessitates purposive sampling techniques because the research question can be answered only with a sample of men having the characteristic of an STD. However, a purposive sample of these men could be assembled by selectively recruiting men from a public STD clinic and then including only those who tested positive; thus this form of sampling essentially becomes a variant of convenience sampling and is still subject to sampling bias, as there are no systematic procedures in place for recruitment and it excludes those men who may have an STD but who have not visited a public health clinic. A preexisting group may not always be available, however. For example, to select a sample of delinquent youths, we may need to use a classroom as the recruitment venue and then recruit only those youths who meet the criterion for delinquency. Purposive sampling must be used with venue-based time sampling as only those people who visit the venue and who meet the pre-established criteria of belonging to the targeted population can participate.

Quota Sampling

Quota sampling mimics the properties of probability sampling by matching known parameters of the population to the sample. This process, of course, is only possible when one or more of the population parameters are known (such as age, race, gender). This technique entails (1) identifying characteristics of the population to be reflected in the sample, (2) determining the distribution of these characteristics in the population (setting the quotas), and (3) selecting the sample based on those characteristics and their proportion in the population. These characteristics are usually sociodemographic factors. Quota sampling can be useful if (1) the researcher determines that demographic factors such as age, gender, and race or ethnicity are critical components of representativeness, and (2) the demographic profile of the population is known. By characterizing the population and matching the sample to these characteristics, researchers can reduce sample bias.

Studies that designate college students as the target population are a good example of an opportunity to apply this technique. Suppose the research question is to identify determinants of binge drinking among undergraduates attending UCLA. Beginning with records from the registrar's office, a researcher could identify the distribution of demographics among the undergraduate population (that is, gender and race or ethnicity). Using these proportions, a matrix can be developed and would contain cells that represent the intersection between gender and race or ethnicity. One cell in the matrix is needed for each possible combination. For example, "Hispanic females" would be one cell. The quota of UCLA undergraduates, then, who are female and Hispanic would be determined based on sample size and the proportion of these characteristics in the undergraduate population (see Box 6.4). The reason for this extensive work is to have a guide for a variant of purposive sampling. The sample will be assembled to match the proportions shown in the matrix that was built from the records obtained in the registrar's office.

BOX 6.4. EXAMPLE OF A MATRIX FOR QUOTA SAMPLING

	Female	Male
African American/ Black	10.0 percent of enrolled students	9.0 percent of enrolled students
Asian	3.5 percent of enrolled students	1.5 percent of enrolled students
Hispanic	8.3 percent of enrolled students	6.2 percent of enrolled students
White	25.7 percent of enrolled students	35.8 percent of enrolled students

The primary problem with this technique is that the research question may or may not be one that lends itself to the assumption that demographic equivalence alone is sufficient to ensure representativeness. Perhaps, for example, binge drinking is a function of sorority and fraternity membership rather than age, gender, or race or ethnicity. In that case, representativeness is best achieved by selecting a sample that mirrors the population with respect to sorority and fraternity membership. Unfortunately, the idea that binge drinking is a function of sorority and fraternity membership may not materialize before the study is conducted; thus the researcher will not know what information should be used to build the selection matrix.

Chain Referral or Snowball Sampling

Just as quota sampling is a specific application of purposive sampling, chain referral or snowball sampling is also a specific application of purposive sampling. Snowball sampling is most useful in identifying and recruiting hard-to-reach populations (such as injection drug users or runaway teens). The basic technique is to begin with a **seed** (the seed is the initial element nonrandomly selected from a population) (a person who qualifies to be in the study and is the start of the chain and helps the chain to grow, thus allowing the sample to grow like a rolling snowball) and perform the interview (or administer any other part of a research protocol). The researcher asks the participant to identify others who meet the eligibility criteria and would possibly like to participate in the study (direct facilitation), or the researchers ask participants to contact others who meet the eligibility criteria so that they can refer them to the researcher (indirect facilitation).

seed
the initial element nonrandomly selected from a population

This form of sampling is effective in accessing hard-to-reach populations and their networks; however, the generated sample is biased because most people recruit those whom they resemble in race, ethnicity, education, income, and religion. This "birds of a feather flock together" phenomenon is referred to as the degree of **homophily** (representing a high degree of similarity between elements in a sample) and introduces a form of selection bias into the sample. Homophily means that members of the sample share common characteristics and may be linked in social networks (two forms of bias in a study sample). Also, unusually well-connected individuals can pose another kind of problem, as they are part of large networks and therefore tend to be oversampled because many recruitment paths lead to them, introducing selection bias. Although snowball sampling provides better access to hard-to-reach populations than traditional convenience sampling or probability sampling, it is still afflicted by biases of unknown size and unknown direction. Thus inferences to the targeted population should not be made based on data from a snowball sample.

homophily
representing a high degree of similarity between elements in a sample

Respondent-Driven Sampling

Respondent-driven sampling (RDS) is a sampling method that combines the network-based methods of snowball sampling with the statistical validity of standard probability sampling methods. Procedures for implementing RDS are similar to snowball sampling, but additional steps must be taken to ensure the RDS process is implemented correctly. First, as is the case in the starting of a snowball sample, seeds or "initial respondents" are identified and recruited to participate. Once they complete the interview or survey, respondents are asked to directly recruit their peers by distributing coupons. Respondents are instructed to give out their coupons only to peers, meaning only to someone they know or are acquainted with and who is a member of the targeted population. Respondents who come into the study must have a coupon; they are then screened for eligibility and asked if they would like to participate. Once they agree and complete the interview or survey, the peer recruitment cycle continues until the desired sample size is reached. Similar to traditional snowball sampling, RDS has the potential to reach members of a hidden population in about six waves. Figure 6.7 shows recruitment chains stemming from ten seeds as part of an HIV-related study in rural Uganda (McCreesh et al., 2012). Seeds are shown at the top of each recruitment network. Symbol area is proportional to network size. HIV serostatus is shown by shading: Black indicates HIV positive; White, HIV negative; grey, HIV status unknown. HIV status was omitted for seeds for confidentiality.

When implementing RDS, it is extremely important that the coupons are numbered to keep track of who recruited whom so that the recruitment

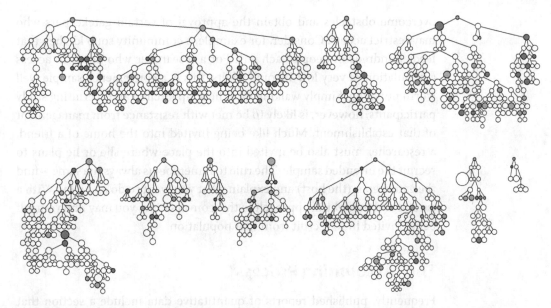

Figure 6.7 Recruitment Networks Showing HIV Infection Status, by Seed
Source: McCreesh et al. (2012).

chains can be analyzed for homophily and other biases. The researchers must collect and record both the serial numbers of the coupons with which the respondents were recruited and the serial numbers of the coupons assigned to each respondent. Also, as part of the research protocol, respondents must be assessed on their numbers of social contacts so each respondent's network size can be estimated. Using the respondent-driven sampling analysis tool (RDSAT) (Respondent-Driven Sampling Analysis Tool, Version 7.1, Ithaca, NY: Cornell University) a mathematical model of the recruitment process can be developed and used to generate weights to compensate for nonrandom recruitment patterns. Through the application of sophisticated statistical modeling techniques, RDS has been shown to produce samples that are unbiased when of meaningful size and allows researchers to control for any effects of differences in network size among respondents. RDS therefore improves on traditional snowball sampling to produce a more representative sample of hard-to-reach populations where inferences to the targeted population can be made and are appropriate once biases are assessed and controlled.

Access Issues

Gaining access to a population is the primary starting point for health promotion research. Irrespective of the sampling technique employed, gaining access to the population may be a challenge; it requires a plan to overcome obstacles and obtain the approval of certain gatekeepers who may restrict access. Consider, for example, a community soup kitchen that feeds hundreds of people each day. For a researcher who needs to access a population of very low-income adults, this is a convenience sample well worth pursuing. Simply walking into the soup kitchen and recruiting study participants, however, is likely to be met with resistance from management of that establishment. Much like being invited into the home of a friend, a researcher must also be invited into the place where she or he plans to recruit the intended sample. The rule to remember is always the same—find the gatekeeper (the host) and explain what you want to do and why. With a careful and thoughtful approach to this conversation, you may find yourself being invited in to recruit from that population.

The "Accounting Process"

Frequently, published reports of quantitative data include a section that systematically accounts for the possibility of sampling bias. For nonprobability samples, such text usually begins by noting how many people were screened for eligibility and how many were found to be eligible. This first step is far less critical than the second step, which involves listing the reasons why eligible people chose not to participate and (possibly) comparing those who refused with those who agreed with respect to key demographic variables such as age, race, and gender. Most important, a participation rate is provided. Low participation rates suggest the possibility that *participation bias* may have occurred; higher rates minimize the possibility of participation bias. Participation bias is introduced into a sample when there may be differences between those who are eligible and participate and those who are eligible and refuse. The probability of participation bias is inversely related to the participation rate. An example of this accounting process follows and is depicted graphically in Figure 6.8.

A convenience sample of adolescent males was selected. The sample was intended to represent a broad cross-section of adolescents residing in low-income neighborhoods of Little Rock, Arkansas. Recruitment sites comprised three adolescent medicine clinics, two health department clinics, and health classes at seventeen high schools. From December 1996 through April 1999, project recruiters screened 1,300 adolescent males to assess their eligibility for participating in the study. Adolescents were eligible to participate if they were male, 14 to 18 years old, unmarried, and reported using alcohol at least once in the previous six months. Of those screened, 515 adolescents were not eligible to participate in the study—the majority (95 percent) did not meet the criterion of alcohol use, and 5 percent did not meet the age criterion. Of the 785 eligible adolescents, 90

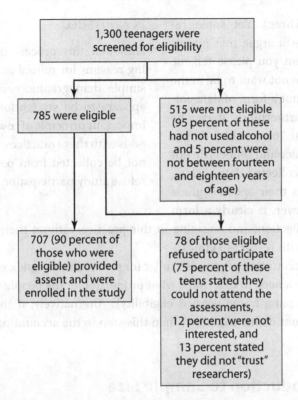

Figure 6.8 An Example of a Figure Used to Represent Recruitment Success

percent ($n = 707$) agreed to participate and subsequently provided their assent. Of the teens who refused participation, the majority (75 percent) stated that their employment schedules would preclude them from making the time commitment (three consecutive Saturdays) for the study. Other reasons cited included lack of interest (12 percent) and a distrust of researchers (13 percent). Differences between those who refused and those who accepted participation were not found with respect to being a racial or ethnic minority ($P =.92$), age ($P =.53$), or level of education ($P = .81$).

Several points from the preceding paragraph warrant explanation. First, the participation rate of 90 percent is high and strongly suggests that participation bias is unlikely. Nonetheless, a reader who continues to suspect participation bias can be assured that refusal was mostly a function of Saturday work commitments. Three demographic comparisons between participants and "refusers" provided further assurance that participation bias was minimal. Although this process of collecting reasons for refusal and making simple demographic comparisons appears to be straightforward, an important principle of research is at odds with these practices: data cannot be collected from people who refuse study participation (see

Chapter Three). Yet some researchers will argue that merely asking, "Can you please tell me why you do not want to be in the study?" is not a form of data collection. Furthermore, it can be argued that "observable" demographics (race and gender) do not qualify as collected data. Asking adolescents their age and grade level, however, is clearly a form of data collection, and engaging in this practice without their assent is a gray area with respect to ethics.

IN A NUTSHELL

Although this process of collecting reasons for refusal and making simple demographic comparisons appears to be straightforward, an important principle of research is at odds with these practices: data cannot be collected from people who refuse study participation.

This accounting process is similar for probability samples, except there may not be a need to determine what proportion of the people was eligible (if the sampling frame defined eligibility). Alternatively, if the sampling frame did not define eligibility, then this step in the accounting process is essential.

An Introduction to Sample Size

As an introduction to the principles that guide sample size determinations, consider the following scenario. A study of 1,000 teens was conducted, and the findings support the hypothesis that teens belonging to gangs will report a higher frequency of marijuana use in the past 30 days. The hypothesis was tested by performing a t-test and had a corresponding t-value of 7.5, which was significant at $P < .01$. Another study was conducted to test the same hypothesis. In this study, the sample size consisted of only 100 teens; however, the statistical findings were nearly identical ($t = 7.4$; $P < .01$). Knowing nothing else about the samples, it is possible to determine which study had the bigger difference between means. This process does not involve mathematics or the use of computers. Instead, it comes down to a simple observation: the large effect ($t = 7.4$) was obtained despite a very low sample size in the second study; thus the effect size (that is, the difference between means for those belonging and not belonging to gangs) had to be far larger in the second study compared to the first.

Without exception, sample size and effect size are interrelated elements of any quantitative study. In the example provided, effect size can be conceptualized as "distance between group means." In the study of 1,000 participants, teens who belonged to gangs smoked marijuana 3.7 days out of the 30 days, on average, and teens who were not in gangs smoked marijuana 1.5 days on average. In contrast, in the study of 100 participants, the effect

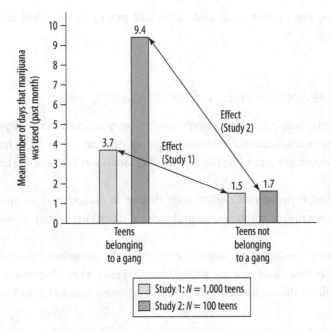

Figure 6.9 Effect Size in Two Similar Studies

size was much greater. The teens who belonged to gangs smoked 9.4 days on average compared with teens not in gangs, who smoked 1.7 days on average. Figure 6.9 provides an illustration of effect size relative to this example. In this figure, effect size is portrayed as a slope. A lack of slope (a flat horizontal line) would represent a complete lack of effect. Conversely, an increasing slope represents an increasingly greater effect size. Note that the slope in the study of a 1,000 teens is quite gentle in contrast to the rather dramatic slope in the study of 100 teens.

An important (and often ignored) point is that effect size is invariant to sample size. Sample size influences the level of statistical significance only (that is, P-value). All things being equal, as sample size increases, significance is more likely to be achieved. (See Box 6.5 for an illustration of this principle.) A larger sample size (along with several other determinants) gives a study an extra boost to find significance for modest to small effect sizes. Conversely, this boost is lacking with small samples (such as $N = 100$); thus only large effect sizes can be detected with small samples. This point leads to a critical principle of sampling: plan for a sample size that is adequate to detect (with statistical significance) the anticipated effect size. A more thorough treatment

IN A NUTSHELL

Plan for a sample size that is adequate to detect (with statistical significance) the anticipated effect size.

of sample size, effect size, and statistical power is provided in Chapter Fourteen.

BOX 6.5. AS SAMPLE SIZE GOES UP, SIGNIFICANCE IS EASIER TO "FIND"

This principle is shown by an example. Consider an experimental program, delivered to high-risk men, that was designed to promote annual cholesterol testing. An index of intent to have a cholesterol test annually was constructed. The highest possible rating was 10.0 and the lowest was 0.0.

Using a pretest-posttest experimental design, with 15 men in each of two groups, the researchers obtained posttest means as follows: Control mean was 6.0; intervention mean was 6.9.

A significance test was conducted to determine whether the observed means were different beyond differences that could be expected by sampling error alone. The researchers used a two-tailed t-test and set their alpha at .05. The P-value achieved was .094; thus the null hypothesis was retained.

One member of the research team had a hard time accepting the finding (this person could not get over the idea that the intervention did not "change" men with respect to the measure of intent). Hence, this person suggested that the sample size "should be doubled and another study should be conducted." After the study was repeated with 30 men assigned to each of the two conditions, the same t-test was conducted (this time N = 60, rather than N = 30). This time the mean in the control group was 6.0 and the mean in the intervention group was 6.9 (exactly the same means that had been found in the study of only 30 men!). However, the obtained P-value in the test of 60 men was .001. The previously disgruntled researcher was now quite satisfied and proceeded to publish the findings.

Summary

Sampling can make or break a research study. The pinnacle of success in sampling is perfect representativeness. Unfortunately, this pinnacle is rarely achieved. The barriers that preclude full achievement are often inevitable. One important example of a barrier is the necessary compromise that must occur to protect the rights of people to refuse study participation. Another important example is extremely practical: researchers are not always granted access to a potential sample of people or organizations, and they may be denied access to useful sampling frames. Once access is

IN A NUTSHELL

The pinnacle of success in sampling is perfect representativeness.

achieved, sampling techniques should be chosen to parsimoniously address the research question and fairly represent the selected priority population. Sampling can select elements comprising "people" or representing organized units (clusters). The selection of people versus clusters is dictated by the nature of the research question. Creative use of these techniques is not only acceptable but also encouraged—as none of the techniques has perfect utility for all research questions.

KEY TERMS

Confounding variable	Primary sampling unit
Design effect	Proportionate
Element	Random selection
Extrapolation	Sampling bias
Homophily	Sampling frame
Interval	Secondary sampling unit
Periodicity	Seed
Population	

For Practice and Discussion

1. Find a journal article that reports an original research study using *nonprobability* sampling. Read this carefully and then answer the following four questions:
   a. What technique was used?
   b. Describe one other technique that could have been used. Explain why.
   c. Was the technique used by the researchers applied correctly? Explain how it was or was not applied correctly.
   d. How well do you think the sample represented the population? Please elaborate.
2. Find a journal article that reports an original research study using *probability* sampling. Read this carefully and then answer the following four questions:
   a. What technique was used?
   b. Describe one other technique that could have been used. Explain why.
   c. Was the technique used by the researchers applied correctly? Explain how this was or was not done.

   d. How well do you think the sample represented the population? Please elaborate.

3. For each of the following three research questions, select the best sampling technique. Be prepared to defend your answers to others.

   a. To determine what portion of African-American, White, and Hispanic adolescents in the United States have a body mass index that is considered to constitute obesity.

   b. To test the hypothesis that women experiencing frequent depression are less likely to be screened for breast and cervical cancer compared to their counterparts not experiencing frequent depression.

   c. To determine the influence of gender, age, and race on exercise behaviors of employees of a community hospital. Note: employees include staff as well as professional positions. Also, the hospital is not willing to provide their list to you.

4. Decision trees are common tools used in planning (if you have never used one, please look up examples on the Internet). Create a decision tree that will unify all of the sampling techniques described in this chapter. Be sure that you annotate this tree to facilitate its use.

References

Abelson, R. P. (1995). *Statistics as principled argument*. Mahwah, NJ: Erlbaum.

Henry, G. T. (1990). *Practical sampling*. Thousand Oaks, CA: Sage.

McCreesh, N., Frost, S., Seeley, S., Katongole, S., Ndagire, T., Tarsh, N., . . . and White, R. G. (2012). Evaluation of respondent-driven sampling. *Epidemiology*, 23(1): 138–147.

Shah, B. V., Barnwell, B. G., and Beiler, G. S. (1997). *SUDAAN: User's manual, release 7.5*. Research Triangle Park, NC: Research Triangle Institute.

CHAPTER 7

MEASUREMENT IN HEALTH PROMOTION

Richard A. Crosby
Laura F. Salazar
Richard R. Clayton
Ralph J. DiClemente

Measurement is an art and a science. However, when too much "artistic license" is taken with regard to measurement, an entire study may suffer. Thus understanding the basic principles of measurement is an obligation for health promotion practitioners and researchers. These principles span a range from metric identification through question-framing and involve a host of considerations that will guide you as you take your research journey.

Measurement is everywhere. It is woven in, on, over, around, and through everything we do. As soon as a baby is born the medical personnel determine "vital statistics"— the height, weight, and Apgar score for the newborn—and record the month, day, year, and time of birth. The time lapsed since birth is used to determine when visits to the pediatrician are scheduled and when certain immunizations are administered. At each postnatal visit, medical staff determine and record the baby's weight and height in order to measure change, and they may take the baby's temperature, measured in degrees. Throughout an individual's life, his or her birthday is celebrated and also used to mark important developmental transitions such as reaching the legal age to drive, to vote, and to drink. Over time, although the specific measures taken may change somewhat, virtually everything in an individual's life is measured. For example, when individuals enter school their attendance or absence is recorded in a student record database, as are their test and achievement scores.

LEARNING OBJECTIVES

- Understand the four metrics of measurement.
- Distinguish a scale from an index.
- Describe and apply methods for judging reliability and validity of scales.
- Identify a hierarchy of preferred measurement techniques.
- Become skilled in wording and framing questions and using methods that reduce bias.
- Distinguish mediating variables from moderating variables.

Each of the measures taken and recorded has a metric. Metrics are standards used to measure tangible (such as weight and, height) and intangible (such as intelligence) phenomena. For example, temperature is measured in degrees Fahrenheit or Celsius, weight is measured in pounds or grams and kilograms, test scores are measured in actual numbers (as in SAT and GRE scores) or in percentiles, and intelligence is measured by a validated IQ test. As you may already know, some metrics are more sophisticated than others. Metrics vary, ranging from what is deemed a nominal scale to an ordinal to an interval and to a ratio scale.

IN A NUTSHELL

Measurement is central to furthering our understanding of health promotion research.

Measurement should be viewed as an essential element of health promotion strategies, campaigns, and programs. Measurement is central to furthering our understanding of health promotion research. Without adequate, reliable, and valid measurement, we cannot know for certain what to target with a health promotion intervention or whether our health promotion efforts are effective. In this chapter, the emphasis is on who and what is measured in public health; when, how, and where the measurements occur; and, most important, why public health phenomena are measured.

Metrics

Perhaps one of the most fundamental aspects of measurement is determining the metric used for variables. A variable is a single measure that, by definition, can take on more than one value. If only one value is possible, then the measure cannot vary and therefore must be a constant. We typically make distinctions among four metrics that can be used to categorize or quantify variables.

nominal

data based on categories that cannot be placed into an order based on preference or any other criteria

Nominal (nominal data are based on categories that cannot be placed into an order based on preference or any other criteria) data are especially common in health promotion research; these refer to phenomena that vary in kind. A nominal metric is used to categorize or group phenomena according to some *attribute*. These attributes constitute mutually exclusive and exhaustive response categories for a variable and by nature are qualitative versus quantitative. For example, before you were born, your mother went through carefully and strategically scheduled measurements. One of those measures determined whether she was pregnant. The answer to the pregnancy test had only two categories—yes or no. One is either pregnant or not pregnant. Similarly, a nominal metric does not include a

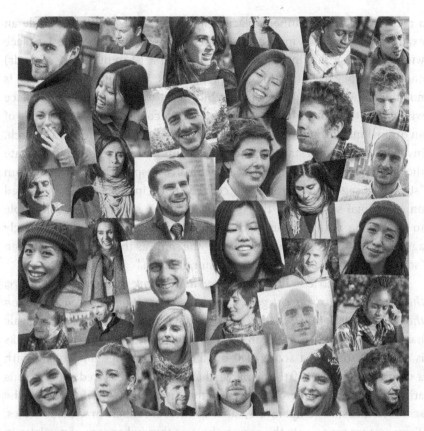

Figure 7.1 People of Various Races and Ethnicities

"more or less" dimension. Something that is measured as "yes or no," "zero or one," or "present or not present" is considered a dichotomy, a specific form of a nominal scale. But, of course, nominal measures may also extend beyond a dichotomy. Race or ethnicity, for example, is a nominal variable that may have many different attributes (see Figure 7.1) and just as many different categories for measuring race or ethnicity. Sex (male or female) and religion are also nominal attributes. It is worth noting that nominal attributes cannot be ranked in any fashion.

The next metric is **ordinal** (ordinal data are based on categories that can be placed into an order of preference). As your mother endured labor, the physician, nurse, and perhaps your father or some other family member might have asked your mother to tell them how bad the labor pains were—say on a scale from low to medium to high. This is called an ordinal level of measurement. It is characterized by transitivity, in which it is clear that high is more than medium which is more than low. Thus the attributes are ranked along a continuum. However, it is worth noting that the distance between ranks is *not* known to be equal. Consider, for example,

ordinal
data based on categories that can be placed into an order of preference

a race in which the runners' placements of 1st, 2nd, and 3rd provide an example of an ordinal metric—the difference in time it took the 1st place winner to cross the line (for example, 2 hours: 12 minutes: 54 seconds) and the 2nd place winner (for example, 2 hours: 12 minutes: 56 seconds) is not the same as that between the 2nd place winner and the 3rd place winner (for example, 2 hours: 13 minutes: 10 seconds). Another example of an ordinal metric, and one used more often in health promotion research, involves presenting a statement to participants and asking them to indicate their level of agreement on a scale with five responses that range from "strongly disagree" to "strongly agree." The participants are thus measured on an ordinal scale. From this example, you can see that it is impossible to determine with certainty whether the difference between "strongly agree" and "somewhat agree" is exactly the same as the difference between "somewhat agree" and "neither agree nor disagree."

interval

data that are continuous; they are not based on categories, and the separation between points on the continuum is always equal

The next metric is **interval** *(interval data are continuous in nature; they are not based on categories, and the separation between points on the continuum is always equal).* Like ordinal measures, an interval scale has transitivity; however, in an interval scale, the distance between ranks is equal. Moreover, a score of 0 on the measure does not equate with a complete absence of the variable that is being measured; rather, it is arbitrary. One example of a measure that uses this type of metric is the scales to measure temperature, such as the Fahrenheit or Celsius scales. Temperature represents the average heat or thermal energy of particles in matter or radiation. One degree Fahrenheit represents precisely 1/180th of the interval between the freezing point (32 degrees) and the boiling point (212 degrees). Thus intervals or distances between degrees are precisely equal, but zero degrees does not reflect a true absence of temperature (heat) for these scales, although it may feel that way for some people. Alternatively, the Kelvin scale, another scale for measuring temperature, does have an absolute zero.

In terms of health promotion research and practice, true interval measures are rare, as many of the constructs are intangible and we cannot determine anything more than the rank ordering of the data. It would be virtually impossible to know with certainty that the difference in the numbers assigned to each of the levels of a construct, such as attitudes toward exercising, reflect the true difference between any two levels. It is important to note that you may see examples of "interval" measurements in health promotion research and practice. Many researchers apply equal intervals to the various levels mainly for statistical analysis purposes; however, in reality these measurements should be classified as ordinal.

ratio

one step better than interval data because they also have a true zero point, a feature not described by interval data

The final metric is **ratio** (ratio data are one step better than interval data because they also have a true zero point, a feature not described by interval data). As your mother went through labor, the physician, nurse, or midwife used what is called a ratio scale of measurement—the number of centimeters that her cervix had dilated so that you could be born. A ratio scale has not only transitivity and equal distance between ranks but also an absolute zero point. Common measures in health promotion, such as "knowledge of heart disease prevention practices," are measured on a ratio metric. Other examples include number of cigarettes smoked per day, number of steps taken in a day, or the number of servings of fruits and vegetables consumed. The advantage of having a measure that is a ratio scale of measurement is that it allows for statements about proportions. In other words, 30 cigarettes smoked per day as compared to 10 cigarettes smoked per day represents a ratio of 3:1. You cannot make these ratio-type statements with the other three types of metrics.

Figure 7.2 provides a graphic depiction of these four levels of measurement. A triangle, circle, and a diamond depict the nominal level. These shapes are distinct—and they cannot be ordered in any meaningful fashion. The ordinal level is shown by taking only one category from the nominal level (a circle) and then ordering these by size (from smallest to largest). As is the case in measurement theory, there is no direct connection between nominal and ordinal measures (nonparametric measures) and the interval and ratio measures (the parametric measures). Numbers therefore depict interval and ratio measures. Note that the interval depiction shows equal

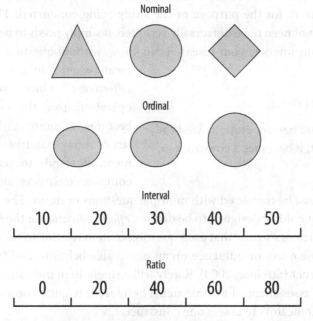

Figure 7.2 A Graphic Depiction of the Four Levels of Measurement

distance between numbers, but no zero point, whereas the ratio includes both (equal distance plus a zero point).

Measuring Constructs

Measuring physical properties such as weight, height, and age is a relatively straightforward process. In essence, it is easy to measure things that are tangible. If all measurement in health promotion research were this easy, then this chapter would be extremely short. Because health promotion research is intertwined with health behaviors and their underlying psychological and psychosocial influences, research questions are frequently centered on intangibles such as self-esteem, depression, self-efficacy, attitudes, perceptions, and beliefs. Although weight exists as a physical entity, self-esteem does not. Indeed, a concept such as self-esteem is not directly observable or measurable, but rather is hypothetical and may be linked to a particular theoretical orientation. For example, scholars theorize that people develop a sense of their own value and that this overall evaluation of their worth or value is influential in shaping some behaviors. Thus self-esteem can be viewed as a concept versus an object. The question becomes, how do we measure something that is not tangible? The answer begins with the brief schematic shown in Figure 7.3.

Because the epistemology of scientific inquiry is built on objectivity, the first step in measuring a *concept* such as self-esteem is to create a formalized definition. In a sense, this *operational definition* will become *the* definition of self-esteem for the purpose of the study being conducted. The definition does not need to be universally accepted; it simply needs to be provided so that consumers of your research can know, without question, what you mean when you use the term *self-esteem*. Once you have operationalized the concept, it becomes a *construct*. The construct now requires measurement. It stands to reason that complex constructs such as self-esteem must be measured with multiple questions or items. The questions or items should be designed to be distinct *effect indicators* of the construct. Effect indicators signify that each question or item relating to the construct infers some effect or influence on an observable behavior and "taps into" the construct (Streiner, 2003). Rarely will a single-item indicator provide a complete assessment of a construct. Therefore it is quite common to use multiple indicators to assess one construct.

IN A NUTSHELL

Once you have operationalized the concept, it becomes a construct.

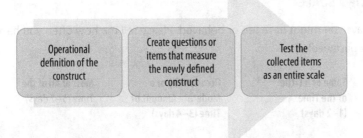

Figure 7.3   Linear Flow Chart of Operational Definition

Self-esteem represents a unitary construct that can be measured by using multiple effect indicators. In this instance, the measure of self-esteem would be called a *scale*—specifically, a measure composed of "theoretically correlated items" (Streiner, 2003, p. 217) measuring the same construct. Examples of scales include the Rosenberg Self-Esteem Scale (Rosenberg, 1989) and the Beck Depression Inventory (Beck, Ward, Mendelson, Mock, and Erbaugh, 1961). Each of these scales has multiple effect indicators that theoretically relate to how self-esteem and depression manifest. For example, one item from the Rosenberg Scale is "I am able to do things as well as most other people."

Although you may encounter instances when other terms are used interchangeably in the literature or in other texts to describe a collection of items or questions, such as scale, test, questionnaire, index, or inventory, it is important to note that in research there are specific distinctions between a scale and an *index*. These two terms should not be used interchangeably, as they mean different things. An index refers to a measure in which the items are considered *causal indicators* because they themselves define the construct and influence the value of the construct (Streiner, 2003). The items in an index typically are heterogeneous and may not necessarily be correlated with each other. The Apgar score, mentioned previously in this chapter, specifically rates newborns on several characteristics—heart rate, respiration, muscle tone, reflex response, and skin color—and is an excellent example of an index. In health promotion research, other examples of indexes are quality-of-life questionnaires, tests that assess levels of physical functionality, and knowledge tests. To illustrate these distinctions, an example of a scale is shown in Box 7.1 and an example of an index is shown in Box 7.2.

BOX 7.1. EXAMPLE OF A SCALE

Below is a list of the ways you might have felt or behaved. Please tell me how often you have felt this way during the past week.

Rarely or None of the Time (< than 1 day)	Some or a Little of the Time (1–2 days)	Occasionally or a Moderate Amount of Time (3–4 days)	Most or All of the Time (5–7 days)

1. I was bothered by things that usually don't bother me.
2. I did not feel like eating; my appetite was poor.
3. I felt that I could not shake off the blues even with help from my family or friends.
4. I felt that I was just as good as other people.
5. I had trouble keeping my mind on what I was doing.
6. I felt depressed.
7. I felt that everything I did was an effort.
8. I felt hopeful about the future.
9. I thought my life had been a failure.
10. I felt fearful.
11. My sleep was restless.
12. I was happy.
13. I talked less than usual.
14. I felt lonely.
15. People were unfriendly.
16. I enjoyed life.
17. I had crying spells.
18. I felt sad.
19. I felt that people dislike me.
20. I could not get "going."

Source: Center for Epidemiologic Studies Depression Scale (CES-D) (Radloff, 1977).

BOX 7.2. EXAMPLE OF AN INDEX

Life-Events Checklist (LEC)

Listed below are a number of difficult or stressful things that sometimes happen to people. For each event, check one or more of the boxes to the right to indicate that: (a) it happened to you personally, (b) you witnessed it happen to someone else, (c) you learned about it happening to someone close to you, (d) you're not sure if it fits, or (e) it doesn't apply to you. Be sure to consider your entire life (growing up as well as adulthood) as you go through the list of events.

Happened to me	Witnessed it	Learned about it	Not sure	Doesn't apply

1. Natural disaster (for example, flood, hurricane, tornado, earthquake)

2. Fire or explosion

3. Transportation accident (for example, car accident, boat accident, train wreck, plane crash)

4. Serious accident at work, home, or during recreational activity

5. Exposure to toxic substance (for example, dangerous chemicals, radiation)

6. Physical assault (for example, being attacked, hit, slapped, kicked, beaten up)

7. Assault with a weapon (for example, being shot, stabbed, threatened with a knife, gun, bomb)

8. Sexual assault (rape, attempted rape, made to perform any type of sexual act through force or threat of harm)

9. Other unwanted or uncomfortable sexual experience

10. Combat or exposure to a war-zone (in the military or as a civilian)

11. Captivity (for example, being kidnapped, abducted, held hostage, prisoner of war)

12. Life-threatening illness or injury

13. Severe human suffering

14. Sudden, violent death (for example, homicide, suicide)

15. Sudden, unexpected death of someone close to you

16. Serious injury, harm, or death you caused to someone else

17. Any other very stressful event or experience

Source: Blake et al. (1995).

Psychometric Properties

Reliability

reliability
the consistency of a measure, directly related to the amount of random error

test-retest reliability
occurs when scores on a measure are consistent over at least two distinct points in time

You can determine the **reliability** of a measure in several ways (reliability refers to the consistency of a measure and is directly related to the amount of random error). First, reliability could be established by administering the index or the scale to a sample at two points in time and looking for a relatively strong correlation in scores for time 1 and time 2. This is known as **test-retest reliability**, which occurs when scores on a measure are consistent over at least two distinct points in time. Notice that the underlying assumption here is that the construct is stable; therefore, a reliable measure should produce the same score at time 2 as it did at time 1 for each person in the sample. Therefore one principle in establishing test-retest reliability is that the construct must *not* be one that undergoes dramatic change over time.

Second, reliability can be established by computing the inter-item correlations between all items constituting the scale. Note that this technique is appropriate for establishing the reliability of a scale because scale items should be tapping into a unitary construct, so they should be intercorrelated. The same is not true for indexes, however. Computing inter-item correlations is not appropriate for establishing the reliability of an index (Streiner, 2003). Calculating the inter-item correlations is called assessing the **internal reliability** of the scale (when the items constituting a measure are correlated with one another, that measure is said to have internal reliability).

internal reliability
the average inter-item correlations for a scale measure

Cronbach's alpha
a statistical measure of internal reliability

We can determine the intercorrelations between items on a scale by employing a statistical procedure that yields the statistic **Cronbach's alpha** (a statistical measure of internal reliability). Cronbach's alpha (α) has a range of 0 to 1, with higher scores representing greater inter-item reliability. Although there are no hard and fast rules, an alpha of .70 or higher is considered sufficient evidence of reliability. It is, however, worth noting that extremely high alphas, such as .95, suggest that there may be redundancy among some of the indicators. In effect, a scale with an alpha close to 1.0 could probably be reduced to fewer indicators. Note that inter-item correlation could be used in conjunction with the test-retest technique. Conversely, it is also noteworthy that the inter-item reliability method can be used in a cross-sectional study, whereas the same cannot be said about the test-retest method because there is only one assessment in a cross-sectional study.

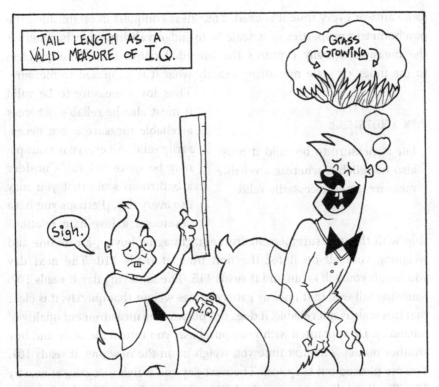

Mincus Reveals a Valid Measure of Chipmunk IQ

Copyright 2005 by Justin Wagner; reprinted with permission.

Third, reliability could be established by using the **split-half method** (a method for assessing reliability in which items from a scale are randomly assigned into sets and then scores from one set are correlated with scores from the other set). Like the inter-item reliability method, this test for reliability could be performed in the context of a cross-sectional study. This analytic procedure begins with dividing the scale into two parallel forms of the measure. For example, an eight-item scale would be randomly divided into two four-item measures. These two shortened forms would then be administered to a sample. The correlation between scores for the two halves is calculated and then used to estimate the reliability of the total measure (Ghiselli, Campbell, and Zedeck, 1981). Similar to inter-item reliability, this method is not appropriate for indexes, as splitting the index into parts would not be meaningful.

> **split-half method**
> a method for assessing reliability in which items from a scale are randomly assigned into sets and then scores from one set are correlated with scores from the other set

Validity

At this juncture you have learned how to judge whether or not a scale is reliable. Again, *reliability* means that a measure consistently provides the same answer every time it is used. Your next conquest in establishing the psychometric properties of a scale is to judge **validity** (that is, whether the measure actually captures the intended construct). Validity refers to the index or scale measuring exactly what it is supposed to measure.

validity

refers to whether the measure actually captures the intended construct

Thus for a measure to be valid it must also be reliable, whereas a reliable measure is not necessarily valid. An everyday example may be quite helpful. Consider a bathroom scale that you may use every day. (Perhaps you have developed a love-hate relationship with this measurement instrument.) Imagine buying a new one and weighing yourself on it for the first time; it reads 110. The next day you weigh yourself again and it reads 115. The following day it reads 107. Knowing full well that nobody gains or loses weight that quickly, it is clear that this scale is not reliable; it does not possess the measurement quality of reliability. Disappointed with your purchase, you return the scale and buy another model. The first time you weigh in on the new one, it reads 101. You are pleased but skeptical. The next day you weigh in, again, at exactly 101. The third day you are again delighted to weigh 101. Clearly, this scale is reliable, but you begin to doubt its validity. Knowing that you have always weighed about 110, and not seeing any obvious signs of weight loss, you finally conclude that the scale is reliable but not valid and return it for a full refund. This vignette provides the basis for the idea that reliability is the first step in a two-step process that must be used to judge the psychometric value of a scale measure. Figure 7.4 provides a visual depiction of this two-step process.

> **IN A NUTSHELL**
>
> For a measure to be valid it must also be reliable, whereas a reliable measure is not necessarily valid.

Like reliability, validity can be established through the application of several different techniques. Two of the most elementary techniques are **face validity** (which implies that the items have been judged by experts as capturing the intended construct) and **content validity** (which implies that experts have concluded that all possible items have been included in the assessment of the construct). Both techniques employ a *jury of experts* (a panel of professionals who possess expertise with respect to the construct or constructs under consideration). Face validity is judged by asking the jury, Does the index or scale appear to measure the construct? Content validity goes a bit further. For scales you would want to ask, Do the items represent the "universe" of all possible indicators relevant for the construct? For indexes, you would want to ask, Do the items represent a census of items underlying the construct? Content validity can be assessed for both scales and indexes, but judgments made regarding the items differ. Scales

face validity

implies that the items have been judged by experts as capturing the intended construct

content validity

implies that experts have concluded that all possible items have been included in the assessment of the construct

Step One: Is it *reliable*? Does it have at least one of these?

- Inter-item reliability coefficient (α) = .70 or greater
- Split-half reliability
- Test-retest reliability

If "No", revise measure.

If "Yes" you may proceed to Step Two.

Step Two: Is it *valid*? Does it have at least one of these?

- Face validity as judged by a jury of experts
- Content validity as judged by a jury of experts
- Construct validity
- Criterion validity

If "Yes," congratulations! You have a psychometrically sound scale.

Figure 7.4 The Two-Step Psychometric Process for Reliability and Validity of Scales and Indexes

assume that there is a universe of potential items from which to draw a sample that represents the unitary construct, whereas items composing an index should be viewed more as a census of items and are dependent on both the underlying theory of the construct and prior research (Streiner, 2003). Nevertheless, for both face and content validity, the support for a measure being valid is a judgment.

A more rigorous method of establishing validity is the use of a test to determine what is known as **construct validity** (when the measure yields a variable that analytically functions in a manner predicted by an underlying theory, construct validity exists). Construct validity refers to the ability of a measure to provide actual findings that are consistent with the underlying theory. For example, to determine construct validity of a measure of attitudes toward the HPV vaccine, you might use the theory of reasoned action. This theory would suggest that attitudes toward the HPV vaccine are related to intentions to be vaccinated. To test this relationship, you could administer your scale, along with a measure of intentions to get the HPV vaccine, to a sample of study participants. Using the data from this study, you would then calculate the correlation between these two measures. If the two measures were positively correlated, then this finding would be strong evidence supporting the convergent validity of your scale that assesses attitudes toward HPV vaccination.

Another method, of even greater rigor, establishes validity by comparing the assessed construct to an actual behavior (such as eating a low-sodium diet, exercising on a regular basis, using contraceptives, receiving the HPV vaccine), or outcome (such as losing weight, increasing aerobic capacity,

construct validity
condition in which the measure yields a variable that analytically functions in a manner predicted by an underlying theory

reducing pregnancy rates, and reducing incidence of cervical cancer). This method is called **criterion validity** (when the measure yields a variable that is analytically associated with its expected outcome, criteria validity exists). The most demanding of the four methods used to judge validity, criterion validity is based on the assumption that the construct should be statistically associated with the expected criterion measure. For example, the theoretical construct of self-efficacy to eat a low-sodium diet would ideally be expected to have a significant relationship with the actual consumption of foods that are sodium free (such as fresh vegetables) or very low in sodium (such as reduced-sodium foods). If the scale assessing this construct were indeed valid, then a statistically significant relationship with sodium intake would provide evidence of criterion validity.

criterion validity
when the measure yields a variable that is analytically associated with its expected outcome

Types of Variables

Unlike people, methods of measurement of variables are not created equal; some methods are inherently superior to others and, in turn, the variables that they measure can be placed in a hierarchy. Although an essential part of and primary means to health promotion research and practice, variables measured by self-report are at the bottom of this hierarchy. Self-reported measures of behaviors, attitudes, beliefs, and other intangible constructs are located at the bottom, due to a host of issues related specifically to self-report measurement, such as social desirability bias, inaccurate recall, and selective recall bias (discussed in greater detail later in this chapter). Next up the hierarchy are variables assessed through direct observation, as this method can, in certain instances, minimize some of the biases associated with self-report (such as weight, height, skill assessment, walkability). Next up are variables assessed through official records (such as medical records, tax records, and data from social service agencies), which are considered quite prestigious in health promotion research because they have less of the biases associated with methods lower in the hierarchy. Finally, at the top is an elite class of variables that are measured by means of biological methods or "biomarkers." These variables have very little bias or error associated with them. This class may be used in health promotion research as outcome variables for health promotion programs and screeners to identify participants for eligibility or perhaps to categorize people into either cases or controls in a prospective study.

In the following sections we describe these methods of measurement and provide examples to illustrate their implementation in health promotion research. As you read this section, please keep in mind what you learned in Chapters Four and Five regarding the roles that variables take in research. For example, outcome variables are the object of prediction in observational research, and dependent variables are the object of interest in experimental research. In observational research, the variables used to predict the outcome measure are either correlates (in a cross-sectional study) or predictors (in all other observational designs). In experimental research, the independent variable is simply assignment to group or condition. These same variables may also take on new roles depending on the context of the research. In some instances, a correlate or predictor variable could be viewed as a **mediating variable**, which "bridges" a predictor variable with an outcome variable via a third measure and helps to explain the association between two other variables. In other instances, it could be viewed as a **moderating variable**, which imposes conditions on the association between a predictor variable and an outcome variable, meaning that depending on the level of this moderator, the association between two other variables can be affected or changed. We will describe these specific attributes in more detail and other issues related to variables and their measurement.

Self-Reported Variables

The majority of measures used in health promotion research use **self-report** (a person's own accounting of her/his beliefs, practices, or intentions) as the method of assessment. Self-report as a data collection method is necessary for many of the variables studied in health promotion research, as we are interested in assessing health-related behaviors, attitudes, beliefs and other intangibles; by definition these variables are not always directly observable (for example, sexual behavior or attitudes toward flu vaccine). Unfortunately, there are several issues related to self-report that can affect the internal validity of the research. For example, self-reported data may be affected by item wording and response format as well as several types of biases such as **social desirability bias** (responding to questions in a way that casts a positive light on the person engaging in the self-report), **inaccurate recall bias** (when people self-report behaviors they may not remember the frequency of these behaviors or even if they have engaged in the behavior at all), and **selective recall bias** (when people self-report behaviors, they may be recalling how often these occurred based on a personally created reality).

To begin, consider item wording and format of the response options. Tobacco use will be used as a case study to illustrate. An example of a question designed to measure lifetime experience with smoking specifies that "ever" smoking includes as little as taking even a puff from a cigarette.

Have you ever tried cigarette smoking, even a puff? (Mark one box.)

☐ Yes

☐ No

mediating variable
variable that "bridges" a predictor variable with an outcome variable via a third measure that better explains the association

moderating variable
variable that imposes conditions on the association between a predictor variable and an outcome variable

self-report
a person's own accounting of her/his beliefs, practices, or intentions

social desirability bias
responding to questions in a way that casts a positive light on the person engaging in the self-report

inaccurate recall bias
when people self-report behaviors they may not remember the frequency of these behaviors or even if they have engaged in the behavior at all

selective recall bias
when people self-report behaviors, they may be recalling how often these occurred based on a personally created reality

There is nothing inherently wrong with this question. One could presume that a "yes" is different from a "no," and that those who have ever smoked may be different from those who have never smoked. However, this is a very gross and imprecise measurement. It tells us nothing about *when* in a person's life they had this experience. Presumably, those who try cigarettes earlier in life rather than later may be different on a number of dimensions: the earlier in life that people try cigarettes, the more likely they are to continue. These are hypotheses that require more precise measurement than *ever* versus *never*. The ever-never dichotomy (nominal variable) does not provide critical information about whether smoking was a transitory behavior or something that continued, increased, and became a chronic behavior pattern. "Yes" or "no" responses to "ever tried smoking?" provide little useful data, certainly not enough information to guide the design or evaluation of a health promotion program.

Recognizing the need to understand how long smoking has occurred, one could ask two questions: one about age at onset of smoking and one about current smoking. In fact, the question about one's first experience with smoking is also a question about ever smoking in one's lifetime. If the person provides an age at onset, it means that he or she has smoked. There is also a subtle difference between the first question and the one that follows. In the "ever-never" question, the investigator is assuming that the person answering the question most likely never smoked. In the following question about the onset of smoking, there is an implicit assumption that the people answering the question have smoked. They are then required to deny the behavior.

How old were you the very first time you smoked even a puff of a cigarette? (Mark one box.)

☐   I have never smoked even a puff of a cigarette

☐   8 years old or younger

☐   9 years old

☐   10 years old

☐   11 years old

☐   12 years old

☐   13 years old

☐   14 years old

☐   15 years old

☐   16 years old

☐   17 years old

☐   18 years old

☐   19 years or older

The second question that will help one develop at least a preliminary picture of the extent of smoking asks about current smoking. In the tobacco field, "current" is defined as the past thirty days or past month.

During the past 30 days, on how many days did you smoke one or more cigarettes? (Mark one box.)

☐   0 days

☐   1 or 2 days

☐   3 to 5 days

☐   6 to 9 days

☐   10 to 19 days

☐   20 to 29 days

☐   All 30 days

This question is more precise than the previous questions. It does provide information about current use of cigarettes. The answers to this question provide an investigator with information about the frequency of use (an ordinal variable). From previous research, we assume that current cigarette use is related to a host of other variables measured at the same time. So, from a health promotion perspective, current cigarette use could be a predictor variable that is associated with some other variable (for example, use of alcohol and other drugs, recent respiratory illnesses, or dependence on nicotine). It could be an outcome variable that is associated with morbidity and mortality.

One of the problems with questionnaire items such as the number of days cigarettes were used is that some people may not organize their memory around the recall period (in this case, the recall period is 30 days), which most likely includes both the current month and the previous month. The calendar month is a much more common organizing framework for memory. However, if the question were about the "past month," what month would we be asking about? If it were March 20, would we be asking about the 19 days of March that have already passed or the entire month of February? Another problem involves the response options regarding the categorization of number of days. Ten to nineteen days, for example, covers a lot of time. One might assume that someone who has actually smoked 10 days (assuming it is possible to remember accurately this number) may be different from someone who has smoked 19 days (assuming again that it is possible to remember accurately this number). Therefore, the preceding question is often coupled with the following question to create a two-question measure of current cigarette use.

On the days that you smoke, how many cigarettes do you typically smoke? (Mark one box.)

☐   I have never smoked even a puff of a cigarette

☐   Less than 1 cigarette per day

☐   1 to 2 cigarettes per day

☐   3 to 7 cigarettes per day

☐   8 to 12 cigarettes per day

☐   13 to 17 cigarettes per day

☐   18 to 23 cigarettes per day

☐   At least 24 cigarettes per day

This is an interesting, but problematic, way to measure current cigarette use. Think about how cigarettes come packaged. A pack contains twenty cigarettes. Notice that none of the categories are easily translated into one-half of a pack or two packs. Regular or heavy smokers may gauge how much they smoke in terms of packs rather than individual cigarettes. Another problem with the question is that it requires the individual answering the question to engage in some mathematical computations. Most of us are not very good at such math. Another major problem with this approach to measuring a simple (but also evidently complex) behavior is the assumption that smokers are consistent from day to day in how much they smoke. This may be true for individuals who have been smoking for some time. For relatively new smokers, however, their pattern from day to day and week to week may be more erratic.

These limitations can be seen most clearly in Figure 7.5. Data in the figure come from an adolescent smoker who was asked the two previous questions—number of days smoked and number of cigarettes per day. She reported that she smoked 20 to 29 days and that she smoked 11 cigarettes a day. She was then asked to keep a daily diary of her smoking patterns.

As shown in Figure 7.5, of the 30 days in the month, the subject smoked for 19 days (30 minus the 11 days that she didn't smoke at all). So, in terms of the categorization, the appropriate answer would have been that she smoked 10 to 19 days, not 10 to 29 days. She smoked on 63 percent of the days in that 30-day period. She did accurately report that she smoked 11 cigarettes a day, but for only 8 of the 30 days in the month. The average number of cigarettes per day was 4.9.

As you can see by now, measurement of a behavior—a behavior with which we are all familiar and, moreover, a behavior that is based on consumption of a discrete commodity (each cigarette in a pack of 20

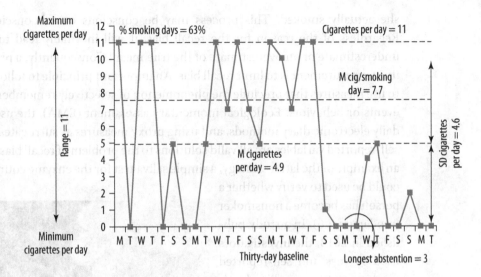

Figure 7.5 A Female Adolescent's Daily Smoking Pattern

cigarettes is not connected to the others in the pack)—is not a simple task. From a public health perspective, these examples should make it clear that our traditional approach to measuring this very important health-related behavior is fraught with limitations.

Of course, measuring a behavior such as tobacco use often requires much more than simply knowing how many cigarettes people have smoked in the past 30 days. Consider, for example, a large-scale tobacco use reduction program (lasting 1 year) that has the ambitious goal of reducing population-level use of cigarettes by 50 percent. Cross-sectional surveys given before and one year after the 1-year program are used to test program efficacy. In both sets of surveys, it is determined that a 12-month recall period is important. This decision is made because the investigator wants to show that effects of the intervention are not fleeting (that is, effects do not wane within a few months after ending the program). The challenge therefore can be summarized as "How can recall bias and inaccurate recall best be avoided?"

Recall bias is introduced into the measurement process when a person wants to remember events in a way that is desirable rather than true. For example, a person who wholeheartedly attempts to break the strong addiction of nicotine dependence may be very likely to remember smoking fewer cigarettes than he or

IN A NUTSHELL

Recall bias is introduced into the measurement process when a person wants to remember events in a way that is desirable rather than true.

she actually smoked. This process may be conscious or subconscious. Regardless of the reason for the recall bias, it will inevitably lead to an underestimate or an overestimate of the true mean. Consequently, a priority in measurement is to limit recall bias. An important principle to follow is to use measures that preclude the phenomenon of selectively remembering events or behaviors. Ecological momentary assessment (EMA), the use of daily electronic diary methods, and using proxy measures as surrogates for self-reported variables are all valid solutions to the problem of recall bias. As an example of the latter strategy, a simple saliva test for the enzyme cotinine could be used to verify whether a person has become a nonsmoker (see Figure 7.6). In a study published in 2013, the investigators used surveys and self-reported smoking status as well as levels of cotinine in saliva samples to identify pregnant active smokers for a smoking cessation program (Smith, Robinson, Khan, Sosnoff, and Dillard, 2013).

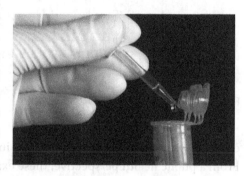

Figure 7.6 Saliva Collection to Test for the Enzyme Cotinine

Inaccurate recall occurs because people simply cannot remember a given event or series of behaviors. This is only a function of forgetting; when aggregated over an entire sample, the inaccuracies may equally underestimate and overestimate the true mean value. Ironically, when these overestimates and underestimates occur with equal frequency the mean will remain unchanged. Although the mean will often remain unaltered, the amount of variance artificially induced into the measure plagued by inaccurate recall could pose a threat to the statistical power of the study. Fortunately, the same solutions used to address recall bias will also reduce inaccurate recall. The pyramid pictured in Figure 7.7 should be used when constructing your questionnaire, as it may guide the selection of question choice, question wording, and time of the recall period.

As shown in the figure, whether people accurately recall any given event or behavior is a function of two factors: how frequently they perform the event and how salient (meaning level of importance in memory) the event or behavior is to them. High salience equates with better recall; however, this may be the case only when the event or behavior is not frequently repeated. For example, using cocaine may be a highly salient event to most people, as it would stand out as a rare experience. Alternatively, for a person who uses drugs on a daily basis, the use of cocaine may not be rare; thus recalling exactly how many times it was used in the past 12 months, for

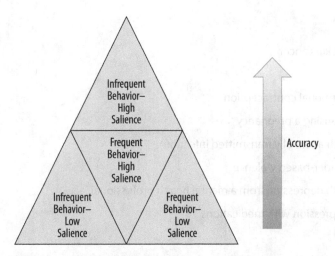

Figure 7.7 Pyramid of Frequency and Saliency of Behavior in Terms of Accuracy of Recall

example, might be difficult or impossible. Therefore, in a population that is not drug-addicted, a simple question would probably yield high accuracy: "In the past 12 months, how many times have you used cocaine?" On the other hand, that same question would most likely yield poor accuracy in a drug-using population (unless cocaine use was a rare occurrence). Inspection of Figure 7.7 reveals that the optimal conditions for accurate recall occur at the top of the pyramid; this is when salience is high (making it easy to remember) but frequency is low enough to make the process of accurate mental recall more reliable. The other triangles of the figure could describe many other potential events or behaviors, but in general, high salience suggests a higher level of recall than events with low salience. Because inaccurate recall introduces error and compromises validity, it is important to see a list of some of the events/behaviors that may well be exempt from this criticism due to their high salience and low frequency (see Box 7.3).

BOX 7.3. SELF-REPORTED EVENTS/BEHAVIORS *LEAST LIKELY* TO LEAD TO INACCURATE RECALL

Having a mammogram

Having a Pap test

Having a colonoscopy

Being diagnosed with hypertension

Having an automobile accident

Being evaluated for skin cancer

Having a root canal

Being prescribed hormonal contraception

Being pregnant or causing a pregnancy

Being diagnosed with a sexually transmitted infection

Being a victim of gender-based violence

Learning to cope with depression from a mental health professional

Being treated for depression with medications

Joining a gym

Joining a formal weight-loss program

Joining an organization dedicated to alcoholics

Being tested for HIV infection

Fortunately, the science of collecting valid self-reported data has greatly improved in recent decades, and several solutions to the problems often plaguing self-reported data are now apparent. This improvement stems primarily from improved technology, with data collection via mobile phones being the most vital of the innovations. For example, researchers in Texas used an existing smartphone application, CycleTracks, developed by the San Francisco County Transportation Authority, to collect information about routes ridden by bicyclists to inform decision making for future biking lanes and routes. Researchers also collected information about age, gender, bicycling frequency, home zip code, work zip code, and school zip code from approximately 300 participants (Hudson, Duthie, Rathood, Larsen, and Meyer, 2012, August). The use of mobile phones may minimize privacy concerns stemming from responding to sensitive questions during a face-to-face interview or via a computer-assisted self-interview in a group setting, either of which may induce study participants to provide responses that are not true, but rather provide responses that would be viewed as favorable by others. These privacy concerns and thus social desirability bias may be alleviated to some degree by collecting sensitive information via a person's own mobile phone. Although the mobile phone does not completely protect against participants' fear of the researchers' subsequently viewing the answers provided, they do protect against fear of other people hearing or seeing their answers, and the mobile phone does afford some degree of anonymity for the participant.

A second solution involves collecting data in very short recall periods to facilitate accurate recall. Inaccurate recall stems from faulty memory and can be greatly minimized when the recall period used to measure the behavior is short (for example, 24 hours versus 30 days, 3 months, or 6 months). This is especially true with behaviors that are quite frequent and/or noneventful. Consider, for instance, the question, "In the past 30 days, how many times have you consumed a meal that contains meat?" For a vegetarian, the answer will be easy, but for all others pondering this question any exact number is likely to be inaccurate. By using mobile phones to text questions to participants daily, we can break down the 30-day observation period into thirty 24-hour periods. Using this data collection method, you can readily see that most study participants would be able to better and more accurately report the number of times they consumed meat.

Selective recall bias, on the other hand, is much more difficult to minimize and stems from people's selective memories pertaining to certain events and their behavior. It may not be purposeful, like social desirability bias; however, using mobile phones and shorter recall periods may minimize it, as people would not have to rely on their memories, which may have been skewed by a variety of factors.

Before we move on, one more important point regarding self-reported measures: beyond simple issues of wording and constructing response options that will serve the question effectively, question-framing involves the actual design of the item. For one, as a standing rule one item should always measure just one variable. The question, "Do you live with your mother and father?" for example, is measuring two variables (lives with mother and lives with father).

A more complex example of why question-framing is so important involves the concept of a **behavioral anchor** (which limits the wording of a question to a very specific situation, increasing the precision of measurement). A behavioral anchor provides a specific behavior relevant to the construct being measured. For example, the theoretical construct of perceived susceptibility is defined as one's subjective perception of the risk of contracting a health condition *given* the existence of a behavioral risk factor. Thus when assessing the likelihood of being infected by a sexually transmitted disease, for instance, it is important to provide a conditional behavioral anchor. The following question exemplifies this principle.

If you had sexual intercourse with a casual sex partner and did not use a condom, how likely is it that you would be infected with an STD?

Note that the question is conditional—it measures perceived susceptibility when a condom has not been used. In the absence of this anchor, the question would measure perceived susceptibility under unknown conditions, thereby providing little value in a study of STD prevention; for

behavioral anchor
limiting the wording of a question to a very specific situation, increasing the precision of measurement

Behavioral Anchors

- **What is the likehood of...**
  - If you do not use a condom
  - If you do not floss every day
  - If you do not use sunscreen every day
  - If you use no birth control
  - If you consume 6 alcoholic beverages per event

Figure 7.8 Behavioral Anchors to Improve Precision of Measurement

example, "If you had sexual intercourse with a casual partner, how likely is it that you would be infected with a STD?" Other examples are presented in Figure 7.8.

Another question-framing issue relates to the **principle of correspondence** (which occurs when action, target, time, and context are all clearly definable in the wording of a question). The premise of this principle is that health behaviors typically have four defining components: action, target, time, and context—which essentially combine to define the health behavior. All four dimensions must be considered when drafting the questionnaire items. For instance, imagine that you are evaluating the outcome of a program designed to promote sunscreen to prevent skin cancer. A questionnaire item that would address all four components would look like the following:

In the past 2 months, have you applied sunscreen a half-hour before every time you went outdoors?

A quick look at the question allows a check on the correspondence:

Action = Applied

Target = Sunscreen

Time = Every time

Context = Outdoors

Changing any one component in this question would result in the assessment of a completely different health behavior. However, there are some health behaviors that do not require specifying all four components. For example, the behavior "taking blood pressure medication daily" does not require a context. As you begin your career in health promotion, prudence dictates that you proceed with caution regarding the inclusion of these four components. With experience, you will find that this task becomes increasingly more intuitive.

principle of correspondence
occurring when action, target, time, and context are all clearly definable in the wording of a question

Variables Assessed by Direct Observation

Because skill is such a central theoretical construct in health promotion, it is increasingly common to measure this construct by observation rather than sole reliance on people's self-reports. And because self-reports may be susceptible to wishful thinking, directly observed measurement, if it is possible, is likely to yield far better precision in your efforts to ensure rigor. A good example can be found in an article published in the *Journal of Adolescent Health* (Crosby et al., 2001). This study measured young women's self-reported level of skill in correctly applying condoms to a penis and subsequently asked each young woman to demonstrate her skill in applying a condom to a penile model. As you might have guessed, self-reported skill level was greatly exaggerated in contrast to young women's actual demonstrated skill. Other health promotion variables that research has shown to have significant discrepancies between actual and self-report are height and weight. This finding was highlighted in a study in the *American Journal of Preventive Medicine* (Nawaz et al., 2001) involving overweight and obese women, in which they found underreporting of weight and overreporting of height. This type of bias can seriously impact the outcome of case control studies, prospective studies, or randomized controlled trials. Directly measuring weight and height with a spring or balance scale, for example, is more accurate yet is noninvasive. It is important to note that direct observation of the health promotion variable may not always be plausible or even possible, but when it is, it can greatly enhance the validity of the measurement.

IN A NUTSHELL

It is important to note that direct observation of the health promotion variable may not always be plausible or even possible, but when it is, it can greatly enhance the validity of the measurement.

One last example taken from environmental health is the level of "walkability" of a neighborhood. Walkability has been found to be associated with body mass index and physical activity levels; therefore, it is an important determinant of obesity. An index has been developed to measure walkability (see http://www.hpe-inc.com/images/pdf/hpe%20walkability%20index%20score%20sheet%20rev%20may%202012.pdf for a copy of the index) and involves direct observation of key causal indicators such as street design (for example, presence of on-street parking, width of pavement, vehicle speed at nonpeak hours), sidewalk design (such as width,

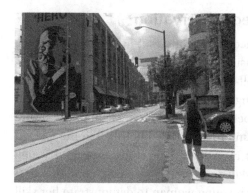

Figure 7.9 Walkability Scores of Neighborhood One

High (Score=88)

Source: Photo courtesy of Francesca S. Clarke

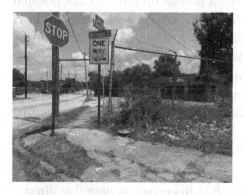

Figure 7.10 Walkability Scores of Neighborhood Two

Low (Score=17)

Source: Photo courtesy of Francesca S. Clarke

pedestrian connectivity, presence and quality of pedestrian features), urban design (such as ratio of building height to street width), land use mix, façade design, and transit-bicycle features. By directly observing these features of a neighborhood and calculating a score, you can have an unbiased measurement of walkability that is superior to neighborhood members' self-reports. Figures 7.9 and 7.10 depict two metropolitan neighborhoods of Atlanta, Georgia in the United States with vastly different walkability scores (88 for Sweet Auburn District, Figure 7.9, versus 17 for Lakewood Heights, Figure 7.10). As shown, you can readily see stark differences, suggesting that the walkability index has validity.

Variables Assessed by Records Review

As health promotion research becomes increasingly more contextual, it is more important than ever to measure variables such as income inequality, social capital, unemployment rates, community rates of teens giving birth, state tax rates on tobacco and alcohol, and traffic fatalities. A good example can be found in a study published by Holtgrave and Crosby (2003). Using only publicly available records, these state-level analyses found that poverty was significantly correlated with rates of chlamydia. Further, the state-level analyses found that income inequality was significantly correlated with chlamydia and AIDS case rates. Finally, it showed that social capital (a variable constructed through public records) was significantly correlated with gonorrhea case rates, chlamydia case rates, and AIDS case rates.

Biologically Assessed Variables

Research regarding sexual risk behavior is often made more rigorous by the addition of one or more biomarkers for actual presence or absence of sexually transmitted infections. A good example is found in a study reported in *Pediatrics* (DiClemente, McDermott-Sales, Danner, and Crosby, 2011). The study used a nationally representative sample and found that more than 10 percent of young adults with a laboratory-confirmed positive STD result reported abstaining from sexual intercourse in the 12 months before assessment and STD testing. Because the STDs assessed were quite unlikely to have existed for 12 months in the young adults, the study provided strong evidence suggesting that reports of abstaining from sex are often fallacious. In the absence of the biological measures, such a conclusion would not have been possible.

Another example is the construct of stress. Stress can be represented as a physiological reaction that involves the release of the hormone cortisol. Both chronic and acute stress have been associated with a host of negative health outcomes, so it is important to consider as a factor in health promotion research. Common ways to measure stress include implementing a measurement index such as the one highlighted in Box 7.2. As shown, it involves having people check off exposures to stressful life events; the more events they experienced, the more stressed they can be expected to be. However, stress is relative, meaning that people differ in their perceptions of what is stressful to them or what causes a stress reaction; although two people can both have the same score on this stress index, in reality one person may not feel as stressed as the other, due to differences in perception. A more accurate measure of stress levels would be to measure the actual cortisol levels via saliva testing, for example. Saliva is a useful biological fluid for assaying steroid hormones such as cortisol; thus salivary cortisol is a better stress indicator not subject to individual perceptions or self-report bias, with increased levels of cortisol correlating positively with increased levels of stress.

Mediating Variables

Mediating variables are those that "come between" or help to explain the nature of a purported cause and its associated effect. The most common example in health promotion involves the cause being a health promotion program and the effect being a change in a targeted health protective behavior. Typically, one or more psychosocial variables come between the cause and the effect, thereby classifying these variables as mediating variables.

For example, a health promotion program that promotes motivation and skill in the selection of low-fat foods might work through the mediators of (1) increased self-efficacy to prepare good-tasting low-fat foods and (2) increased outcome expectancies regarding the benefits of eating a low-fat diet. In this example, note that the mediators are both cognitive; thus they would be assessed via self-report.

Because some mediating variables may exist beyond the cognitive level, they may also be assessed by records review or direct observation, or biologically. For example, suppose a state embarks on a comprehensive large-scale campaign to reduce the amount of tobacco consumption. The health promotion campaign involves a substantial increase in the state excise tax on cigarettes; a universal prohibition on smoking in restaurants, bars, and other public places; the dissemination of effective prevention programs in schools; and the funding of effective smoking cessation interventions in health insurance plans and in worksites. All of this would be presented as an integrated strategy via an aggressive public awareness and marketing campaign. A targeted outcome of the antismoking campaign might be a change in social norms (a community-level measure) regarding smoking, so that smoking becomes a behavior that is frowned on. In this instance, affecting social norms is one mediating variable that allows the intent of the campaign to be translated into lowered tobacco consumption. At the policy level, the passage of state legislation that substantially increases taxes on cigarette sales might work through the possible mediating variable of making cigarette use too costly (a variable that could be assessed via in-state sales records).

In addition to explaining how a health promotion program works, mediating variables can also be found in observational research. For example, it has been shown in numerous studies that women who experience gender-based violence tend to have higher rates of sexually transmitted infections (STDs) including HIV (Cohen and Maclean, 2004). An important question that must be understood is: why? Aside from experiencing direct vaginal penetration by an infected partner, experiencing physical abuse or emotional abuse would not "cause" an STD. Research has identified several mediating variables that help to explain this relationship, such as fear of condom use negotiation, alcohol and substance use, and self-efficacy to negotiate condom use. Identifying modifiable mediating variables that further our understanding of and help explain complex associations involving negative health outcomes is critical to developing more effective health promotion programs.

Moderating Variables

Moderating variables, as the name suggests, are those that change the nature of the relationship between two variables, making it stronger, weaker, or null. It is useful here to think about the potential moderating variable as the "third variable"

IN A NUTSHELL

Moderating variables, as the name suggests, are those that change the nature of the relationship between two variables, making it stronger, weaker, or null.

when a significant bivariate association has been established between two other variables. For example, if the bivariate relationship between exercise and mental health was statistically stronger among Whites compared to Blacks, then race would be considered the moderating variable. If the relation were stronger among those who were from rural rather than suburban and urban areas, then place of residence would be the moderating variable. Social support is a classic example of a moderating variable in the health promotion literature, in which perceptions of high levels of social support serve as a buffer (that is, moderator) against experiencing the negative effects of stress on health outcomes. Thus it is important to consider which modifiable variables in health promotion could potentially moderate effects of traumatic events and other stressors on negative health outcomes so that health promotion programs can target those variables. Furthermore, some variables may moderate the effectiveness of health promotion programs. For example, imagine that a health promotion program was effective in reducing fat consumption (as shown by a bivariate association between the "group" variable and the levels of fat intake variable), but only for women. For men, the association between the program and the outcome of reduced fat consumption was nonsignificant. Thus gender serves as the moderating variable. It is important to consider what variables may serve as moderators of program effectiveness because doing so provides far greater precision in estimating the potential value of the intervention to public health. Because moderating variables may exist at or beyond the individual level, they may be measured by self-report, direct observation, review of existing records, or through biological assessments.

Summary

Achieving rigor in measurement can be a vast undertaking. Once the level of measurement (nominal, ordinal, interval, or ratio) for any given variable is determined, the next task is to decide how the variable will be used. Essentially, the research team must determine what variables will be designated as predictor variables (or correlates, if a cross-sectional design has been used), mediating variables, moderating variables, and outcome variables. Once all the necessary variables have been identified, the task becomes one of determining how each will be measured. For variables that represent constructs, the additional task is to create an operational definition of the concept being measured. Although variables such as age, gender, income, and education level are relatively easy to measure, the assessment of variables such as smoking frequency or self-esteem may pose tremendous challenges to the research team. This challenge brings several issues to the table. Among these issues are the length of the recall period, the wording of the question(s), the response alternatives, and the technique that will be employed to actually collect the data. Although long-standing techniques such as paper-and-pencil questionnaires may serve the research question well, advances in technology have created a host of new options that may add to the validity of the measure. Moreover, these innovations may be very useful for assessing the context of behavior rather than simply the behavior in isolation.

KEY TERMS

Behavioral anchor

Construct validity

Content validity

Criterion validity

Cronbach's alpha

Face validity

Inaccurate recall bias

Internal reliability

Interval

Mediating variable

Moderating variable

Nominal

Ordinal

Principle of correspondence

Ratio

Reliability

Selective recall bias

Self-report

Social desirability bias

Split-half method

Test-retest reliability

Validity

For Practice and Discussion

1. Locate three journal articles that each report findings from a study that used at least one scale measure. What were the Cronbach's alpha values

for each scale in each article? What do the values mean? Which, if any, of the articles gave information about validity? If none of the articles offered evidence of validity, what does that mean?

2. Mincus and Dincus conduct a study and find that chipmunks who eat low-fat nuts tend to be more depressed than those eating the really fatty nuts. They do, however, determine that this relationship applies only to female chipmunks. Select the bolded term from this chapter that best describes this finding. Defend your answer with a brief explanation of two or three sentences.

3. Using the principle of correspondence, compose three measureable objectives for behavior change. Be sure that each of these objectives meets all four criteria, and provide annotations that defend your work.

4. Working with at least one other person who is also learning from this textbook, go online to locate and download the codebook from any public use dataset. A codebook is essentially a copy of the questionnaire that was used to collect the data. Go through this codebook for at least 10 pages of question items and label each one with either a (1) for nominal, (2) for ordinal, (3) for interval, or (4) for ratio. Ask your colleague(s) to complete the same exercise using the same 10 pages. Then compare your answers with those of your colleague(s) and resolve any discrepancies by rereading the appropriate pages from this chapter.

References

Beck, A. T., Ward, C. H., Mendelson, M., Mock, J., and Erbaugh, J. (1961). An inventory for measuring depression. *Archives of General Psychiatry, 4*, 561–571.

Blake, D. D., Weathers, F. W., Nagy, L. M., Kaloupek, D. G., Gusman, F. D., Charney, D. S., and Keane, T. M. (1995). The development of a clinician-administered PTSD scale. *Journal of Traumatic Stress, 8*, 75–90.

Cohen, M., and Maclean, H. (2004). Violence against Canadian women. *BMC Women's Health, 4*(1), S22.

Crosby, R. A., DiClemente R. J., Wingood, G. M., et al. (2001). Correct condom application among African American adolescent females: The relationship to perceived self-efficacy and the association to confirmed STDs. *Journal of Adolescent Health*; 29:194–199.

DiClemente R. J., McDermott-Sales J., Danner F., and Crosby R. A. (2011). Association between laboratory-confirmed STDs and young adults self-reported abstinence: Findings from a national probability sample. *Pediatrics, 127*, 208–213.

Ghiselli, E. E., Campbell, J. P., and Zedeck, S. (1981). *Measurement theory for the behavioral sciences.* New York: Freeman.

Holtgrave, D. R, and Crosby, R. A. (2003). Social capital, poverty, and income inequality as predictors of gonorrhea, syphilis, chlamydia and AIDS case rates in the United States. *Sexually Transmitted Infections, 79*, 62–64.

Hudson, J., Duthie, J., Rathood, Y., Larsen, K., and Meyer, J. (2012, August). Using smartphones to collect bicycle travel data in Texas. U.S. Department of Transportation. Report no: UTCM 11–35–69. Grant no: DTRT06-G-0044.

Nawaz, H., Chan, W., Abdulrahman, M., Larson, D., and Katz, D. (2001). Self-reported weight and height. *American Journal of Preventive Medicine, 20*(4), 294–298.

Radloff, L. S. (1977). The CES-D scale: A self-report depression scale for research in the general population. *Applied Psychological Measurement, 1*(3), 385–401.

Rosenberg, M. (1989). *Society and the adolescent self-image* (rev. ed.). Middletown, CT: Wesleyan University Press.

Smith, J., Robinson, R., Khan, B., Sosnoff, C. and Dillard, D. (2013). Estimating cotinine associations and a saliva cotinine level to identify active cigarette smoking in Alaska Native pregnant women. *Maternal and Child Health Journal*, 10.1007/s10995–013–1241-x.

Streiner, D. L. (2003). Being inconsistent about consistency: When coefficient alpha does and doesn't matter. *Journal of Personality Assessment, 80*(3), 217–222.

CHAPTER 8

QUALITATIVE RESEARCH STRATEGIES AND METHODS FOR HEALTH PROMOTION

Laura F. Salazar
Alejandra Mijares
Richard A. Crosby
Ralph J. DiClemente

Health promotion research is undertaken to understand risk and protective factors for disease outcomes and related health risk behaviors. The goal is to reduce risk and enhance protection so that public health can be improved. Although the predominant paradigm used for this research is quantitative, qualitative research is an essential part. Qualitative research complements and extends quantitative methods by providing context and additional layers of understanding.

As iterated throughout this book, the overarching purpose of scientific inquiry is to generate knowledge. In the context of health promotion, scientific inquiries are undertaken to generate knowledge specifically regarding prevalence and incidence of disease, risk factors for disease and health-risk behaviors, etiologic factors, theoretical perspectives, and effectiveness of health promotion programs. The long-term goal of these scientific inquiries is to prevent morbidity and premature mortality. As described in Chapter One, conceptualizing and implementing these scientific inquiries entails embarking on a journey through a nine-step research process.

As with any journey, however, there are always many decisions to make and myriad options from which to choose. To some degree, each leg of this research journey will have consequences (both good and bad), and, depending on the path taken, may result in reaching a crossroad

LEARNING OBJECTIVES

- Distinguish between basic philosophies of a qualitative research paradigm compared to a quantitative paradigm.

- Describe five characteristics that comprise the qualitative mode of inquiry.

- Delineate the four purposes that can be served by qualitative research for health promotion.

- Compare and contrast the tenets of phenomenology, ethnography, grounded theory, and ethnoscience.

- Describe the different types of triangulation and identify the purposes each type serves.

- Explain four different types of observation as a data collection methodology and provide one example of each type.

or even reaching a dead end. Thus it is important to consider each decision point and plan your journey carefully. Of course, because you may not have been on this type of journey before, we don't expect you to travel alone. We have attempted to be your tour guide for this journey, walking you through the research process, helping to identify salient points of interest, and issuing warnings of any potential dangers. In the spirit of being the best tour guides possible, however, we must acknowledge that so far we have taken you on this journey using only one mode of transportation. Let's assume that for this analogy you have been primarily traveling by car. As you can imagine, traveling cross-country by car will provide quite a different experience than going by train. Therefore, because we want you to have the fullest experience possible, it is time to get off the road and see how the countryside looks from the seat of a passenger train.

IN A NUTSHELL

A methodological paradigm is a discipline's view of which research techniques and practices are promoted and should be practiced. A discipline's methodological paradigm has strong implications for how the discipline as a whole will progress.

paradigm
model, pattern, or example that may be influential in shaping the development of a discipline

In this journey analogy, the mode of transportation refers to the methodological paradigm applied to the research process. From the Greek word *paradeigma*, **paradigm** means model, pattern, or example; however, this rather simple definition can be expanded to encompass a worldview that may be influential in shaping the development of a discipline. A methodological paradigm is a discipline's view of which research techniques and practices are promoted and should be practiced. A discipline's methodological paradigm has strong implications for how the discipline as a whole will progress.

positivism
the view that serious scientific inquiry should confine itself to the study of relations existing between facts that can be directly observed

The approaches, methods, designs, and perspectives described thus far mostly fall under a paradigm termed **positivism**. Positivism is the view that serious scientific inquiry should not search for ultimate causes deriving from some outside or unidentifiable source, but rather must confine itself to the study of relations existing between facts, which are directly accessible to observation. Science or knowledge is based on the exploration of natural phenomena, in which properties and relations are observed and are verifiable. Consequently, positivism involves the use of methods that should be objective and involves testing theories through the generation and falsification of hypotheses in order to assemble "facts" (see Chapter Two for more details). In the end, relations can be supported, disconfirmed, or falsified. As you can extrapolate from this description of positivism, positivistic inquiries lend themselves to the use of quantitative modes of inquiry.

Given that the research questions, designs, and methods described thus far can be labeled as positivistic, if we stopped and did not go any further, then we would have presented a skewed view of health promotion's paradigm. It would ostensibly appear that health promotion research was ideologically bound by research methods (for example, experimental designs, random sampling, quantitative data, inferential statistics) that many of us have been conditioned to view as the epitome of rigor and as "real" research (Glesne and Peshkin, 1992). Although much health promotion research uses these methods, designs, and data justifiably, as a discipline we are not bound by them. Indeed, much health promotion research uses epistemologies that are supported by an **interpretivist** paradigm (Glesne and Peshkin, 1992).

interpretivist
the view that reality is socially constructed because each individual perceives, understands, experiences, and makes meaning of reality in different ways

In contrast to positivism, interpretivism views the world as a multiplicity of realities in which each individual perceives, understands experiences, and makes meaning of that reality in different ways; thus reality is socially constructed. Research in this paradigm focuses on studying individuals' lives and their significance. The overall aim within this paradigm is to understand others' experiences and relate them to one's own reality (Colangelo, Domel, Kelly, Peirce, and Sullivan, 1999). Thus an interpretivist paradigm is supported through the use of qualitative modes of inquiry. Just as positivism and interpretivism differ, their modes of inquiry also differ. Quantitative and qualitative modes of inquiry differ in the assumptions made about the generation of facts, in their purposes, in their approaches, and in the role of the researcher. These differences are highlighted in Table 8.1.

In viewing Table 8.1, is it important to note that there is no judgment attached to the underlying assumptions of the two modes, and there shouldn't be; rather, differences are illuminated to assist in making decisions regarding the research process. One approach is not necessarily better than the other in this instance, and one approach should not be considered more scientific or more rigorous than the other—just different. There are some similarities as well. We strongly advocate that both are not only compatible but also complementary, allowing the capture of diverse data that can provide contextually richer, more complete understanding of the phenomenon under investigation. Nevertheless, it is important to learn how the two modes differ along the dimensions presented in Table 8.1.

In this chapter, we provide an overview of qualitative research purposes, strategies, and methods so that you can glean a better understanding of when and how to conduct qualitative research. We will describe what constitutes qualitative research and several major purposes within health promotion for which qualitative inquiry is conducive. We describe four

Table 8.1   Predispositions of Quantitative and Qualitative Modes of Inquiry

Quantitative Mode	Qualitative Mode
Assumptions	
Social facts have an objective reality	Reality is socially constructed
Primacy of method	Primacy of subject matter
Variables can be identified and relationships measured	Variables are complex, interwoven, and difficult to measure
Etic (outsider's point of view)	Emic (insider's point of view)
Purpose	
Generalizability	Contextualization
Prediction	Interpretation
Causal explanations	Understanding of perspectives
Approach	
Begins with hypotheses and theories	Ends with hypotheses and grounded theory
Manipulation and control	Emergence and portrayal
Uses formal instruments	Researcher as instrument
Experimental	Naturalistic
Deductive	Inductive
Component analysis	Searches for patterns
Seeks consensus, the norm	Seeks pluralism, complexity
Reduces data to numerical indices	Makes minor use of numerical indices
Abstract language in write-up	Descriptive write-up
Researcher Role	
Detachment and impartiality	Personal involvement and partiality
Objective portrayal	Empathic understanding

Source: From C. Glesne and A. Peshkin, *Becoming Qualitative Researchers: An Introduction*, copyright © 1992. Published by Allyn & Bacon, Boston. Copyright © by Pearson Education. Reprinted by permission of the publisher.

main qualitative strategies, which are somewhat analogous to research designs in quantitative terms, and we identify the data collection methods most appropriate. Keep in mind as you read through this chapter that unlike traveling by car, this train ride requires no seat belt. So relax and enjoy your trip!

What Constitutes a Qualitative Mode of Inquiry?

Essentially, there are five characteristics of qualitative research that make it "qualitative": (1) it is naturalistic, (2) the data are descriptive, (3) there is concern with process, (4) it is inductive, and (5) meaning is the goal (Bogdan and Biklen, 1998). In any given qualitative research study it is not necessary to have all five features weighted equally to signify that the research is

IN A NUTSHELL

Essentially, there are five aspects of qualitative research that make it "qualitative": it is naturalistic, the data are descriptive, there is concern with process, it is inductive, and meaning is the goal.

qualitative, or to even have all five of the characteristics. For example, imagine that a qualitative researcher studying homeless women wants to understand the circumstances of their lives and what led them to become homeless. He or she may collect descriptive data, be concerned with the process, and be focused on revealing the meaning of the participants' experiences. Yet he or she may conduct in-depth interviews with the women in a coffee shop rarely visited by homeless women. Some qualitative research will emphasize certain features more so than others, but for practical purposes, ideally, qualitative research should attempt to encompass all five characteristics.

Naturalistic

Qualitative research is **naturalistic** as opposed to observational or experimental. Naturalistic and experimental differences can be quite distinct; however, distinctions between naturalistic and observational are more subtle. Although both designs involve a lack of manipulation or control, naturalistic signifies that the data are collected in the natural setting, such as a person's home or school, whereas observational research can occur in an artificial setting. Furthermore, it is the setting in which the research takes place that provides the data, and it is the researcher who serves as the mode for data collection. The data are collected in a manner that is also natural (such as observing or conversing). Because qualitative research is concerned with contextualization—meaning that the results must be placed and interpreted within the setting where the research took place, to aid understanding—naturalistic approaches provide a high level of context. In a study of people who experienced chronic pain and who were receiving treatment for opiate addiction at a methadone clinic, qualitative interviews were conducted with patient participants at the clinic (Marie, 2013). Although we cannot say for certain, had the researcher attempted to take the participants into a different setting, such as a university, conducting the interviews in an artificial setting could have had an impact on the results.

naturalistic
within the context of research, naturalistic pertains to when data are collected in a natural setting or environment

Descriptive Data

Qualitative research uses data that are descriptive (Bogdan and Biklen, 1998). Qualitative data can take several different forms, such as words, pictures, video, notes, charts or records, and narratives. Data are not represented in numerical terms. If some numerical interpretation is provided, it is usually minor and may be presented to emphasize a pattern in the data. Written results may contain participants' quotes, interview transcripts, field notes, photos, and so on and provide a rich, in-depth analysis centering on interpretation. This approach, of course, contrasts with a quantitative mode, in which data are expressed in numerical forms, statistical analyses are performed to describe the data and to test hypotheses, and the results are presented in statistical terms with little or no context.

As an example, Melville and colleagues conducted a qualitative research study of patients visiting an STD clinic to determine the emotional and psychosocial impact of receiving a positive genital herpes diagnosis (Melville et al., 2003). In-depth interviews were conducted with 24 clinic patients onsite. A sample of the data is provided in Box 8.1 and a sample of the write-up from the published article is provided in Box 8.2. As shown, the data are words composing the transcription of the interview, and the results represent the researchers' interpretations and understanding of the participants' words.

BOX 8.1. TEXT TRANSCRIBED VERBATIM FROM AN INTERVIEW WITH A PATIENT FROM AN STD CLINIC

I: Thinking back to when you first found out you had genital herpes, how did you feel at the time? This would have been not when you and I talked the other day, but when you first heard your results. And I'm assuming you talked to them on the phone, is that correct?

P: Yeah, I called in. How did I feel? Uh . . . I don't . . . can you stop this for a second?

I: Sure.

P: Okay.
       (Tape stops.)

I: So you're not even sure how you actually felt?

P: I knew I had something, but in a way I was relieved to find out what it was, because as bad as it could be . . .

I: Right, I understand that.

P: And I guess a part of me could move on now. I could figure out what I needed to do.

I: As opposed to someone saying, "No no you don't have anything." And yet you know you have these weird symptoms?

P: Yeah.

I: Okay. So part of you was relieved and part of you was . . . ?
       (Pause)

P: You know I think I had a little bit of anger too, because I think I know who it was. I remembered back to this whole incident and I'm pretty sure, so I had a little bit of anger with that. So relief and I don't know . . .

I: Herpes is a source of stress for some people but not for others. Did your discovering that you had herpes cause you enough stress to affect your daily behavior—for example, your work, friends, and relationships? If so could you please explain in as much detail as possible?

P: No it hasn't really. It hasn't changed. The relationship a little bit. I'm putting off . . . I have a girlfriend but I'm putting off going over to her house. I know I need to tell her, but I'm not sure exactly how to go about that. So that's stressful, that could be classified as stressful. But as far as work goes, no.

I: But it sounds like from what you said before though that part of it was confirming and a relief to hear that you had something. That would be a relief of some kind of stress as opposed to creating stress. And having to tell someone about it—that's a whole different category that needs to be addressed at some point.

P: And as far as my life goes, I've been through a lot and I'm used to rolling with what comes at me. So I don't really feel all that much stress.

I: Maybe this is minor compared to some other things?

P: Yeah.

I: Self-concept is broadly defined as how you view yourself as a person. Did any of the feelings you experienced when you first discovered you had herpes change your self-concept in any way?

P: Wow. I think it makes me feel like, How am I going to get something going in a relationship as far as being with somebody? I don't understand how I could talk to someone about this, I really don't. I think in a way it's closed me—I'm already pretty closed as it is—but I think it's closed me a little bit more. Out of fear—I guess bottom-line rejection.

I: Do you recall if the discovery affected your daily moods at all?

P: I don't really recall. Maybe it'd be better if you had a list of questions—I'd get a chance to think about them before I came in.

    (Laughter)

P: No. I don't think so.

I: Did it affect your feelings of body image and sexual attractiveness?

P: Maybe body image. I'm not sure about sexual attractiveness. That's really a mind thing I think. I think attractiveness is really a mind thing. I think it's the same.

I: Has it affected your sex drive?

P: No.

I: Has it affected your desire for long-term sexual relationships?

P: Has it affected my desire for long-term sexual relationships? I don't know. I still have that desire, it's just what am I going to do with this?

I: After the tape is off, we can talk more about this and your sex partners.

P: Okay.

I: Has it affected your ability to relate to your partner?

P: Yes.

I: Yeah, you mentioned that you haven't gone to her house.

P: Yeah, I'm staying away. I have to tell her, I can't just . . .

I: How long have you been with her?

P: Uh, two months, three months.

I: Some of the initial effects experienced by people who newly discover they have herpes change with the passage of time. Can you compare the answers that you just gave me to the feeling you have today? For example, how do you feel about learning that you were positive for herpes type 2?

P: How do I feel?

I: Well for example, when you first heard your results part of you felt relieved because you suspected and now it was confirmed. And another part of you was angry because you were thinking who gave it to you and it brought that up. So now that you've had some time since you first heard your results, what are your feelings now? Are they different from that day?

P: Yeah, I think now I'm more, not resigned but like resigned to move on. There's not really anything I can do about that now. It's water under the bridge. But I need to move on.

I: That's the impression I have too. So in terms of stress affecting your daily behavior, that sounds like it's still just affecting your relationship with your girlfriend?

P: Yeah, work is going, it's really going well.

I: Has there been any change in your self-concept in any way?

P: Well I have a pretty good self-concept for someone who just did a lot of time. But I think as far as—I don't understand the question. I'm trying to ramble on.

I: Since finding out that you have herpes, you talked about how initially it did affect your self-concept a little bit. But I'm hearing from the way you are talking about things, it's probably not affecting you as much anymore. In fact, if I could put forth what I'm picking up, is that maybe in the beginning it was something you thought about a lot, but now it's on the back burner and it comes up when you think about seeing your girlfriend because then you have to talk about it. But otherwise it's not really bothering you.

P: Very good, very good!

I: Is that where you are?
     (Laughter)

P: Yeah. Part of me puts it off into the back and then when the opportunity arises when she'll call me up and I'll make excuses.

I: Oh good. We're going to have a lot to talk about when the tape is off.

P: Okay okay.

I: For many people, having herpes causes problems at some points in life but not at other times. After you knew you had herpes up till now, do you recall specific situations that may have intensified any negative feelings attached to your having herpes?

P: Something negative that is attached?

I: Yes.

P: I would think that outbreaks would be negative. That would be a hard time to deal with it. But I can't really think of anything else.

BOX 8.2. SAMPLE RESULTS WRITE-UP

Fear of telling a current partner was a frequent psychosocial response associated often with fear of rejection, present even for participants who knew that their current sex partner had herpes. One man (32, STD) said, "I thought she was going to freak out and run away from me. Scared that she was going to run off and leave me forever." Another man (37, STD) reported that his initial thought was, "Oh my gosh, I'm positive, and if I tell him, he probably, you know, might reject me for this. Then I thought, oh no he's had herpes so he's certainly not going to do this to me. But there's always the possibility. So there was this little thinking that went on subconsciously....I waited a couple of days and then told him, because I think I had to go through my own little process of dealing with that."

Source: Melville et al. (2003), 282.

Process-Focused

Qualitative research entails a focus on the process involved with a particular phenomenon rather than solely on the outcome (Bogdan and Biklen, 1998). Again using the research study of homeless women as an example, one focus of the research could be to understand the process through which women came to be homeless. How did these women become homeless? What happened in their lives that brought them to this point? Other examples from health promotion could be, How do young women negotiate condom use with their partners? What processes do they go through to protect themselves? And why do some young women think they are overweight? How do they come to view themselves in this way? What is the impact of thinking they are overweight? In the qualitative study mentioned previously with participants recruited from a methadone clinic, the purpose was to address the structures and pathways of *how* the individuals developed the two conditions of addiction and chronic pain (Marie, 2013). In one last example, Scorgie et al. (2013) examined *how* violence and related human rights abuses affect the lives of female, male, and transgender sex workers in Kenya, South Africa, Uganda, and Zimbabwe. As sex work is a criminal offense in these countries, the researchers specifically wanted to understand the strategies sex workers use to cope with or avoid violations, or to seek formal redress.

Inductive Approach

inductive logic
deriving general patterns from observations that may eventually become hypotheses or theories

Qualitative research is inductive. As you may recall from Chapter Two, **inductive logic** involves deriving general patterns from your observations that may eventually become hypotheses or that may constitute a theory. This approach contrasts with deductive logic, the approach most often used in quantitative inquiries, which involves testing specific hypotheses that were derived from general ideas. The process underlying qualitative research is considered inductive because, in very simple terms, you begin by making observations and gathering data, then you describe the data, and finally you attempt to interpret the data. The interpretation is much like working on a puzzle and typically involves putting seemingly abstract pieces together so that they make an understandable whole. This process is ongoing, dynamic, and emerging. After making initial observations and deriving initial patterns, you might go back and gather more observations, and you might even revise your initial conclusions. In this sense, the process is inductive, but you may at times use deduction. Not surprisingly, considering this type of research process, qualitative research has also been compared to patchwork quiltmaking and filmmaking (Sterk and Elifson, 2004).

Finding Meaning Is the Goal

Essentially, the task of qualitative research is to find meaning in the observations and experiences of the participants, which brings us to the fifth feature of qualitative research. The perspective of the participants is the main concern. For example, Plattner (2013) wanted to understand how young children in Botswana conceptualized AIDS, HIV, and condoms. Children aged 4 to 7 years were asked to draw a picture about AIDS and tell a story about the drawing; this was followed by three questions in which participants were asked to explain what AIDS, HIV, and a condom meant to them. Plattner found that most children were able to draw a picture of AIDS and tell a story about it. For one boy, "AIDS is these sores over this person's body [points to the dots in the drawing]. You do not have to touch him otherwise you will get the disease. This person also touched someone with the sores and got AIDS. He is going to die if he does not go to the hospital to get pills." HIV was more difficult to describe for most children, but for slightly more than half, it was related to some illness, with some equating it with AIDS and some simply with death. Results were mixed in terms of what condoms meant: the older children indicated that condoms could prevent AIDS or illness, whereas the younger ones felt that condoms were dirty and could make you sick.

Understanding the perspective of the participants in their natural surroundings in some way that is meaningful is the main goal of qualitative research. Although this may seem like an easy task, interpreting the experiences of other people is rather difficult. As with any research, qualitative or quantitative, researchers bring their own experiences, values, and biases with them that may color or influence the interpretation. The main difference (refer to Table 8.1), however, between providing meaning to qualitative research and quantitative research is that in the former, the researcher typically acknowledges his or her values and biases and also understands that the process is subjective. Conversely, in quantitative research, the researcher when collecting and interpreting the data makes an assumption of objectivity. This implies that the researcher is detached and impartial for all aspects of the research, including the interpretation. You should consider, however, whether researchers truly detach themselves from the process just because they are implementing an experimental design, administering quantitative measures, and performing statistical analyses.

Purposes for Qualitative Research in Health Promotion

Although there may be an infinite number of purposes for which qualitative research can be used and should be used in health promotion research, we shall focus on four general purposes. First, qualitative inquiry is useful for conducting exploratory research where little is known about a particular health issue. Second, qualitative inquiry can be used in health promotion research to increase the depth and validity of quantitative inquiries. In this instance, qualitative research is combined with quantitative approaches and utilizes triangulation. Third, before a large-scale randomized trial is implemented, qualitative research can be used as a precursor to implementing a health promotion program and then provide additional information during the evaluation. Finally, qualitative inquiry can be used as an alternative when other methods are precluded.

For Exploratory Research

As you may recall from Chapter Four, investigations of certain health phenomena generally evolve through a two-stage process: exploratory and conclusive. The exploratory stage entails research questions that will shed light on an issue for which little is known. "In this early stage [of the process], observations are needed to provide investigators with data to define health issues, to begin to understand the etiology of those health issues, to formulate theories, to reveal relevant factors, and to identify potential relationships." There is purpose to exploratory research, and its purpose corresponds strongly with a qualitative mode of inquiry. Because not much is known yet during the exploratory stage, it would be difficult to develop any hypotheses a priori that warrant testing. It may not be prudent at this stage to launch a large-scale research study using large samples and geographically diverse locations. Exploratory research lends itself quite nicely to a qualitative mode, in which you could begin to gather observations using a naturalistic approach within a limited geographical context, and data collected are not structured and formalized but descriptive. Interpretation of the data centers on defining the patterns grounded in the data and making sense of it all. Perhaps preliminary hypotheses or even a theory could emerge from the data at this point.

Let's illustrate this point by referring back to the research study involving patients with herpes who were asymptomatic. At the time the study was conceptualized little was known about how varied asymptomatic people's reactions would be to receiving a positive herpes diagnosis. Also, the serological test (western blot) used to detect antibodies to herpes simplex virus was becoming readily available and was emerging as a useful screening tool for diagnosing large numbers of people. The researchers felt that it was important to understand the emotional and potential psychosocial responses people may have to receiving a diagnosis, so that counseling strategies could be devised that would address these responses. Therefore a qualitative study was conducted to ascertain a relatively small number (24) of people's responses to receiving a positive diagnosis. The results suggested a theory of both short-term and ongoing responses and their relations as well as the influence of other factors (such as social support or knowledge about herpes) on those responses—both negative and positive. The theory that Melville et al. (2003) generated from the data is graphically depicted as a model in Figure 8.1. In viewing the model, one can see the nature of the relationships among the variables and that the variables are such that quantitative measurements could be derived and a quantitative research study could be employed to test the model on a larger scale. This example of exploratory research helped to advance the field to the next stage so that conclusive research could be conducted.

Referring back to Table 8.1, we can see that the purposes of qualitative research, which are parallel to the purpose of exploratory research,

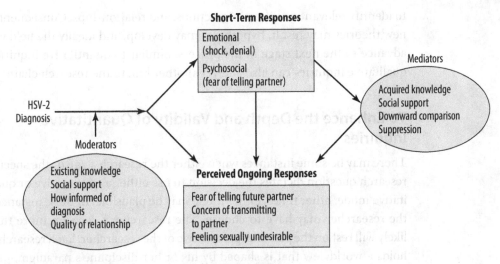

Figure 8.1 Model of Psychological Responses to a Serological HSV-2 Diagnosis

are **contextualization**, interpretation, and understanding of perspectives. Determining whether or not the interpretation of those experiences will generalize to others is not the goal. Once an understanding of perspectives is reached, depending on the situation, future research can use other modes of inquiry to see whether these experiences generalize to others. Suppose, for example, that you are interested in understanding better the role parents may play, beyond the genetic component, in contributing to the obesity of their children. You could choose a setting such as small rural town or even a particular school district that may have unusually high rates of obesity for the inquiry. Your approach in understanding the daily lives of the families who reside in the setting could entail not only observing, interviewing, and interacting with parents and trying to determine how they view their lives, but also identifying the historical, social, political, and environmental influences that interact and shape their reality. Once meaning is derived and a complex picture of the phenomena is obtained, then perhaps a larger-scale study that is more on the conclusive side can be justified and implemented.

When using a qualitative mode of inquiry, another caveat may be in order: this process is inherently complex, and trying to reduce or simplify the complexity of people's lives is not the goal. The researcher must "do justice to that complexity, to respect it in its own right" (Glesne and Peshkin, 1992, p. 7). For researchers using a qualitative mode of inquiry, it helps if they immerse themselves and take an insider's point of view. An insider's point of view is referred to as **emic** and should entail using multiple methods such as interviewing, observation, focus groups, and so on. The result will reveal the complex nature of the phenomena in question and help

contextualization refers to research that seeks to provide an understanding based on the experiences of the participants in a particular social setting

emic an insider's point of view

to identify relevant qualities, interactions, and relationships. Consequently, new theories may result, hypotheses may develop, and ideally the field will advance to the next stage in the process. Similar to quantitative inquiries, qualitative inquiries can also add yet another link to the research chain.

To Enhance the Depth and Validity of Quantitative Inquiries

There may be some instances when either the research stage or the specific research question dictates the decision to use either a quantitative or qualitative mode; other times, either mode may be plausible. In these instances, the researcher may have to choose. The researcher's decision more than likely will rest on the personal perspective of the researcher. Each researcher holds a worldview that is shaped by his or her discipline's paradigm, personal experiences, and other socialization processes; thus as researchers our own ideals and values shape our research. More important, however, is that regardless of how or why the decision is made to adopt a certain approach, we do not want to present this decision as a conflict. The two approaches are not necessarily incompatible, and choosing which approach to use in your research does not have to be viewed as an "either-or" decision.

triangulation
the combination of multiple researchers, theories, methods, and data sources in a study

Many times in health promotion research both modes are useful, compatible, and, indeed, desirable. In fact, as opposed to endorsing or adopting only one approach, researchers should aspire to **triangulation** when planning any research study. Triangulation is very useful to help "overcome the intrinsic bias that comes from single-method, single-observer, and single-theory studies" (Denzin, 1978). The underlying assumption in using a triangulation design is that the weaknesses of one approach are counterbalanced by the strengths of another. For example, conducting interviews with health care providers regarding a certain health promotion topic may yield detailed information about providers' experiences with patient care. But these interviews would be limited to providers' perspectives. Including observations of the clinic setting (that is, patient-provider interaction, physical environment) could highlight new insights about the patient-provider communication and the setting.

Triangulation can serve two important purposes: confirmation and completeness. Triangulation for the purpose of *confirmation* can increase validity of results. Researchers can confirm the results of multiple data sources by using methods that converge at one point (or yield the same conclusions). However, when triangulation yields conflicting results, it doesn't necessarily mean that one set of results is wrong or both are wrong. In fact, it may mean that both findings are correct, but a deeper and more complex analysis is warranted. Conflicting results may occur because "different types of inquiry are sensitive to real-world nuances" (Patton, 2002, pg. 556). Inconsistent findings should be viewed not as a problem but rather as an opportunity, as this inconsistency may point the researcher toward a deeper understanding of the phenomenon being studied. In addition, researchers may triangulate data sources in order to conduct a more *complete* analysis. A phenomenon that is studied from multiple perspectives, and using multiple methods, theories, and data sources, is likely to produce a more complete interpretation and understanding of the various aspects of that phenomenon.

For example, let's imagine that you were conducting an evaluation of three models of HIV patient care. As part of your evaluation you decide to conduct interviews with various types of HIV health workers (such as physicians, case managers, and the like) and focus groups with HIV-positive patients receiving care through each of the three patient care models. Then you triangulate your analysis of health worker interviews to *confirm* findings (for example, multiple health workers discussed the same and/or similar barriers and facilitators to providing HIV care), and provide a *complete* picture of barriers and facilitators experienced by different types of providers. For instance, case managers' perspectives of HIV care could highlight the importance of emotional support of patients in retention in care, whereas physicians' perspectives of HIV care could highlight the use of electronic medical records in managing patient care. Both findings are important to completing the "patchwork quilt" of your study. Along with these data sources, focus group data of patient experiences with care could be triangulated with providers' perspectives of patients' barriers and facilitators to care. Triangulation of these data could prove to be very fruitful if, say, providers perceived one HIV patient care model to be better than standard of care but patients who received care through that HIV care model indicated they were dissatisfied with the care they were receiving. If focus groups with patients had not been conducted, it might have been assumed that the HIV care model that providers preferred was running smoothly and the best model. In this case, triangulation could help glean a more accurate picture.

IN A NUTSHELL

Whether the purpose of your research is confirmation or completeness, the beauty of triangulation is that it provides the researcher with multiple ways to design and analyze any study.

Whether the purpose of your research is confirmation or completeness, the beauty of triangulation is that it provides the researcher with multiple ways to design and analyze any study. There are four types of triangulation: (1) investigator, (2) theoretical, (3) data, and (4) method.

Each type has benefits and disadvantages, but all are intended to help researchers have more valid and complete results.

investigator triangulation
the use of multiple researchers or analysts to increase the internal reliability and validity of research findings

Investigator triangulation can occur (1) by using a multidisciplinary research team that has varied, yet relevant expertise (this is increasingly common in health research where physicians, epidemiologists, behavioral scientists, and economists can all contribute to one study); and (2) by having multiple coders and/or analysts in one study. Investigator triangulation can help reduce the effects of bias from having one researcher, but if not managed adequately, it can also increase bias.

theoretical triangulation
the use of multiple theories or frameworks in one research study

Theoretical triangulation can be performed when two different theories are used to analyze or test one hypothesis. This not only helps researchers organize large amounts of data in meaningful and systematic ways but also pushes researchers to think through their data in ways that are more profound and that they may not have considered (Thurmond, 2001).

data triangulation
the use of several data sources to inquire about a specific phenomenon

Data triangulation is helpful when inquiring about a specific phenomenon, and there are three types: (1) time, (2) space, and (3) person. Time triangulation refers to the study of one phenomenon at various time points. For instance, in a study you might collect data on blood pressure at different times of the day and week. It is important to note that longitudinal studies cannot be triangulated, because they aim to recognize changes over time. Space triangulation refers to the collection of data in two or more sites and aims to test the sites for consistency. Person triangulation uses data from individuals, groups, or collectives to gain a more comprehensive view of a specific phenomenon or problem. For example, in a study of HIV treatment adherence, interviews with multiple stakeholders (for example, physician, nurse, clinic administrator, patient) may yield a more comprehensive picture of the issues affecting patient adherence then just interviewing one type of stakeholder (Halcomb and Andrew, 2005).

method triangulation
the use of multiple data collection strategies to answer the same research question

Method triangulation. There are two types of **method triangulation**: (1) within methods and (2) between methods. Within methods triangulation uses multiple data collection strategies from the same type of approach or paradigm, for instance, conducting interviews with providers and patients, and conducting observations of provider-patient interaction to answer the same research questions. Within methods triangulation aims to assess internal reliability. Alternatively, between methods triangulation refers to the use of both qualitative and quantitative approaches (commonly referred to as mixed-methods approach) to answer the same research questions, for example, conducting face-to-face interviews and administering a quantitative survey. Between-methods triangulation can also be classified as simultaneous or sequential. **Simultaneous triangulation** occurs when both qualitative and quantitative data are collected and analyzed at the same time. In this approach, the datasets are not equally weighted in terms of significance, meaning that results from one type of data are viewed as the main findings whereas the other type of data is meant as a complement to the main findings. **Sequential triangulation** is helpful when there are multiple phases to a study. The results of one approach are used to inform the other approach. The sequence used (that is, qualitative, then quantitative, or quantitative, then qualitative) depends on the intent and needs of the study (Morse, 1994).

As an example, Nakkash et al. (2003) used sequential triangulation of methods (quantitative and qualitative) and data sources (community members and coalition members) in their development of a cardiovascular disease prevention program. They first conducted a household survey (a quantitative method) using a representative sample from the community (the first data source) in which the program was to be implemented. The survey was designed to assess knowledge, attitudes, and behaviors related to cardiovascular disease and to identify risk factor levels. They also asked participants from the household survey to participate in focus groups (a qualitative method) to identify the facilitators and barriers to achieving healthy lifestyles as well as intervention ideas. A coalition consisting of key informal and formal community leaders (the second data source) was assembled. The researchers conducted natural group discussions (a qualitative method) with the coalition members to understand the relevancy, feasibility, affordability, acceptability, and sustainability of proposed intervention activities. The researchers made the following comments regarding their use of triangulation in developing the community-based program:

> The advantages far outweigh the disadvantages. The intervention activities developed as a result of the triangulation of data methods and sources are community specific, relevant, and affordable. As a result, they are more effective and sustainable. This combination of intervention activities could not have been developed in the absence of any one piece of information. Effective and sustainable interventions are, in fact, cost-effective. Thus, the cost-intense disadvantage is ultimately diminished in an assessment of efficiency. Practitioners are encouraged to obtain information from a variety of methods and sources in the development of community-specific interventions.
>
> [Nakkash et al., 2003, p. 738]

Although some researchers may admit that carrying out a sophisticated quantitative study while also conducting in-depth qualitative

simultaneous triangulation
the use of qualitative and quantitative data collected and analyzed at the same time

sequential triangulation
method in which the results of one approach are used to design and implement another approach

research is rife with challenges and may be difficult for many, essentially all research is rife with challenges. Given the breadth of experiences described by Nakkash et al. (2003) and their subsequent endorsement of triangulating in retrospect, it would be hard to argue that using a combination of approaches should not be attempted or at least considered. If the researcher's perspective endorses more of a quantitative view, then he or she could use triangulation of data sources. Furthermore, if multiple methods are desired, the researcher could use triangulation of investigators (that is, a multidisciplinary approach) and collaborate with researchers who are experts in qualitative methods, thereby expanding the methods used. There are myriad ways to use triangulation, but you may have to be creative. Needless to say, the result will be a more in-depth understanding and increased validity of your findings.

IN A NUTSHELL

There are myriad ways to use triangulation, but you may have to be creative. Needless to say, the end result will be a more in-depth understanding and increased validity of your findings.

As a Precursor to Implementing Health Promotion Programs

Another way in which qualitative research may be useful is before the health promotion program (HPP) is implemented. Methodological issues related to the implementation of the program are best determined beforehand through the use of qualitative research. These include issues such as

- Recruitment strategies (for example, the best way to recruit)

- Participants' perceptions of randomization (for example, thoughts of being in a control group)

- Retention of participants (for example, strategies to stay in contact with participants)

- Compensation (for example, the amounts or the type that are appropriate)

- Logistical issues (for example, the most convenient time to have the HPP)

Given the time and resources involved in developing an HPP, it would be judicious to conduct some qualitative research to ensure that the program will be well received and that the research to evaluate it can be conducted successfully. For example, Salazar, Holtgrave, Crosby, Frew, and Peterson (2005) conducted a qualitative research study to examine attitudes and beliefs about obtaining a hypothetical HIV/AIDS vaccine (in this instance, the vaccine would be considered an HPP) among men who have sex with men (MSM). The purpose of the research was to understand their perceptions of and opinions about vaccination, given the commercial availability of an HIV/AIDS vaccine, and also to understand the salient issues critical to their decision-making process. Because as of this writing several HIV vaccines are undergoing Phase II and Phase III clinical trials, understanding the barriers to and facilitators toward getting vaccinated is necessary to ensure widespread uptake of a vaccine that may be approved in the future. For a vaccine to truly protect people, there must be widespread acceptance of the vaccine. Limited motivation to obtain vaccination would have a great impact on the success of a vaccine program. Therefore the qualitative inquiry was conducted with 24 MSM to better understand their motivation to participate in an HIV/AIDS vaccine program. The interviews were transcribed and analyzed. The main issues that emerged from the data are shown in Table 8.2.

Numerous studies have been conducted that have examined patient characteristics such as race, marital status, and age as influencers of enrollment in cancer trials (Roberts, 2002); other studies have examined barriers to participation such as concerns with the trial setting, a dislike of randomization, general discomfort with the research process, complexity and stringency of the protocol, presence of a placebo or no-treatment group, and potential side effects (see Mills et al., 2006). Although these studies have provided much-needed information that is helpful for researchers implementing a randomized controlled trial (RCT) of cancer treatments, Roberts (2002) felt that a clear understanding of how trials were being presented to potential volunteers was lacking. Roberts wanted to understand the process that oncologists went through in their presentation of options to potential study volunteers. In other words, she wanted to know what type of information was being presented as well as how it was being presented. She audiotaped interactions between oncologists and their patients who had been diagnosed with breast cancer. The interaction represented the communication between the oncologists and their patients as they discussed the patient's options for adjuvant therapy. She analyzed the transcripts and found much variation in the way oncologists presented information regarding the clinical trial option. Her qualitative analysis suggests that differences in the way physicians present information for the same clinical trial can lead to differential response rates. This information could not have been gleaned using a quantitative mode of inquiry.

When implementing an RCT, it is just as important to understand the potential volunteer's perspective as it is to understand the physician's

Table 8.2   Emergent Themes Related to Getting a Future HIV/AIDS Vaccine

Factors and Description	Illustration
Knowledge Factors	
Vaccine strategy	"Is it made with a piece of the HIV virus?"
	"Do they actually inject you with HIV?"
	"What symptoms or damage would it prevent?"
Clinical trial research	"First of all that it's solid and that it works 100 percent."
	"Very little side effects where it would not affect our daily lives."
	"How many people were in the study; what was the make of the study as far as males, females; different ethnic groups; what were their sexual practices, were they straight or gay (sexual orientation); and how long did the study last?"
	"How does this drug work on different ethnic groups?"
Vaccine attributes	"We have to realize that medicine costs money, and our health has an economic consequence."
	"Is it something that I would only need to take once?"
	"Can it be put into a pill?"
	"I'd like to know who sponsored it and who stands to make a profit."
	"Does the vaccine have FDA approval?"
Racial differences	"It makes a big difference to me if it was tested in Acorra, Cameroon, where it's all Black people, with a high HIV percentage rate, or if it was tested on White gay males in Chelsea, in New York."
Encouraging Factors	
Knowledge about AIDS vaccine	"I would be cool with it if there were no side effects."
Perceived high risk	"If I were dating someone who was HIV positive, I may take the vaccine."
Cost	"If all the research states that it works fine, no adverse reactions, I don't see why I would not take it as long as I could afford it."
Discouraging Factors	
Harsh side effects	"I can't really think of a reason why I would not want to take this vaccine other than side effects that would affect my body that would stifle my daily progress or my daily functions in my life."
Low perceived risk	"If I have sex, which might be rarely, it is safe sex and I don't put myself in the situation where I would need the vaccine."
Backlash effect	"Because our people take it and think 'Oh God, it's a cure and let me go throw my rubbers away, I can get back out there and do whatever I want.'"
Cost prohibitive	"Something that was really expensive . . . like $1,500 or $5,000."

perspective. How do certain people perceive the details of participating in a trial? Knowing and understanding this viewpoint may provide information needed to ensure adequate enrollment and reduce participation bias. Moreover, ethical guidelines stipulate that patients who participate must be adequately informed, but how do you gauge or measure whether participants have been adequately informed? Not surprisingly, we advocate that qualitative research methods are an appropriate way to answer some of these methodological and ethical questions.

Because qualitative research is about the process, it is also helpful to use during the implementation of the RCT and afterward so that the researchers can better understand how the health promotion intervention worked. What activities resonated to the participants, and what activities did not? Why did the participants change their attitudes or alter their behavior? If the program was not effective, then why did participants think it didn't work? What was it about the intervention that evoked the observed changes? Even if the program was effective, what did they like about it? All of these questions could be asked of the participants, and their responses could reveal patterns that would give researchers a much more in-depth understanding of their intervention. In fact, an entire textbook has been dedicated to describing various process evaluations that have used qualitative methods and strategies for answering many of these questions (see Steckler and Linnan, 2002). Clearly, it is critical to know whether the program worked, but equally important is to know why and how it worked. Incorporating a qualitative approach into an evaluation will help to supplement, validate, explain, and illuminate or possibly reinterpret the quantitative data gathered from the participants. The result will be more comprehensive and have a multidimensionality that could not otherwise have been achieved without triangulation (Miles and Huberman, 1994).

IN A NUTSHELL

Incorporating a qualitative approach into an evaluation will help to supplement, validate, explain, and illuminate or possibly reinterpret the quantitative data gathered from the participants.

As an Alternative Method When Other Methods Are Precluded

In certain jurisdictions of the United States there are laws that restrict the type and nature of educational programs and subsequent inquiries to evaluate those programs. For example, the state of Louisiana dictates the type of sex education programs that can be implemented in the schools and proscribes the nature of questions students can be asked. For health promotion researchers who are interested in prevention of pregnancy and STDs among adolescents in Louisiana, not only must they adhere to abstinence-only education, but they also must restrict their evaluations of these programs to content other than sexual beliefs and behavior.

Clearly, this presents a challenge to program evaluators who are seeking to determine the effectiveness of abstinence-only educational programs in this jurisdiction. Thus alternative ways of investigating students' experiences with the program must be devised. Of course, this legislation does not preclude the use of surveys or quantitative instruments per se; however, it does limit to a large degree what can be surveyed. One alternative in this instance would be for program evaluators to query participants about their experiences with the program and what value the program had for them. Yoo, Johnson, Rice, and Manuel (2004) took this approach when they conducted a qualitative evaluation of a sexual abstinence program implemented in southern Louisiana. Researchers conducted semistructured interviews with principals, teachers, and peer mentors and facilitated eight gender-stratified focus groups of students who had participated in the program. By using qualitative methods, Yoo et al. were able to garner "valuable insights for future improvement in abstinence-only programs" (p. 329). For example, they were able to learn that all respondents indicated that the program should be taught in lower grades (the program had been implemented in grades seven through nine) and that responses to the program were mixed: some felt it was of no value and some felt it provided needed information and skills (Yoo et al., 2004). It should be noted, however, that although this inquiry provided participants' opinions about the program and stayed within the boundaries of the law, it still does not provide a behavioral indication of program effectiveness.

As health promotion practitioners and researchers, we must always work within laws and follow policy guidelines as they pertain to program content and the research. In those instances when certain content cannot be measured or surveyed, a qualitative approach can provide an alternative to quantitative approaches and yield valuable information that would otherwise have been omitted.

Qualitative Research Strategies for Health Promotion Research

Up to this point, we have discussed the features of qualitative research and the instances in health promotion in which qualitative research is warranted; however, we haven't provided a clear discussion of the different types of qualitative research. Essentially, unlike quantitative research, qualitative research does not have specific designs per se; rather, qualitative research has varying strategies that can be thought of as different philosophical orientations providing a general direction for implementing the research. The research strategy can also be thought of as the "tool" for accomplishing a particular research task.

IN A NUTSHELL

Qualitative research does not have specific designs per se; rather, qualitative research has varying strategies that can be thought of as different philosophical orientations providing a general direction for implementing the research.

These various orientations have historical roots in different disciplines such as anthropology, philosophy, education, zoology, and sociology. The strategy selected is dictated largely by "the purpose of the study, nature of the research question, and the skills and resources available to the investigator" (Morse, 1994, p. 223).

Because qualitative strategies are too numerous to describe in great detail, we cover four basic strategies that can be useful for conducting qualitative research in health promotion. Morse (1994) has outlined these four basic qualitative strategies: (1) phenomenology, (2) ethnography, (3) grounded theory, and (4) ethnoscience. Each of these qualitative strategies offers "a particular and unique perspective that illuminates certain aspects of reality more easily than others and produces a type of results more suited for some applications than others" (Morse, 1994, p. 223). To illustrate the differences among these strategies, Morse used a hypothetical research scenario involving travelers arriving and departing at an airport. Her conceptualization of each strategy is presented in Table 8.3.

Note the differences among the strategies in the nature of the research question, recommended sample sizes, the types of results that could be gleaned, and the types of qualitative methods appropriate for the research question. As we go through each of the strategies in more detail, it may be helpful to apply another hypothetical research example derived from health promotion. For example, a phenomenon that has been highlighted in the literature, sensationalized in the media, and persists is the notion of living on the "down low." The term "down low" has a negative connotation; it has been applied mostly to African-American men and refers to their maintaining an outwardly heterosexual lifestyle while also surreptitiously engaging in sexual intercourse with other men. Of course, this phenomenon is not unique to African-American men. There are also numerous examples of men of other races and ethnicities who also live double lives or remain in the closet for fear of social ostracism; however, men who have sex with other men represent the highest-risk population for HIV, which in turn may place their female partners at risk. Given that Blacks compose only 12 percent of the total U.S. population but 44 percent of new HIV infections in 2010 (Centers for Disease Control and Prevention, 2012), conducting qualitative research on the phenomenon of living on the down low may

Table 8.3 A Comparison of Strategies in the Conduct of a Hypothetical Project: "Arrivals and Departures: Patterns of Human Attachment"

Strategy	Research Question or Focus	Participants/Informants[a]	Sample Size[b]	Date Collection Methods	Type of Results
Phenomenology	What is the meaning of arriving home?	Travelers arriving home; phenomenological literature; art, poetry, and other descriptions	≈ 6 participants	In-depth conversations	In-depth reflective description of the experience of "what it feels like to come home"
Ethnography	What is the arrival gate like when an international plane arrives?	Travelers, families, others who observe the setting, such as skycaps, rental car personnel, cleaning staff, security guards, and so forth	≈ 30 to 50 interviews	Interviews; participant observation; other records, such as airport statistics	Description of the day-to-day events at the arrival gate of the airport
Grounded theory	Coming home: Reuniting the family	Travelers, family members	≈ 30 to 50	In-depth interviews: observations	Description of the social psychological process in the experience of returning home
Ethnoscience	What are types of travelers?	Those who observe the setting daily—skycaps, rental car personnel, cleaning staff, security guards, and so forth	≈ 30 to 50	Interviews to elicit similarities and differences of travelers, card sorts	Taxonomy and description of types and characteristics of travelers
Qualitative ethology	What are the greeting behaviors of travelers and their families?	Travelers and their families	Units—numbers of greetings—100 to 200	Photography, video, coded	Descriptions of the patterns of greeting behaviors

[a] Examples only.
[b] Number depends on saturation.

Source: From J. Morse (1994), "Designing Funded Qualitative Research," in N. K. Denzin and Y. S. Lincoln (Eds.), *Handbook of Qualitative Research*, Thousand Oaks, CA, Sage, p. 225. Copyright 1994 by Sage Publications, Inc. Reprinted with permission.

help researchers to understand African-American men's perspectives and perhaps devise programs or structural interventions that can lead to a reduction in gay-related stigma to eliminate men's feeling they have to live on the down low.

Phenomenology

Within an interpretivist paradigm, **phenomenology** refers to an analysis made by phenomenological investigation rather than the typological classification of a class of phenomena. Stemming from the discipline of philosophy, phenomenological investigations focus on interpreting "the meaning of events and interactions to ordinary people in particular situations" (Bogdan and Biklen, 1998, p. 23). The emphasis is on understanding the ways in which people construct their realities; that is, an attempt is made to reveal what perspective they hold and how they interpret events that happen. Phenomenology focuses on people's subjective experiences and interpretations of the world. That is, the phenomenologist wants to understand how the world appears to others.

phenomenology
philosophical discipline focused on the study of consciousness and the way in which one perceives and interprets events and one's relationship to them in terms of behavior

As a research strategy, phenomenology is subjective and relies heavily on trying to understand the participants' point of view. You may be wondering at this point: how can a research approach that is subjective also be considered as scientific research? As we have stated previously, quantitative modes of inquiry attempt to be objective, and it is that objectivity that serves as a gauge of methodological rigor. Conversely, in the phenomenological interpretivist approach, subjectivity is treated as "a topic for investigation in its own right, not as a methodological taboo" (Holstein and Gubrium, 1994, p. 264). So within this approach, subjectivity is the underlying mode and is embraced.

The method to accomplish phenomenological inquiries may be in-depth conversations and interviews with participants. For researchers using this strategy, however, gaining access to another person's point of view implies that in doing so the researcher may have some influence on the participant's perspective. Nonetheless, there is great utility in this approach, as it involves the collection of data that can provide an in-depth understanding of a phenomenon. Consequently, we may learn something that in turn may be useful for improving some aspect of the human condition. For example, Chiaranai (2013) conducted a phenomenological study with Thai heart patients to understand what it meant for them to live with chronic and debilitating illness. Interviews with participants revealed that they used religious and cultural beliefs, such as karma as a tool to rationalize the occurrence of their heart failure experience, and *kreng jai* as a cultural desire not to disrupt the happiness of others. These beliefs could affect these patients' quality of life if, for example, patients don't ask for help when they need it because they don't want to "disrupt the happiness of others."

Applying phenomenology to our example of men living on the down low would be very useful for gaining insight into the lives of these men. Our research question could be "What is the meaning of living a double life or on the down low?" and could be approached by engaging men in conversations about cultural and religious beliefs regarding sexual orientation, homosexuality, being an African-American man, how they view their lifestyle, and how they make sense of their lifestyle. Our emphasis would be on describing the structures (their opinions, values, beliefs, attitudes) of participants' reality that help to explain and interpret the meaning they have attached to their reality. In this example, one hypothetical result could be the following: "For African-American men living on the down low, their secretive behavior means keeping their families intact while fulfilling their sexual lives that makes them happy and ultimately a better husband or partner."

Ethnography

ethnography
a social scientific description of a people and their culture

Ethnography is a qualitative strategy that has its origins in cultural anthropology, the study of human beings in relation to their social interactions and culture. Derived from the Greek term *ethnos*, meaning a people, a race, or a cultural group, and the term *graphic*, meaning descriptive, ethnography is a systematic description of people and the cultural basis of their behaviors, attitudes, norms, and beliefs (Peacock, 1986). In this context, culture refers to the "acquired knowledge that people use to interpret experience and generate social behavior" (Spradley, 1979, p. 4). Culture is therefore relative and can be interpreted from more than one perspective, such as an outsider's or an insider's point of view. As a qualitative research strategy, ethnography focuses on providing a detailed and accurate description of values, behaviors, practices, and beliefs of a given group of people rather than explanation; however, the description should be in terms of the native's point of view rather than from the researcher's. Yet doing ethnography does not entail only studying people and observing their behavior; rather, the ethnographer must go beyond the gathering of observations and facts and learn what they mean. This experience requires researchers to immerse themselves in the culture under study and not only observe the behavior, artifacts, and emotions but also try to understand

IN A NUTSHELL

Because ethnography is also concerned with meaning, it is similar to phenomenology, but differs in that its purpose has a much greater scope and culture is the guiding framework used to interpret and attach meaning to the experiences.

the meaning attached to them from an insider's perspective. Because ethnography is also concerned with meaning, it is similar to phenomenology, but differs in that its purpose has a much greater scope and culture is the guiding framework used to interpret and attach meaning to the experiences.

To conduct ethnography, researchers should triangulate multiple data collection methods, such as naturalistic observation, interviews with key informants, gathering of artifacts, and examination of archival data. In this way, they can capture a full description of those aspects of culture that shape people's experiences, behavior, beliefs, and emotions. For example, Menard, Kobetz, Diem, Lifleur, Blanco, and Barton (2010) conducted an ethnographic study with Haitian women living in Miami about *twalet deba* (a Haitian feminine hygiene practice). *Twalet deba* is of concern because it could increase women's risk of STDs. Exploring the reasons Haitian women do *twalet deba* and the context in which these practices occur is important for developing HPPs. In Phase I of this study, researchers conducted participant observation (over a 2-year period) and interviews with key informants about gynecological health beliefs, hygiene practices, and home remedies used for these practices. In Phase II, researchers conducted observations at *botánicas* (Haitian health retail stores) and interviews with *botánica* owners and employees regarding the availability and use of ethnomedical remedies. Results from this study indicated that Haitian women's beliefs about gynecological health and sexual pleasure were powerful motivators for regularly engaging in feminine hygiene practices that increase a woman's vaginal dryness and tightness, while also increasing their risk for STDs. Menard et al. described the use of ethnographic methods as "critical for collecting personal sensitive data that are necessary to inform future intervention" (2010).

Getting back to our hypothetical example, if we were to apply ethnography to the study of men living on the down low, we would be interested in describing what life is like for men who live this way. In this situation, we might have to enlist the assistance of an informant, someone who could be a source of information to help communicate knowledge regarding the experience and serve as a teacher to the researcher. We could conduct interviews with men and perhaps locate venues where they may go to meet other men, while observing and taking notes. We would also want to consider interviewing other relevant participants such as a wife or girlfriend or other members of the community, who may play a cultural role in this lifestyle. We would attempt to describe their lives in relation to the culture in which they are embedded. This attempt at description involves a translation process, which entails "discovering the meanings of one culture and communicating these meanings to people in another culture" (Spradley, 1979, p. 205). In this example, one hypothetical result could be something like the following:

> African American men, who live on the down low, view being gay as religiously immoral and also as detrimental to a person's standing in the community—as many people in the African American community support the view that homosexuality is a sin and taboo, and gay men are viewed as being less than men. They do not describe themselves as gay, as this would contradict their notion of male identity and upset their lives and their families' lives. Instead, personal and social self-preservation requires that they adhere to the cultural norm of heterosexuality. Thus they fulfill their need for male sexual contact in secret. They justify this behavior by saying it is only an indulgence in male fantasy; it is not a betrayal nor is it hurtful to their wives, because they are not sleeping with other women.

Grounded Theory

grounded theory
a general methodology for deriving a theory or theories from data systematically gathered and analyzed

Essentially, **grounded theory** is a general methodology for deriving a theory or theories from data systematically gathered and analyzed (Strauss and Corbin, 1994). Grounded theory has been described as a marriage between positivism and interpretivism. First conceptualized as a strategy by two sociologists, Glaser and Strauss (1967), grounded theory is best used for understanding phenomenal processes (Morse, 1994). By processes, we mean that what is being studied or understood is dynamic and may entail stages or phases but may also involve "reciprocal changes in patterns of action-interaction and in relationship with changes of conditions either internal or external to the process itself" (Strauss and Corbin, 1994, p. 278). Because theory development is the main focus of this qualitative strategy, it differs in its central purpose from other qualitative strategies in which meaning and describing are the core purposes. The brilliance of this qualitative approach lies in its logic: explicitly link empirical data to the creation and elaboration of a theory. As you may recall from Chapter Two, we stated that intuition, previous knowledge, or Baconian inductivism were ways in which theory can be developed. Although similar in concept to Baconian inductivism, grounded theory is a unique and superior way in which theory development should be approached—through research. "A theory is not the formulation of some discovered aspect of a preexisting reality 'out there' . . . rather theories are interpretations made from given perspectives as adopted or researched by researchers" (Strauss and Corbin, 1994, p. 279).

To use grounded theory as your approach, you must gather and analyze data in a systematic way; hence grounded theory possesses some features of positivism. The system entails an iterative process sometimes referred to as constant comparative analysis, in which first data are used to generate a theory and then subsequent data are compared against the initial theory. At the beginning of the process, an assumption is made that the initial theory will be provisional; if necessary, changes and modifications can be made as new data are generated and analyzed and new patterns and themes emerge. Key to this process is the use of multiple perspectives when gathering and analyzing the data. If you refer back to Table 8.2, note that approximately 30 to 50 participants are recommended when undertaking this approach. Moreover, when using this approach researchers should distinguish the type of theory they are trying to develop. Substantive theory, which is derived from research in one substantive area (for example, short-term and ongoing psychosocial reactions to herpes diagnosis), and formal theory, which is more general and has broader applications (such as social cognitive theory), are the two overarching categories of theories. The former typically serves as a springboard to the development of the latter. Both types of theories can be developed using grounded theory; however, the approach is better suited to the development of substantive theory.

For example, Canales and Geller (2004) conducted a grounded theory study in which they examined mammography decision making across the breast cancer screening continuum: women who consistently got yearly mammograms, women who were inconsistent or failed to get a mammogram, and breast cancer survivors. They were able to develop a theory titled "Moving in Between Mammography," which described the decision-making process and identified several factors that influenced their behavior (Canales and Geller, 2004). Applying a grounded theory strategy to our hypothetical example, we could use this strategy to develop a psychosocial theory that attempts to explain the psychological, psychosocial, and sociocultural factors that influence the behavior of men on the down low. Using Canales and Geller's theory as inspiration, we could title our theory, "Between Straight and Gay," and potential influencers could be impulsivity, risk-taking, social anxiety, cultural norms, social support, and religiosity.

Ethnoscience

Ethnoscience is related to cognitive anthropology and strives to understand how people understand and organize their own reality. Ethnoscience

ethnoscience
a discipline, closely related to cognitive anthropology, that focuses on the relationship between human culture and human knowledge, cognitions, and perceptions

goes beyond studying the behavior of a particular culture by attempting to identify the culturally derived classification systems that people use to make sense of their reality. Each person's classification system comprises cognitive categories that provide some order and understanding to life experiences. The main objective of an ethnoscience inquiry is to reliably represent these cognitive categories; that is, to reveal a cogent classification system used by people to process and understand behavior, events, emotions, and things—a taxonomy of sorts. Each culture has its own indigenous classification system. Consequently, people from different cultures have markedly different perceptions of any given set of behaviors, events, emotions, or things. Bottorff et al. (1998) conducted a qualitative ethnoscience study to examine the breast health practices of South Asian women living in Canada. They conducted in-depth interviews with 50 women, which were analyzed and used to develop a taxonomy that represented relationships among emerging cultural themes and domains. They found that women held four central beliefs regarding breast health practices, ranging from beliefs about taking care of their breasts to beliefs about accessing services.

IN A NUTSHELL

Each culture has its own indigenous classification system. Consequently, people from different cultures have markedly different perceptions of any given set of behaviors, events, emotions, or things.

In our hypothetical example, an ethnoscience study would focus on developing a reliable classification system that the men use to explain their lifestyle. A taxonomy could be developed that would classify men according to their underlying cultural beliefs. An example of this taxonomy could be several domains of beliefs that represent the explanations of their lifestyle choice, such as "cultural taboos against being gay," "homophobia," and "endorsement of the sexual double standard for men that permits promiscuity and adultery."

Qualitative Data-Collection Methods for Health Promotion Research

As we have described four main qualitative strategies, you may have noted that each strategy was associated with a particular data-collection method or methods. Primary data-collection methods can include observations and in-depth interviews as well as personal and official documents, photographs, recordings, drawings, e-mails, and informal conversations. For example, in Table 8.3, phenomenology was associated with in-depth conversations, whereas grounded theory used in-depth interviews and observations. Thus the strategy selected by the investigator is connected to a specific method for data collection (Sterk and Elifson, 2004). In this section, we describe and discuss two data-collection methods widely used to conduct qualitative inquiries: interviewing (whether one-on-one or in focus groups) and participant observation. The advantages and disadvantages of each method are highlighted in Table 8.4.

Interviewing

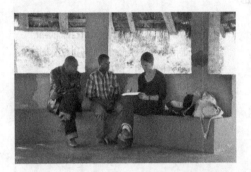

Figure 8.2   Volunteer for NGO Conducting a Field Interview
Source: Photo courtesy of Jeff Walker/CIFOR licensed under BY-NC-ND 2.0. https://creativecommons.org/licenses/by-nc-nd/2.0/.

In general, interviewing can take several different forms, ranging from unstructured to structured, and may involve interviewing an individual, a dyad, or a group (that is, a focus group). The first form of interviewing we will discuss is the **unstructured interview**, which can be thought of more as an informal conversation than a formal interview (as depicted in Figure 8.2). When using this method, there are no specific questions asked; rather, topics emerge and flow from the conversation. Of course, the interviewer must prepare a plan to discuss certain general topics related to the research; however, the process is provisional in that certain topics may not get discussed and there is no set order to the discussion (Babbie, 2004). This form of interview is used frequently in phenomenological investigations or other inquiries in which the investigator is interested in understanding the meaning behind participants' experiences, events, practices, or behavior. It would be difficult to construct specific questions a priori.

The goal of this type of interview is to explore and to probe the interviewee's responses so that an in-depth understanding of the phenomena can be reached. This process places a major emphasis on the details of the interviewee's life experiences and social behavior. The interviewer attempts to engage the interviewee in conversation about the interviewee's attitudes, interests, feelings, concerns, and values as these relate to the research topic. Because this interview is an interaction, the interviewer and the interviewee jointly construct meaning; meaning is rarely revealed as an epiphany by the interviewee, although it may happen. A skilled interviewer allows participants to describe their experiences and explore their thoughts and opinions

unstructured interview
a conversational interviewing method in which no specific questions are asked, but topics emerge and flow from the conversation

Table 8.4 The Pros and Cons of Data Collection Methods

Pros	Cons
Interviews	
Allows for clarification	Reactive effect: interviewer's presence and characteristics may bias results
High response rate	Expensive
Able to gather in-depth information and pursue hunches	Requires strong interviewing skills
Can tailor the line of discussion to the individual	Slowest method of data collection and analysis
Easier to reach those who are considered unreachable (the poor, homeless, high status, mobile, etc.)	Responses may be less honest and thoughtful
May be easier to reach specific individuals	Interviewer should go to location of respondent
More personalized approach	Respondents who prefer anonymity may be inhibited by personal approach
Easier to ask open-ended questions, use probes, and pick up on nonverbal cues	May reach only a smaller sample
	Difficult to analyze and quantify results
Focus Groups	
Generate fresh ideas	Moderately time consuming
Allows clarification	Moderately expensive
Efficiency of getting information from a number of people	Subject interpretation
Provides immediate sharing and synthesis	High cost per participant
Works well with special participants	Lack of confidentiality
Less expensive and faster than personal interviews	Respondents who prefer anonymity may be inhibited by personal approach
Personalized approach	Input may be unbalanced because some group members dominate
Group members stimulate each other	Group members and interviewer can bias responses
	May be difficult to analyze or quantify data
Observations	
Setting is natural, flexible, and unstructured	Requires skilled observer
Evaluator may make his/her identity known or remain anonymous	The evaluator has less control over the situation in a natural environment
Evaluator may actively participate or observe passively	Hawthorne effect—if group is aware that they are being observed, resulting behavior may be affected
Can be combined with a variety of other data collection methods	Observations cannot be generalized to entire population unless a plan for representativeness is developed
Generates relevant, quantifiable data	If observer chooses to be involved in the activity, he/she may lose objectivity
Most useful for studying a "small unit" such as a classroom, coffee shop, or clinic waiting room	Not realistic for use with large groups

about the research topic. Because of this dynamic, it is critical that the interviewer try to establish rapport with the participant and create a sense of trust; however, building trust and establishing a respectful relationship in which the interviewee feels comfortable may be affected by other issues, such as gender and race, which may play a role in this process (Fontana and Frey, 1994).

In conducting this type of interview, interviewees should be given a considerable amount of latitude to expand on the topics because it is they who are "knowledgeable, have a meaningful perspective to offer, and are able to make this explicit in their own words" (Sterk and Elifson, 2004, p. 137). It truly is a conversation taking place between the interviewer, who is an active participant, and the interviewee. Although there is a predetermined topic of interest, the conversation or interview should be viewed as spontaneous and unstructured. A caveat must be stated, however. Even though the interview should be viewed as a conversation, the interviewer must focus on listening to the interviewee. Rather than trying to appear to be interested, the interviewer should be genuinely invested in what the interviewee has to say (Babbie, 2004). In fact, Lofland and Lofland (1995) recommend adopting the role of the "socially acceptable incompetent" (p. 56) when interviewing, as the interviewer may appear "ignorant" and is trying to learn as much as he or she can about the culture or topic in question.

It is prudent to begin the conversation with less sensitive, benign topics and then gradually ease the conversation toward more sensitive and complex issues. For example, if a researcher were to have a "conversation" with a man who lives on the down low, he or she would want to start the conversation with a discussion of what it is like to be an African-American man in today's society, what his experiences were growing up, and what life is like for him in the present. Because this is a highly personal and sensitive topic, it might be best, if possible, to match the interviewer's gender and race with those of the interviewee (for example, male and African American). This matching may facilitate the establishment of rapport. Once trust has been established (this could take from several hours to perhaps several interview sessions over the course of several days), the conversation could be steered toward more sensitive topics such as sexual behavior.

During the interview or the conversation, it is also beneficial if the interviewer is cognizant of any responses that would allow for more in-depth probing. **Probing** takes many forms, but basically entails an effort on the part of the interviewer, either verbally or nonverbally, to elicit more details, to guide the dialogue, to iterate the meaning of something said by the interviewee, or to allow the interviewee to feel comfortable in preparing his or her response. Probes perform these functions while also allowing the interviewer to establish a relationship with the interviewee and indicate

probing
an interviewing technique in which the interviewer uses verbal or nonverbal communication in order to collect more information or make the interviewee more comfortable

IN A NUTSHELL

Probing takes many forms, but basically entails the interviewer's effort either verbally or nonverbally to elicit more details, to guide the dialogue, to iterate the meaning of something said by the interviewee, or to allow the interviewee to feel comfortable in preparing his or her response.

the desire to understand what the interviewee is saying (Fontana and Frey, 1994). For example, the interviewer could ask a directive question such as "Could you tell me a little more about that?" The interviewer could also use the echo probe, in which he or she paraphrases what the interviewee has just said. This indicates to the interviewee that the interviewer is listening to what he is saying. The interviewer could also simply use comments such as "Uh-huh," "I see," "Yes," or "Mm." Nonverbal probes are also effective; these include nods of the head or simply remaining silent to give the interviewee time to reflect or prepare his next thought. In any event, the function of the probes is to motivate the participant to communicate more fully and to help him focus on the general topics while keeping the communication flowing.

semistructured interview

an interview method that uses a series of open-ended questions that are typically asked of all participants in a predetermined order

A more structured type of interview than the unstructured interview is the **semistructured interview**, which uses open-ended questions that are typically asked of all participants in a predetermined order. The questions are considered directive and are used to ascertain specific topics related to the research. The interviewer should read the question exactly as it is worded to avoid changing the intent of the question in addition to asking all of the questions that apply. Although the interviewer is encouraged to use probes, the probes should be as neutral as possible to avoid introducing bias into the process. For example, if the interviewer asks a question and the participant says, "I don't know," or "I am not sure," one type of neutral probe, called a "clarification probe," that could be used in this instance is, "There are no right or wrong answers to these questions; we are only interested in finding out how you feel about this."

Although there is more structure to this form of interview, the open-ended questions still allow the participant to elaborate and provide significant details on his or her experiences. Thus this type of interview is well-suited for grounded theory and ethnography, when little is known about a certain issue but the research question has a definite direction. For instance, semistructured interviews were used in a study of fourteen Mexican and Mexican-American women living at a shelter for battered women. The study sought to describe the barriers experienced by these women when attempting to negotiate condom use with their abusive partners. Several questions from the semistructured interview guide were: Tell me what you know about HIV/AIDS. What can a person do to keep from getting HIV/AIDS? What do you do to keep from getting HIV/AIDS? Tell me what you think or know that is good about condoms. How does your partner respond when you ask him to use a condom? Themes of physical, psychological, and sexual abuse of the women who requested condom use emerged, as did the influence of power and control exerted over their public, private, and sexual interactions (Davila and Brackley, 1999). As another example, imagine that you are conducting an evaluation of a family planning program in India. As part of the program, nurses received training on family planning counseling and IUD insertion techniques. So you design a study in which you use semistructured interviews to investigate whether and how the capacity to provide IUD services has changed since the training and to determine the barriers experienced by nurses when providing family planning services. An example of a semistructured interview guide that could be used in the study is presented in Box 8.3.

BOX 8.3. SEMISTRUCTURED INTERVIEW GUIDE FOR FAMILY PLANNING PROGRAM EVALUATION

1. What are some of the concerns or misconceptions that you hear from your patients regarding the IUD as a method of contraception?

2. In what situations do you recommend IUDs to your patients?

3. In what situations do you avoid recommending IUDs to your patients?

4. Since your IUD insertion training, what has prevented you from inserting IUDs?

5. In what way did the IUD training prepare you to solve or prevent clinical difficulties when inserting or removing IUDs?

6. In the past 12 months, have you experienced any challenges with stock out issues for any contraceptive methods at your clinic?

7. What have you done in situations where a contraceptive method is not available?

8. In the past 12 months, what are some of the new family planning initiatives you have seen implemented at your clinic? (For example: changes in schedules, new publicity, educational information.)

9. In your opinion, what measures have improved the satisfaction of patients?

10. What measures have helped you do your work more effectively?

11. What changes can still be made to improve the quality of the family planning services at your clinic?

12. What support do you receive from the clinic leadership with regards to family planning services?

Focus Groups

focus group

an interviewing method in which the interviewer interviews a small group of people at the same time; typically, it involves a homogeneous group of strangers

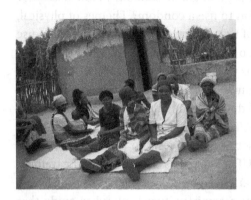

Figure 8.3   A Focus Group

When the interviewer interviews a small group of people at the same time, it is termed a **focus group**. Focus groups typically involve between 6 and 12 individuals (on average 8) who are a homogeneous group, but who do not usually know each other (for an example, see Figure 8.3). A homogeneous group is one in which participants have similar characteristics that are chosen based on the research question, such as gender, age range, socioeconomic status, education level, or race/ethnicity. The size will depend on the research topic, the age of the participants, and how detailed the discussion needs to be. With too few participants, you may not be able to generate a good discussion or have diverse opinions; with too many, the discussion may be difficult to manage. Participants for the focus group should clearly be chosen on the basis of the research topic. For example, if we were to conduct a qualitative inquiry as formative research to designing an health promotion program to prevent teen alcohol and drug use, we would choose participants for the focus group that were similar in age, gender, and ethnicity to the targeted intervention population. Recruiting for focus groups typically involves using nonprobability techniques such as convenience sampling (see Chapter Six). Although the results may not be generalizable, they can still provide very useful information. In contrast to the one-on-one interview, the emphasis of the focus group is not necessarily on each participant's individual experiences, beliefs, and attitudes; rather, it is the interaction between participants that is of interest to the investigator.

Focus groups have been used extensively in advertising and marketing research, in which researchers have gathered information about new product ideas, name changes to existing products, or customers' opinions about existing products (Brilhart and Galanes, 1998). In health promotion, focus groups are used quite frequently to provide information about interventions, salient health issues, or health care needs; to identify interests, topics, or concerns of the targeted population; or to develop new scale measures. Focus groups can be unstructured, with the moderator—the person facilitating and conducting the focus group—announcing the topic to be discussed and allowing the participants to respond freely. This should entail participants presenting their own views and then also responding to the views expressed by the other group members. Focus groups can also be semistructured, with the moderator using a guide to cover questions and specific topics presented in some order.

Depending on the topic, there are instances in which the group should be stratified by gender, age, or some other relevant characteristic. For example, Cameron et al. (2005) conducted four online focus groups (similar in structure to a regular focus group; however, online focus groups are conducted in a chat room via the Internet) with internet-using teens to discover their experiences with, exposure to, and perceptions of sexually oriented websites and sexually explicit websites. Because of the sensitive nature of the topic, the researchers stratified each group by gender and age to ensure that participants felt comfortable responding to sex-related content and to ensure that the topics presented were developmentally appropriate.

One advantage of using a group interview as opposed to conducting individual interviews is the group dynamic. People reacting to each other tend to create a synergy that is much greater than what could be created on an individual basis. Thus the method is synergistic and holds the potential for generating additional topics and information that might otherwise have been missed. Other advantages include its flexibility, low cost, and speedy results (Krueger, 1988). Yet there are some disadvantages. At times, there may be one group member who tends to dominate the conversation or who may intimidate other group members. This is a difficult situation that must be addressed skillfully by a trained moderator. Clearly, because there is the group dynamic, the moderator has less control of the situation as compared with individual interviews. There is also the issue of confidentiality. The moderator can assure the participants that whatever is discussed "within the group stays within the group," but the same cannot be said for the participants. If the topic is sensitive, then precautions should be taken, such as having participants agree to maintain confidentiality in the informed consent form and also agree to explicit protocol guidelines before the focus group begins (Sterk and Elifson, 2004).

Whether the interviews are semistructured or unstructured, or conducted with an individual or with a group, there are some basic issues for the qualitative researcher to consider. For example, how many participants or focus groups should be conducted? Table 8.3 provides some general guidelines for sample size depending on the research question and the strategy; however, most qualitative researchers agree that these are meant as guidelines and should not be used in the same manner as sample size estimation performed in power analyses. Essentially, the number of participants or the number of focus groups is sufficient when the selected participants represent the range of potential participants in the setting, and at the point at which the data gathered begins to be redundant—that is, when consistent themes are repeated. This latter point of data redundancy and repetition is also referred to as data saturation. It is at this point that the investigator should feel confident in knowing that an adequate sample size has been reached or a sufficient number of focus groups has been conducted.

All interviews and focus groups conducted should be audio recorded with the permission of the interviewee(s). Of course, audio recording or, in some instances, video recording interviews does not preclude the interviewer from taking notes during the interview or writing notes after the interview. Once the interview or focus group is completed, the audio recording can be transcribed verbatim to begin the process of data analysis. In fact, we recommend having a note-taker during an interview or focus group so that the interviewer or moderator can concentrate their attention on the participants. Also, notes have proven to be very important if there are technical difficulties. In many cases the notes can become your data! To help you when conducting interviews, in Box 8.4 we provide a summary of some basic ground rules that can be useful whether you are conducting a one-on-one or a focus group.

BOX 8.4. GROUND RULES FOR INTERVIEWING

- Greet the respondent at the beginning of the interview in a culturally appropriate manner.
- Explain the purpose of the interview and obtain informed consent.
- Explain how the information will be recorded. Ask for permission to audio record or video record the session if you plan to do so.
- Arrange comfortable seating to facilitate communication.
- Start with a topic that is not sensitive and is important to the respondent. This helps create an informal, friendly atmosphere, facilitating a natural flow of ideas and opinions.
- Be an active listener; look at your informant's face (not at your interview guide), and always behave in a culturally sensitive way.
- Pick up phrases that the informant uses and use these to phrase your questions.
- Avoid giving opinions or judgments about what the informant says, and treat her as an equal.
- Jokes, or friendly gestures toward any small children present can help break the ice.
- Use open-ended questions rather than closed ones that allow for only "yes" or "no" answers.
- Avoid asking leading questions.

- Follow the flow of the discussion, but make sure that all the topics are covered.

- Ask probing questions to clarify points or to encourage more explanation.

- Respond to any issues raised by your informants that are not on your interview guide, and probe on these as well.

- Thank the informant at the end and give her time to ask more questions.

Source: World Health Organization.

Observation

To emphasize the importance of observation as a research method to the overall research enterprise, one need mention only one name—Charles Darwin. His meticulous attention to detail, copious notes, and commitment to extended and lengthy periods of observation resulted in his formalization of a biological theory of evolution, with his assertion that natural selection was the main underlying mechanism. Needless to say, the impact of his research on science, society, religion, education, and politics is immeasurable, and his work is considered by many as scientifically revolutionary. Yet interestingly, rather than study his subjects under controlled settings using manipulation and randomization, Darwin's research method was naturalistic observation. Clearly, observation as a scientific method has great utility. In addition to generating new theories, observation can be used to supplement other data-collection methods, such as interviews, to provide an expanded understanding of some phenomenon or to provide "insight into the social context in which people operate" (Sterk and Elifson, 2004, p. 142).

Participant observation is a specific type of naturalistic observation in which the researcher observes people in their own setting. To do this, however, the investigator must first identify an appropriate setting and then gain access to that setting. Whether the setting is public or private, there typically is some gatekeeper, a person with the power and authority to control access, with whom the investigator should negotiate to gain access. For public settings, identifying a gatekeeper may be more difficult, or one may not exist. The investigator must also consider the ethics of observing people who are in the public realm without their informed consent. For example, how would you feel if you were out at a coffee shop or at a bar with your friends and you happen to notice a person sitting off in the corner taking notes and watching what you and your friends did? We are not contending that observing people in a public setting is unethical or wrong.

participant observation
a type of naturalistic observation in which researchers enter the world of the people they want to study

Table 8.5   Potential Roles of Investigators Conducting Observations

Type of Participation Observation	Level of Involvement	Limitations
Complete Participant	Role of researcher covert; high level of integration with population	Loss of objectivity; potentially biased results; ethical considerations
Participant as Observer	Role of research overt; high level of integration with population	Loss of objectivity; potentially biased results due to observer effects
Observer as Participant	Role of researcher overt; low level of integration with population	High degree of objectivity; potential loss of perspective when interpreting results
Complete Observer	No integration with population; can directly or indirectly observe setting	High degree of objectivity; substantial loss of perspective when interpreting results

complete participant

role in which the researcher behaves as though his role is that of a participant rather than a researcher

participant as observer

role in which the investigator identifies as a researcher while interacting with the participants in the social process

observer as participant

role in which the investigator identifies as a researcher but enters the social setting periodically for brief periods to conduct the observations

In fact, many sociological and anthropological studies of public settings have been conducted in this way (for example, Lofland, 1973; McCoy et al., 1996; Monaghan, 2002; Tewksbury, 2002); however, there are other important issues to consider, and these issues must be weighed against the importance of the research and the balance of ethics and methodological rigor. For example, the investigator must decide what role he will adopt when making observations and whether or not to be covert or overt. Gold (1958) outlined four potential roles, moving from the more involved and covert to the completely detached and overt. These roles are listed in Table 8.5.

The first role is that of the **complete participant**, with the researcher acting not as the researcher, but more as a participant. It is considered covert because participants in the setting do not realize this person is researching them. Acting in the role of a participant may also raise methodological problems because the investigator interacts with the participants, which may have an effect on the dynamics of the setting, the participants' behavior, or both. Because of these considerations (ethical and scientific), the decision to adopt the role of the complete participant should be well justified.

In other instances, it may be practical to adopt the second role, that of the **participant as observer**, in which the investigator is overt, in that he identifies as a researcher while interacting with the participants in the social process. This role avoids some of the ethical issues in the complete participant role, but some of the methodological issues remain; for instance, observer effects. The advantage of both roles is they provide a unique insider's perspective that assists in the interpretation of what is being observed.

The third role is that of the **observer as participant**, in which the investigator's main role is that of the observer. She identifies as a researcher but enters the setting periodically and for brief periods of time to conduct the observations. In this role, the ethical issues are rectified; however, because of the higher level of detachment than in the first two roles and the lack of involvement in the setting and with the participants, it may be more difficult to garner the perspective of the participants and provide accurate interpretation to the observations.

Finally, the fourth role is that of the **complete observer**, in which the researcher observes the social process without ever becoming a part of it. In this role there is some variation in the level of detachment. Observations can be made directly by researchers as they passively observe the setting, or in some instances researchers may remain completely outside of the setting. In this instance, they may opt to use equipment such as video recorders to make the observations. This role is more along the lines of an "objective" researcher, with ethical issues and observer effects minimized; however, the researcher does not have the benefit of understanding from the perspective of an insider. Thus he may not interpret the findings in a way that accurately captures the participants' perspectives. The complete-observer role is more suited to qualitative ethology, in which the participants' perspectives are not the main focus of the inquiry.

complete observer
role in which the researcher observes the social process without becoming part of it

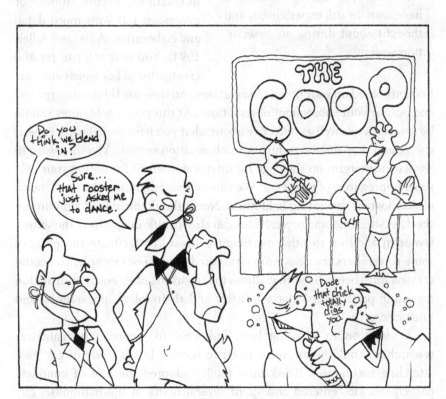

Mincus and Dincus as "Complete Participants" for Their Chicken Study

Once the researcher has identified the setting, gained access, and worked through the issues of what role to adopt, it is time to begin observing. How, what, and when you record your observations depend on the nature of the study, whether or not there is freedom to take notes as the observations are being made, and the stage of the research process. Note taking is generally the mode used to record observations. The process of note taking can require some level of expertise and may be approached systematically. In the initial stage of the research process, observations should be more broad and descriptive. These initial observations serve as a guide to identify the key aspects of the setting, people, and behaviors that are of interest. This may involve unstructured note taking in a free form, with the researcher trying to home in on the most relevant aspects of what is going on and record not only the actual observation but also her interpretation of the observation (Babbie, 2004).

IN A NUTSHELL

Field notes should be descriptive as well as reflective about what you have seen, heard, experienced, and thought about during an observation session.

As the research progresses, the investigator may begin to narrow the focus and record observations of fewer people, interactions, events, times, or processes, but with more detail and elaboration (Adler and Adler, 1994). You may want to try and create a list of key words and participants based on your initial observations and then use this list to organize and outline your subsequent observations. At this point, field notes should be descriptive as well as reflective about what you have seen, heard, experienced, and thought about during an observation session. You may want to leave wide margins on the page for interpretations or for noting your personal impressions of the event. We cannot overemphasize the importance of detail when generating field notes. Notes should include at a minimum the date, site, time, and topic. Notes can also include diagrams of the setting layout in addition to other pertinent context. To facilitate the process, some researchers create a more structured guide. For example, you could create a form beforehand that allows the recording of essential information regarding participants' characteristics and their roles, appearances, and interactions.

In addition to knowing how and what to record, the qualitative researcher should be aware of when to record. In his study of gay men attending bathhouses, Tewksbury (2002) adopted the role of complete participant. He "entered and spent several hours in the bathhouse, circulated with and among patrons, and carefully observed others, their activities, movements, interactions, and the use of the physical features of the environment. Field notes were written during periodic retreats (usually every 10 to 15 minutes) to one of the private rooms available for rent to patrons" (pp. 84–85). Although it is recommended to take field notes while observing, in this instance, because of his covert role, Tewksbury was not at liberty to take field notes while he was observing. Moreover, even if it is possible to take notes while the events are occurring, it may not be feasible to observe everything, let alone record everything. To solve this problem, Spradley (1979) recommends using an approach that entails first making a condensed account of what occurs while it is occurring, followed up with an expanded account in which the researcher fills in the details that were not recorded on the spot. This approach ensures that relevant observations are not missed because of note taking. In addition, Spradley asserted that his "ability to recall events and conversations increased rapidly through the discipline of creating expanded accounts from condensed ones" (p. 75).

Many qualitative researchers also suggest maintaining a **fieldwork journal** that will assist later on in the data analysis and may become an important data source (Spradley, 1979). This process for recording thoughts and ideas is sometimes referred to as "memoing" and can provide a picture of how the study evolved. Similar to conducting interviews, field notes should be transcribed verbatim on a regular basis. Transcribing the field notes allows the researcher to begin the process of identifying preliminary themes and helps pinpoint the right time to end the study. As was the case with interview data, the study should be ended at the point of data saturation, when later themes and patterns are consistent with earlier findings and no new themes have emerged.

fieldwork journal
a journal the researcher uses to record feelings, reactions, ideas, fears, and problems that arise during the course of the study

Summary

This chapter is unique: it is the only chapter in this book that adopts the interpretivist perspective, which should be viewed as having great importance and relevance to health promotion research and practice. Qualitative research can address research questions that cannot be addressed by quantitative approaches. Because it is contextual, it provides a more thorough understanding of the phenomena that may be missed with a quantitative strategy. Furthermore, one of qualitative research's greatest strengths is that it can be used to generate testable hypotheses, theories, or both. Qualitative research encompasses varying strategies, uses multiple methods (in other words, triangulation), and involves data-collection methods that are integrated with the setting and the researcher. Qualitative data are descriptive and comprise text and images, so data analysis cannot be performed using standardized procedures and techniques; rather, the analysis is iterative, subjective, and subject to the researchers' professional intuition and views.

Like quantitative research, although there is no manipulation, the nature of qualitative research may still necessitate attention to certain ethical issues. Contrary to what some may believe (that qualitative research is "easier" than quantitative research), qualitative research involves a personal commitment and voluminous amounts of data; thus qualitative research may not be for the faint of heart. Nevertheless, qualitative research has contributed to the overall research enterprise in substantive ways and will continue to do so.

KEY TERMS

Complete observer	Naturalistic
Complete participant	Observer as participant
Contextualization	Paradigm
Data triangulation	Participant as observer
Emic	Participant observation
Ethnography	Phenomenology
Ethnoscience	Positivism
Fieldwork journal	Probing
Focus group	Semistructured interview
Grounded theory	Sequential triangulation
Inductive logic	Simultaneous triangulation
Interpretivist	Theoretical triangulation
Investigator triangulation	Triangulation
Method triangulation	Unstructured interview

For Practice and Discussion

1. Select one qualitative study that you have read this semester and discuss the strategy that was used, the research question, who the participants were, and the data collection mode. Identify the strengths or weaknesses of the study and make suggestions as to how you would improve the methods.

2. Formulate a research question that would be better addressed with a qualitative approach than a quantitative approach. Select the most appropriate research strategy, recruitment method, sample size, and

data collection technique(s) for your research question. Prepare a rationale that supports your choices.

3. Triangulation can serve multiple purposes. Discuss the benefits of triangulation and design a study that would benefit from utilizing several forms of triangulation. Provide details of how you would implement each type and the rationale for each.

4. Semistructured interview guides are typically used for focus groups. Pick a research topic of your choice that you could investigate with focus groups. Describe the research question and the targeted population and create a semistructured interview guide for the focus groups.

References

Adler, P. A., and Adler, P. (1994). Observational techniques. In N. K. Denzin and J. S. Lincoln (Eds.), *Handbook of qualitative research* (pp. 377–392). Thousand Oaks, CA: Sage.

Babbie, E. R. (2004). *The practice of social research* (10th ed.). Belmont, CA: Wadsworth.

Bogdan, R. C., and Biklen, S. K. (1998). *Qualitative research in education: An introduction to theory and methods* (3rd ed.). Boston: Allyn and Bacon.

Bottorff, J. L., Johnson, J. L., Bhagat, R., Grewal, S., Balneaves, L. G., Clarke, H., and Hilton, B. A. (1998). Beliefs related to breast health practices: The perceptions of South Asian women living in Canada. *Social Science & Medicine, 47*(12), 2075–2085.

Brilhart, J. K., and Galanes, G. J. (1998). *Effective group discussion* (9th ed.). Boston: McGraw-Hill.

Cameron, K. A., Salazar, L. F., Bernhardt, J. M., Burgess-Whitman, N., Wingood, G. M., and DiClemente, R. J. (2005). Adolescents' experience with sex on the Web: Results from online focus groups. *Journal of Adolescence, 28*, 535–540.

Canales, M. K., and Geller, B. M. (2004). Moving in between mammography: Screening decisions of American Indian women in Vermont. *Qualitative Health Research, 14*(6), 836–857.

Centers for Disease Control and Prevention. (2012). Estimated HIV incidence in the United States, 2007–2010. *HIV Surveillance Supplemental Report, 17*(4).

Chiaranai, C. (2013). A phenomenological study of day-to-day experiences of living with heart failure. *Journal of Cardiovascular Nursing.* doi:10.1097/jcn.0000000000000105

Colangelo, L., Domel, R., Kelly, L., Peirce, L., and Sullivan, C. (1999). Positivist and interpretivist schools: A comparison and contrast. Retrieved February 16, 2005, from www.edb.utexas.edu/faculty/scheurich/proj2/index.htm.

Davila, Y. R., and Brackley, M. H. (1999). Mexican and Mexican American women in a battered women's shelter: Barriers to condom negotiation for HIV/AIDS prevention. *Issues in Mental Health Nursing, 20*(4), 333–355.

Denzin, N. K. (1978). *The research act: A theoretical introduction to sociological methods* (2nd ed.). New York: McGraw-Hill.

Fontana, A., and Frey, J. H. (1994). Interviewing: The art of science. In N. K. Denzin and J. S. Lincoln (Eds.), *Handbook of qualitative research* (pp. 361–376). Thousand Oaks, CA: Sage.

Glaser, B. G., and Strauss, A. L. (1967). *The discovery of grounded theory: Strategies for qualitative research.* Chicago: Aldine.

Glesne, C., and Peshkin, A. (1992). *Becoming qualitative researchers: An introduction.* White Plains, NY: Longman.

Gold, R. L. (1958). Roles in sociological field observations. *Social Forces, 36,* 217–223.

Halcomb, E., & Andrew, S. (2005). Triangulation as a method for contemporary nursing research. *Nurse Researcher, 13*(2), 71–82.

Holstein, J. A., and Gubrium, J. F. (1994). Phenomenology, ethnomethodology, and interpretive practice. In N. K. Denzin and J. S. Lincoln (Eds.), *Handbook of qualitative research* (pp. 262–272). Thousand Oaks, CA: Sage.

Krueger, R. A. (1988). *Focus groups: A practical guide for applied research.* Newbury Park, CA: Sage.

Lofland, J., and Lofland, L. (1995). *Analyzing social settings* (3rd ed.). Belmont, CA: Wadsworth.

Lofland, L. (1973). *A world of strangers.* New York: Basic Books.

Marie, B. S. (2013). Coexisting addiction and pain in people receiving methadone for addiction. *Western Journal of Nursing Research.* doi:10.1177/0193945913495315

McCoy, C. B., et al. (1996). Sex, drugs, and the spread of HIV/AIDS in Belle Glade, Florida. *Medical Anthropology Quarterly* (New Series), *10*(1), 83–93.

Melville, J., et al. (2003). Psychosocial impact of serological diagnosis of herpes simplex virus type 2: A qualitative assessment. *Sexually Transmitted Infections, 79,* 280–285.

Menard, J., Kobetz, E., Diem, J., Lifleur, M., Blanco, J., and Barton, B. (2010). The sociocultural context of gynecological health among Haitian immigrant women in Florida: Applying ethnographic methods to public health inquiry. *Ethnicity & Health, 15*(3), 253–267. doi:10.1080/13557851003671761

Miles, M. B., and Huberman, A. M. (1994). *Qualitative data analysis: An expanded source book* (2nd ed.). Thousand Oaks, CA: Sage.

Mills, E. J., Seely, D., Rachlis, B., Griffith, L., Wu, P., Wilson, K., . . . Wright, J. R. (2006). Barriers to participation in clinical trials of cancer: A meta-analysis and systematic review of patient-reported factors. *Lancet Oncology, 7*(2), 141–148. doi:10.1016/s1470-2045(06)70576-9

Monaghan, L. F. (2002). Opportunity, pleasure, and risk: An ethnography of urban males heterosexualities. *Journal of Contemporary Ethnography, 31*(4), 440–477.

Morse, J. (1994). Designing funded qualitative research. In N. K. Denzin and J. S. Lincoln (Eds.), *Handbook of qualitative research* (pp. 220–235). Thousand Oaks, CA: Sage.

Nakkash, R., Afifi Soweid, R. A., Nehlawi, M. T., Shediac-Rizkallah, M. C., Hajjar, T. A., and Khogali, M. (2003). The development of a feasible community-specific cardiovascular disease prevention program: Triangulation of methods and sources. *Health Education and Behavior*, 30(6), 723–739.

Patton, M.Q. (2002). *Qualitative research and evaluation methods* (3rd ed.). Thousand Oaks, CA: Sage.

Peacock, J. L. (1986). *The anthropological lens: Harsh light, soft focus*. New York: Cambridge University Press.

Plattner, I. E. (2013). Children's conceptions of AIDS, HIV and condoms: A study from Botswana. *AIDS Care*. doi:10.1080/09540121.2013.772278

Roberts, F. (2002). Qualitative differences among cancer clinical trial explanations. *Social Science and Medicine*, 55, 1947–1955.

Salazar, L. F., Holtgrave, D., Crosby, R. A., Frew, P., and Peterson, J. L. (2005). Issues related to gay and bisexual men's acceptance of a future AIDS vaccine. *International Journal of STDs and HIV*, 16(8), 546–548.

Scorgie, F., Vasey, K., Harper, E., Richter, M., Nare, P., Maseko, S., and Chersich, M. F. (2013). Human rights abuses and collective resilience among sex workers in four African countries: A qualitative study. *Global Health*, 9(1), 33. doi:10.1186/1744–8603–9–33

Spradley, J. P. (1979). *The ethnographic interview*. Orlando: Harcourt Brace Jovanovich.

Steckler, A., and Linnan, L. (Eds). (2002). *Process evaluation for public health interventions and research*. San Francisco: Jossey-Bass.

Sterk, C., and Elifson, K. (2004). Qualitative methods in community-based research. In D. Blumenthal and R. DiClemente (Eds.), *Community-based research: Issues and methods* (pp. 133–151). New York: Springer.

Strauss, A., and Corbin, J. (1994). Grounded theory methodology: An overview. In N. K. Denzin and J. S. Lincoln (Eds.), *Handbook of qualitative research* (pp. 273–285). Thousand Oaks, CA: Sage.

Tewksbury, R. (2002). Bathhouse intercourse: Structural and behavioral aspects of an erotic oasis. *Deviant Behavior*, 23(1), 75–112.

Thurmond, V. (2001). The point of triangulation. *Journal of Nursing Scholarship*, 33(3), 253–258.

Yoo, S., Johnson, C. C., Rice, J., and Manuel, P. (2004). A qualitative evaluation of the Students of Service (SOS) program for sexual abstinence in Louisiana. *Journal of School Health*, 74(8), 329–334.

PART THREE

APPLICATIONS OF HEALTH PROMOTION RESEARCH

CHAPTER 9

CONDUCTING OBSERVATIONAL RESEARCH

Richard A. Crosby
Laura F. Salazar
Ralph J. DiClemente

As described in Chapters One and Four, observational research is an important link in the chain of research evidence. Whether conducted as a forerunner to randomized controlled trials (RCTs) or as a definitive form of study, observational research is very much the "bread and butter" of evidence in health promotion. Indeed, observational research constitutes the vast majority of early- and mid-level work in any chain of research evidence. Given the low cost and relatively short time commitments of some forms of observational study, graduate students and entry-level researchers are particularly likely to take on a project that is observational rather than experimental. This chapter will prepare you to plan, implement, and provide executive oversight of observational research.

Without question, research is an expensive and time-consuming endeavor. However, observational research is inherently far less demanding than experimental research. Thus some scholars in the field of health promotion exclusively engage their efforts in observational research. If you are a student, you will most likely use one of the observational research designs described in Chapter Four for your capstone, thesis, or dissertation project. This is not at all a compromise, as observational research has made some of the most important contributions to health promotion practice. For example, have you ever considered how all of the behavioral theories were developed?

LEARNING OBJECTIVES

- Acquire the basic principles involved in gaining access to a study sample.

- Understand the difference between passive and active recruitment.

- Explain the tenets of effective recruiting and systematic recruiting.

- Delineate and describe assessment issues as they pertain to cross-sectional and prospective studies.

- Identify effective methods of promoting retention in prospective studies.

IN A NUTSHELL

Whether conducted as a forerunner to randomized controlled trials or as a definitive form of study, observational research is very much the "bread and butter" of evidence in health promotion.

Indeed, all of the behavioral theories you have ever learned about in the field of health promotion have been developed based on observational research. Observational research methods have been greatly refined over the past two decades, thereby allowing researchers to construct theoretical pathways of cause-and-effect, which, in turn, are often used to generate theory.

The ultimate caveat with observational research is that rigor must be high. Several textbooks have provided a litany of conceptual issues that must be addressed to ensure this rigor (for example, Huck and Cormier, 1996; Shi, 1997; Sim and Wright, 2000). Unfortunately, the "nuts and bolts" of conducting observational research (that is, the steps that can and should be taken to avoid these conceptual problems) have often been neglected. Indeed, the process of conducting observational research is far from straightforward, and the number of potential pitfalls is endless. This chapter addresses multiple concerns relevant to the conception, design, and implementation of observational research in health promotion.

Researchers typically confront four distinct types of issues when conducting observational research. The first is gaining access to a sample. Access alone, however, is not enough; effective recruitment strategies are paramount. Next, issues related to assessment are critically important to the preservation of rigor. Finally, studies that follow people over time must have built-in mechanisms to ensure that attrition in the cohort is minimal. These four issues are important to constantly bear in mind, so we have developed an acronym—GLAD—to aid you in remembering this basic set of "rules":

Gain access to a sample.

Learn how to recruit effectively and systematically.

Assessment-related issues must be addressed and minimized.

Develop protocols to reduce attrition.

Gaining Access to a Sample

As noted in Chapter One, the first step in the research process is to define the study population. This task, however, is highly dependent on gaining access to the targeted population. For example, imagine that you have identified runaway or perhaps street youth as the study population, as depicted in Figure 9.1. You have two options. You could hire staff to recruit a sample of youth from various street locations, or you could centralize the process by working in a shelter or community center that assists runaway youth. The first option may be quite labor intensive, given that you would need

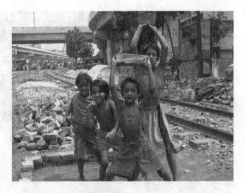

Figure 9.1 Street Youth

to locate and efficiently intercept and screen a massive number of youth on the streets to find even a few (with luck) who are runaways or homeless. The second option seems more attractive, yet this option requires something that may be difficult to secure: administrative buy-in from the shelter or community center.

Whether the point of access is a shelter or a public venue, there are **gatekeepers** (in other words, people who are in positions to grant or deny access, such as a board of directors or an executive director who control access (see Figure 9.2). Research ideas may sometimes be looked at with great suspicion by gatekeepers, so gaining their approval to conduct the study may be a challenging (and time-consuming) process. The goals of the research and the goals of the gatekeepers may be not only quite different but also incompatible. For example, the shelter for runaway youth may view its primary goal as providing a temporary safe haven where youth can receive referrals to social services. Given this mission, concerns about the proposed observational research may arise and could engender questions such as:

gatekeepers
people in positions of authority to grant or deny access to a potential population of study volunteers

- How will youth who take part in this study benefit from participating?
- What assurances can you offer that the youth will not feel coerced into participating?
- What type of questions will you be asking? Will these questions be personally invasive?
- Will your assessments be anonymous?
- How will your study help us? How will it help the community?

Naturally, addressing these issues in a satisfactory manner is a prerequisite to gaining access to the population; however, this could be a complicated response, as such concerns are not addressed easily. For

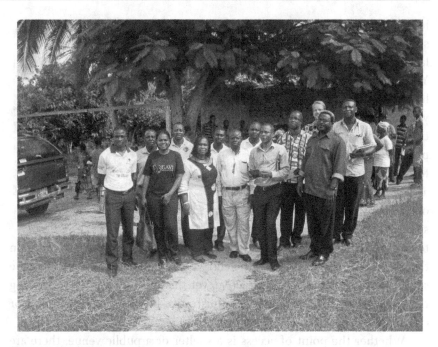

Figure 9.2 Gatekeepers

example, in responding to how the youth will benefit, one problem is that you are not providing a health promotion program; thus the research will not provide direct benefit to the youth. Also, you cannot guarantee that the youth will *not* perceive the "offer to participate" as coercive. Given that they are street youth or runaways, your local IRB must grant a waiver of parental consent. Furthermore, your research questions may necessitate assessing substance abuse and sexual behaviors and may be considered invasive or sensitive. If your study is prospective, then you will need to ask youth for contact information so you can locate them again in about 30 days. For these youth who are transient and/or homeless, this will be a major challenge. Finally, the expected findings from your study may have very little relevance to the provision of services.

How can these problems be brought to a successful resolution? The answer lies in the second step of the research process (formulating the research question), the fifth step (determining what variables should be measured), and potentially the sixth step (sampling). For example, you may need to formulate a research question that addresses a unique need of the shelter or the immediate community. This does not diminish your original intent in any way; it simply adds to the magnitude of your project. Next, you may need to either justify or remove planned measures from your assessment. However, removing some measures may diminish the quality and scope of your research. Based on a delicate balance between gaining access and asking the "right" questions in the assessment, researchers must be prepared to make compromises, but only to a point. The point at which the required compromises jeopardize the ability of the research process to generate rigorous findings should be the terminal point

IN A NUTSHELL

The point at which the required compromises jeopardize the ability of the research process to generate rigorous findings should be the terminal point of the negotiation.

of the negotiation. It may be preferable to identify a different population rather than conduct a study that does not meet your needs. For this reason, the search for a population that can be properly accessed may be a time-consuming and labor-intensive task.

To further illustrate the potential complications of gaining access to a sample, consider this real-world example. In an NIH-funded study of condom effectiveness (Crosby et al., 2012), the research team needed to access a sample of 1,200 study volunteers who were HIV-negative but likely to be infected (and reinfected) with sexually transmitted infections STDs. The study protocol required that volunteers be tested for chlamydia, gonorrhea, and trichomoniasis at baseline (that is, the first assessment in an observational study that serves as the "basis" for further comparisons), 3 months after baseline, and 6 months after baseline. Although these STDs can all be tested with urine specimens (meaning the study did not have to be clinic-based), there was a need to treat anyone testing positive in order to look for subsequent acquisition of the infection. Thus the study design inherently demanded that the sample be accessed through a clinic that can treat STDs. Moreover, using public clinics that treat primarily low-income populations was determined to be preferable because these clinics traditionally have a high-risk patient base. Unfortunately, the average inner-city public clinic that treats STDs is unlikely to have enough throughput of patients (that is, the actual number of patients coming into the clinic) to generate a sample of 1,200 people willing to engage in a 6-month study. Therefore the decision was made to use clinics in three different states. This created the need to forge relationships with three different clinic directors and their respective supervisors in order to obtain permission and support to conduct the study on their premises. Each clinic director wanted something different from the research project. One asked only that the study results be reported to the clinic staff on an annual basis. Another asked that the study provide STDs education and prevention materials to the general patient population. The third asked for a sharing arrangement regarding STDs test results obtained through the study. After meeting each director's needs, researchers obtained IRB approvals for each respective clinic and developed working relations between the study staff members and the clinic staff. As "guests" in these clinics, the study staff and the principal investigator were dependent on the good will of the clinic staff (particularly the nurses) to obtain the needed recruitment goals. Despite cultivating these relationships year after year, they never fully met their recruitment goals. One reason for this shortcoming was that nurse referrals in two of the clinics dropped off after the second year of the study, thereby crippling recruitment efforts. As guests of the clinic, the staff were not able to rectify this "referral burnout" experienced by the nurses. This real-world case illustrates that even under seemingly favorable conditions, accessing a sample is a complex task.

There are times when gaining access to a sample requires a compromise in the sampling plan. In this context, compromise must involve achieving a balance between the goals of the research and the values of the gatekeepers. This can be done through communication to obtain a mutual acceptance of terms—often involving variations from an original goal or desire. In the example with youths, shelter administrators may insist that youths be recruited into the study only during the daytime hours on Saturday and Sunday (they may feel strongly that other times of the week are "just too busy"). Furthermore, they may insist that only kids aged 16 and older can participate. The research team must respect the negotiation and make every effort to accommodate these requests, but requests that are perceived by the team to jeopardize the rigor and scope of the research merit further negotiating effort on the part of the research team. Providing decision makers with a carefully delivered explanation and rationale of the sampling needs may go a long way toward achieving a successful resolution so that everyone is satisfied.

Recruiting Effectively and Systematically

Chapter One described the importance of rigor. Rigor is lost in small, sometimes seemingly unimportant, aspects of a study. Recruitment is a good example of an opportunity for rigor to decrease substantially. The primary concern is that a low *participation rate* (sometimes called a *cooperation rate*) may lead to *participation bias*, also called *selection bias* (in other words, the sample is not representative of the population). This problem is not always a consequence of the selected sampling technique although it can be; rather, it stems from poor planning or poor implementation of a recruitment protocol. Incidentally, there is no universally accepted criterion for defining a "low" participation rate. One often-applied standard, however, is the use of a 70-percent or greater participation rate. Thus, for recruitment to be "successful," no more than 30 percent of those eligible can refuse participation. Yet, because all research is voluntary, refusal rates exceeding 30 percent are not uncommon, depending on the research question and population.

Understanding two key principles can set the stage for successful recruitment in health promotion research: (1) strategies have been devised to promote effective recruitment (that is, to yield a high participation rate), and (2) recruiting efforts should always be systematic. The importance of *effective* and *systematic* recruitment cannot be overstated. Chapter Six described a number of sampling options commonly applied to health promotion research. Sampling plans (also known as sampling protocols) are the result of carefully matching a sampling option with the research question(s). Unfortunately, the best-laid plans may fall apart if a large number of those eligible (that is, people who were sampled and met the inclusion criteria) refuse to enroll in the study. This problem may be a direct consequence of ineffective recruiting. Furthermore, plans may fall apart if some of the eligible "would-be" volunteers are recruited more vigorously than others. This problem may be a direct consequence of recruiting efforts that are not systematic.

Effective Recruiting

Although research methods are used to answer health promotion research questions, studies of the various methods employed (that is, research about conducting research) have been neglected. For example, it would be quite enlightening to know the relative importance of three factors involved in the recruitment process: (1) the amount of financial incentive being offered and its effect on participation rate, (2) the effect of timing and setting on recruitment success, and (3) the correlation between the recruitment approach and recruitment success. Unfortunately, empirical evidence addressing these questions is scarcely found in the published literature. In this chapter, we rely on anecdotal evidence (from our own studies and studies conducted by colleagues) to provide some guidance in effective recruiting.

First, **incentives** are provided to people to motivate them to participate. Incentives are important for research studies; these can take the form of cash, vouchers, gift cards, or tangible goods, but their value should be commensurate with the amount

incentives
items useful for attracting study volunteers; typically cash, vouchers, gift cards, or tangible goods

IN A NUTSHELL

The value of the incentive should be commensurate with the amount of time and effort required to fulfill the requirements of the study.

of time and effort required to fulfill the requirements of the study. For example, spending 3 to 4 hours to answer a lengthy questionnaire deserves a much larger incentive than that offered for taking a 15-minute survey. The amount of compensation may be established in part by local standards. It should be noted that in addition to being considered coercive, high-value incentives may create **participation bias**, which means the results will be nonrepresentative due to a disproportionate number of participants who might be using the research study as a form of extra income. Incentives, however, do not always need to be merely financial. The concept of contributing to science is not at all an unrealistic incentive in populations experiencing high rates of disease burden.

participation bias
a bias that manifests when people enroll in a study for reasons unrelated to volunteering to benefit science

Second, success in research, as it is in life generally, is all about timing. Timing is important because it can influence recruitment efforts. For example, people may be more receptive to participating when they are not under stess and when they feel that they have time on their hands. Also, people at a medical clinic may be more easily recruited while they are in a waiting room and are essentially a captive audience rather then when they have finished their appointment. Thus the timing of when potential participants are approached is everything. In fact, the first author of this chapter achieved high participation rates (90 percent) in studies of men attending sex resorts by recruiting during the daytime hours (near a swimming pool) rather than in the evenings and nights when a primary concern of the men was engaging in sex (Crosby and DiClemente, 2004).

Third, the recruiting approach can be an important determinant of success. Of course, a "one-size-fits-all" approach does not exist. The best approach is one that matches the needs of the potential volunteers. For example, if you were conducting a street-based qualitative study of low-income (or no-income) people in a developing nation, one approach to recruiting would be to offer to conduct the interview over a long meal that is provided at a local restaurant. In many cultures, the offer of food is symbolic of friendship, trust, and companionship; the gesture alone may thus inspire goodwill and thereby prompt people to volunteer.

active recruiting
involves the research team's actively and directly seeking study volunteers

Recruiting approaches can also be deemed as *active* or *passive*. **Active recruiting** occurs when investigators seek out participants, whereas in **passive recruiting** participants seek out investigators as a result of some advertisement (flyers, radio and television announcements, newspaper ads, newsletters, and internet banner ads). Active recruiting is best used when the investigator wants to have optimal control regarding fidelity to the sampling technique and fidelity to the eligibility criteria. All potential volunteers are first approached and asked about their willingness to be screened for study eligibility. Those deemed eligible are then solicited for study enrollment. This works very well when a relatively large population of likely volunteers (who are also eligible) can be easily accessed. However, it is less well-suited to studies that involve access to rare populations, such

passive recruiting
involves the research team's waiting for potential volunteers to inquire about study enrollment

as persons living with a long-term disease, persons with genetic disorders, or persons with severe mental illness. In these more hidden populations, advertising and referrals are a much more productive approach for the study team than active recruitment methods. For example, Tucker et al. (2011) used active recruitment in their qualitative study of social networks of female sex workers in South China. Researchers collaborated with local sex worker advocacy organizations, which provided lists of potential participants who were identified during syphilis/HIV outreach campaigns. Researchers then contacted the potential participants to participate in interviews. The data suggested that "*laoxiang* [social network member] ties may establish healthy behavioral norms, create relationships with outreach group members and physicians, and help to create a local environment conducive to sexual health" (Tucker et al., 2011).

An example of passive recruitment can be found in the Chemicals, Health, & Pregnancy study (CHirP). The researchers used posters, a website, online and print advertising, media coverage, and study booths at baby "trade shows" to recruit participants. The researchers found that "the recruited study population was less ethnically diverse, more affluent and more educated than the background population of pregnant women in Vancouver" (Webster et al., 2012, p. 435).

Another contemporary example of passive recruitment can be found in conjunction with federally funded research designed to test potential AIDS vaccines in human volunteers. Recruitment protocols for these studies require a passive approach (using multiple forms of media to promote the study to massive numbers of people).

Because passive recruitment removes the investigator from the recruitment process, it becomes problematic to determine how many people were solicited for study participation. Indeed, a methodological benefit of active recruiting is that determining a true participation rate and refusal rate is possible; the same cannot be said for passive recruitment. Another important advantage with active recruitment is that if data are available, comparisons can be made between those who participate and those who refuse.

BOX 9.1. EXAMPLE OF A RECRUITMENT BROCHURE

You're Invited!

You are invited to participate in a study that will investigate concerns people may have about accepting an AIDS vaccine if one ever became available for use in the United States. To be eligible you must

- Be 18 years of age or older

- Be able to read and understand English
- Not knowingly be positive for HIV (the virus that causes AIDS)

Enrollment in the study means that you will agree to participate in a 1-hour interview (on the day of enrollment) and another 1-hour interview 2 months after the first. After each interview, you will be provided with $35 to compensate you for your time. All information that you provide will be confidential.

If you would like to learn more about this study, please contact:

Study Director
402 Main Street, Room 390
Washington, MO 30111
Phone: (234) 555–1234

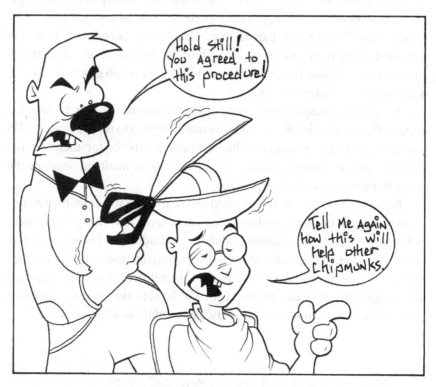

Mincus and Dincus Use Passive Recruitment for Their Study

Copyright 2005 by Justin Wagner; reprinted with permission.

Systematic Recruiting

A rigorous study will follow a strict recruiting protocol. All potential volunteers should be treated in the same manner. This sameness is just as important as the content of the protocol. One common practice to ensure consistency is to provide research staff with recruitment scripts. Scripts should be short enough that staff can recite the script naturally, not artificially, and long enough so that they accurately portray the study. Box 9.2 displays several examples of recruitment scripts applied to health promotion research. One of the best examples of this kind of commitment to a protocol can be found in phone surveys—in these protocols, research staff are reciting recruitment scripts verbatim. To ensure that staff do not drift from the script, supervisors should intermittently monitor (and correct) staff performance. The importance of this supervision cannot be overstated.

BOX 9.2. EXAMPLES OF RECRUITMENT SCRIPTS

"We are conducting a study that will help us learn about the HIV prevention needs of African-American women. Would you be willing to provide us with 30 minutes of your time?"

"The Wyoming State Department of Health has commissioned a study of farm injury prevention. Part of that study involves interviewing the teenage children of farm families. You qualify to participate in the study. If you are interested, I can explain the process to you in detail."

"I am recruiting study volunteers who are willing to help me and others who work with me to learn about the reasons why men do not always use condoms. Because you have been diagnosed with an STD today, you qualify to be in the study. Are you interested in helping us? The information you provide could be very useful in the eventual design of an education program."

"To improve the quality of our health care services, we are asking clients to consider volunteering for a 2-year study. We would ask you some questions today and then contact you by phone 3 times during every 6 months. The questions and phone calls are intended to provide us with data regarding how you make decisions whether or not to be seen by a doctor in our clinic. We are trying to improve our services as much as possible. Would you consider helping us out?"

Assessment Issues Must Be Addressed and Minimized

Assessment-related issues refer to screening, enrollment, and (if the study is prospective) follow-up.

A rigorous study will need to document:

- How many people were screened for eligibility
- How many of those screened were eligible
- Of those who were eligible, how many enrolled and participated

In prospective studies, it is equally important to include

- How many returned to the first planned follow-up assessment
- How many returned to the second planned follow-up assessment and those that followed

Maintaining these records is, of course, labor intensive. Ideally, a study director (someone who is always "on duty") should keep these records by using a daily diary. However, the records may also require the use of forms. If the local Institutional Review Board (IRB) permits it, documentation could include asking people who refused to participate why they refused and also collecting basic demographic data (age, gender, race) to compare nonvolunteers to volunteers. Some local IRBs, however, may prohibit any data collection among nonvolunteers. The ultimate goal of this data collection is to build a table that empirically addresses the potential for participation bias. Table 9.1 provides an example of this type of evidence. Notice that the table provides a head-to-head comparison of volunteers and nonvolunteers. The data make clear that volunteers were significantly less likely than nonvolunteers to be Black or African-American and significantly more likely to be White. Also, volunteers were significantly more likely than nonvolunteers to be unemployed and significantly less likely to be retired.

Regardless of whether it is the screening assessment, the baseline assessment, or follow-up assessments in question, the selected assessment method must be implemented with great fidelity. Just as a sampling plan can be foiled by poor recruiting, an assessment method can be compromised by poor implementation. Three key issues are paramount: (1) avoiding response bias, (2) avoiding undue respondent fatigue, and (3) facilitating accurate recall. Unlike measurement issues (see Chapter Seven), these three issues pertain to daily oversight of the research. In essence, the rigor of the study will rise and fall as a function of the effort expended in ensuring that real-life conditions of assessment are optimized.

> **IN A NUTSHELL**
>
> Just as a sampling plan can be foiled by poor recruiting, an assessment method can be compromised by poor implementation.

Avoiding Response Bias

response bias
a bias that manifests when people do not provide honest or accurate self-reported data

Response bias, which occurs when respondents do not answer honestly or accurately, can take several forms. One common concern is that study participants will "play to" or "play against" their perception of the

Table 9.1 A Comparison of Volunteers and Nonvolunteers

Characteristic	Number (%) Volunteers (N = 1,000)	Number (%) Nonvolunteers (N = 400)
Age		
18–29	90 (9.0)	40 (10.0)
30–39	450 (45.0)	160 (40.0)
40–49	410 (41.0)	160 (40.0)
50 and older	50 (5.0)	40 (10.0)
Race		
American Indian or Alaskan Native	12 (1.2)	12 (3.0)
Alaskan or Pacific Islander	95 (9.5)	40 (10.0)
Black or African American	**455 (45.5)**	**200 (50.0)**
White	**438 (43.8)**	**148 (37.0)**
Ethnicity		
Hispanic	290 (29.0)	120 (30.0)
Non-Hispanic	710 (71.0)	280 (70.0)
Employment		
Full-Time	770 (77.0)	320 (80.0)
Part-Time	70 (7.0)	30 (7.5)
Unemployed	**110 (11.0)**	**6 (1.5)**
Retired	**50 (5.0)**	**44 (11.0)**
Sex		
Male	490 (49.0)	210 (52.5)
Female	510 (51.0)	190 (47.5)

Note: Bold entries represent differences that are significant at P < .05.

study hypotheses. For example, if a male participant suspects that the study is designed to test whether people are more likely to be abusive toward a sex partner during periods of intoxication, then his hunch may have a conscious or subconscious effect on how he responds to the questions. He may answer in a way that falsely supports the hypothesis—or falsely fails to support it. One strategy that is sometimes used to avoid this form of bias is to avoid providing information to participants about the study hypotheses. IRBs will occasionally approve consent forms that do not fully disclose the purpose of the study. Of course, the recruitment script and even the questions being asked should be constructed to avoid bias. Most importantly, research staff must be skilled in the art of responding to any questions volunteers may ask without appearing impolite or unconcerned when they do not directly answer questions that would betray the hypotheses.

Another common form of bias stems from **social desirability**. Social desirability manifests when participants respond in ways that will be viewed

social desirability
a bias that manifests when study volunteers try to please the researchers by exaggerating or fabricating their self-reported behaviors

favorably by the researcher. This form of bias is easy to understand for anyone who has ever sat in a dental chair and been asked, "How often do you floss?" Most people are tempted to inflate their answer to please the hygienist or dentist and to create the impression that they practice excellent dental hygiene. In observational research that addresses health behavior, study volunteers may experience a similar need to please the person conducting the interview. Fortunately, this problem can be addressed by informing participants that the "best answer" is an honest answer. If administering an online survey, messages can be delivered throughout the survey to remind respondents that their responses are confidential and will be grouped with the other respondents. Although this seems simple enough, encouraging honesty sometimes requires a completely nonjudgmental atmosphere (especially in face-to-face interviews). For example, if someone is asked, "How many sex partners have you had in the past three months" and the answer provided is "about three dozen," then the person conducting the interview must not react any differently to this response than if the response had been "two."

Avoiding Undue Respondent Fatigue

respondent fatigue

a phenomenon evidenced when, after some amount of time, study volunteers no longer provide accurate self-reported data

Respondent fatigue typically happens toward the end of a study or survey. It is simply a phenomenon wherein respondents tire of answering questions or being in the study, and it can result in inaccurate responses. Although research is the backbone of science, conducting research with people also requires simple attention to their needs. One important principle to keep in mind is that the research and the questions are probably not as interesting to the study participants as they are to the researchers. In fact, the questions may be perceived as tedious. Apart from constructing clear questions and devising interesting response formats (see Chapters Seven and Thirteen), the researchers conducting the assessment must be attuned to the energy and interest level of the respondents. Are people attentive during the entire assessment period or does their attention wane after the first 10 minutes? If their attention does wane, then what can be done to get them back on track? Do people need a break at some point during the process? Does providing food help? Attending to these questions is the responsibility of the research staff and is similar to being a good host who ensures the comfort and enjoyment of his guests. The goal is to create an environment that is comfortable and ask people to complete a reasonable task without undue constraints. The same goes for online surveys—building in a process that enables respondents to leave the survey temporarily and complete it at a later time helps reduce fatigue, increase completion of items, and reduce missing data.

Along with alleviating fatigue, the research staff must also engage in a form of **quality assurance** (that is, ensuring that there are no missing data). One of the worst fates suffered by a data set is the absence of answers—to any number of questions—from a substantial proportion of the participants. Depending on the arrangements agreed to in the consent process, members of the research staff may, for example, review completed questionnaires before respondents leave the setting. A polite request to "please consider providing responses to questions 76 through 89 on the last page" (for example) may be met with cooperation. This small prompt may make the difference between including and excluding a participant's data from the final analysis. Less forward strategies include asking participants, before they leave, to please be sure they have answered all of the questions except for those that don't apply or those they purposefully chose not to answer. Of course, participants should also be informed (perhaps at several points in the assessment process) that the research staff would be happy to clarify any of the questions that may be confusing or problematic to answer. This offer, though, must never be taken lightly by the research staff because "clarification" can easily become a source of bias if the staff member strays from the written, spoken, or recorded question. Defining words and modestly paraphrasing questions are two practices that may be safe. If the survey is being self-administered either online or on a computer, programming can be implemented that will prompt respondents to fill in an answer if they skipped an item or conduct automatic quality assurance checks on certain items.

> **quality assurance**
> the steps taken to monitor study activities to promote adherence to study plans

IN A NUTSHELL

A polite request to "please consider providing responses to questions 76 through 89 on the last page" (for example) may be met with cooperation. This small prompt may make the difference between including and excluding a participant's data from the final analysis.

Facilitating Accurate Recall

Health promotion research often asks people to recall past events. Infrequent events that have high salience generally do not pose a problem (for example, the events that occurred on September 11, 2001). Typically, it can be expected that events with high saliency and low frequency facilitate the most accurate recall (see Chapter Seven). As an example, consider someone who has had sex twice in the past six months (high salience). Recalling the details of these two events may be relatively easy. Conversely, someone who has experienced more than a hundred sexual events in the past six months may be challenged to recall with a high degree of accuracy any details of these one hundred events. Events may be frequent but lack salience, leading to low accuracy in recall. For example, asking study participants who regularly eat eggs to recall the number of eggs they have consumed (low salience) in the past 30 days would probably lead to inaccuracies in recall.

The most challenging scenario occurs when the behavior under study is low in salience and is relatively frequent. Such a challenge may require the use of shortened recall periods, calendars marked with key dates, and verbal probes if the assessment is given in a face-to-face format.

Implementing short recall periods may be extremely useful. It is not at all unusual for health promotion research studies to use a one-day recall period (for example, "What are the foods that you consumed yesterday?") or a last-event recall period (for example, "The last time you ate out at a restaurant, what did you order?"). Of course, the risk of this truncated assessment period is that the "one day" or "last event" may not represent the true nature of the health behavior of the person being assessed.

Research staff may also increase accurate recall by starting each assessment with a large calendar. In settings where the staff member can interface with participants individually, the session can begin by helping participants fill in key dates. To illustrate, imagine asking questions designed to assess how many alcoholic beverages people consume in a typical month. To facilitate accurate recall, a staff member might ask, "Have you had any special events in the past month that were celebrated by having a party?" Another question might be, "In the past month, there were four weekends." (Show these by pointing at the calendar.) "On any of these weekends, did any sporting events occur that you watched while drinking—and if so, which ones?" Another example might be, "In the past month, was there a time in your life when you were extremely stressed or depressed? Can you please indicate those days on the calendar for me?" Any affirmative answer can be followed up to elicit a date, which is then recorded on the calendar. This entry may serve as a benchmark for the person when asked to recall how many drinks had been consumed. Notice that the questions are not the issue here; rather, the goal is to train research staff in the art of conducting an assessment that will maximize the odds of procuring accurate recall from the participants.

Finally, in face-to-face interviews (see Figure 9.3), verbal probes can greatly facilitate accurate recall. For example, to assess how many sex partners someone had over the past 6 months, the interview would begin with the basic question and if the initial answer is somewhat unclear, proceed with probes. A hypothetical example follows:

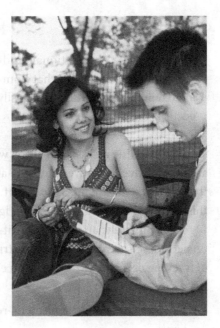

Figure 9.3 Face-to-Face Interview

Interviewer: In the past 6 months, how many different people have engaged in sexual intercourse with you? (Sexual intercourse means that one person's penis is placed into the mouth, vagina, or rectum of another person.)

Participant: Uhhh, umhh, I would have to say between 10 and 12 people. On second thought, umhh, make that 15.

Interviewer: This kind of counting can be difficult—I noticed you initially said "10" and finally said "15." Please think about why you raised your answer—did you raise it too much? Or perhaps not enough?

Develop Protocols to Reduce Attrition

The advanced version of recruitment is retention. Retention and attrition are simply opposite sides of the same coin. **Retention** is calculated as the number of people who completed a follow-up assessment divided by the number of people who completed the baseline assessment. **Attrition** is simply the number of people not completing a follow-up assessment divided by the number of people who completed the baseline assessment.

retention
the proportion of people in a sample who complete all of the scheduled assessments

attrition
the number of people in a study who fail to complete all of the scheduled assessment

IN A NUTSHELL

In prospective observational studies, retention is so vital that complete failure of the study may easily occur if the retention rate is low.

In prospective observational studies, retention is so vital that complete failure of the study may easily occur if the retention rate is low. Prospective data are complete only when at least two time points have been covered by the study. A baseline assessment alone will not answer research questions that are prospective in nature. Thus the attrition of any one participant negates the value of her baseline assessment. Of course (as described previously in this book), as attrition rates grow, rigor shrinks.

Unfortunately, attrition is inevitable: in general, the longer the follow-up period, the greater the rate of attrition. To minimize attrition, a number of tracking procedures have proven effective. These procedures include the following:

1. Hiring a full-time recruitment-retention coordinator to track participants

2. Requesting friendship contacts—participants are required to provide the name, telephone numbers, and addresses of two confidants

3. Providing monetary compensation for completing follow-up assessments

4. Ensuring confidentiality of data and identifying information (in other words, all data will be maintained, offsite, in a locked cabinet that is limited to access by key staff only, with only code numbers used on data forms)

5. Providing appointment cards indicating the time and date of the follow-up assessments

6. Providing reminder phone contacts a week before as well as 48 hours prior to their scheduled follow-up assessment

7. Mailing thank-you cards to participants for attending their follow-up assessments

8. Mailing "touching base" cards, such as birthday cards and holiday cards (there are many holidays throughout the year that provide an opportunity to maintain contact with participants)

A broad range of strategies have been designed to maintain the study cohort. Implementing them in a timely fashion, treating participants with courtesy and respect, providing assurances of confidentiality, and maintaining frequent contact to identify changes in locator information all enhance retention. We will discuss two of these strategies in greater detail.

Mobile Phone Contacts

The type of maintenance contact that occurs between research staff and study participants will be a function of the agreement with the IRB and the language in the consent form. The mobile phone is an essential tool for ongoing contact with study participants; therefore, it is clearly important to gain permission from the IRB to ask volunteers for a reliable phone number in prospective studies. At this juncture, you should be aware that all prospective studies inherently lack the ability to be anonymous simply because names must be used to gain repeated contact. After the baseline assessment is complete, research staff members have two essential obligations: (1) collect accurate contact information and (2) provide any promised incentives for study participation. Both tasks can be performed with one goal in mind: to establish rapport with participants in order to inspire them to come back! Merely asking for a phone number would be wasting an opportunity to build rapport. The occasion should instead be used to learn when and how to contact participants. Many of the participants may be unlikely to use their mobile phone as a phone per se, instead using it primarily as a texting device. Others may use their mobile as a way to communicate with people via internet-based tools such as Facebook and Twitter or e-mail. Thus collecting contact information should be a carefully conducted process (and it should occur before the incentive payment is made). Here is an example of how this contact information-gathering process might work:

> **IN A NUTSHELL**
>
> All prospective studies inherently lack the ability to be anonymous simply because names must be used to gain repeated contact.

Staff Member: I would like to contact you a few times before we meet again in three months. It would be very helpful to me if you would let me know how most people you know usually reach you—for example, phone, text, e-mail, Facebook.

Participant: I usually don't answer the phone, but I am pretty quick to text people back whenever possible. I do not e-mail at all, but I do have a Facebook account.

Staff Member: OK, good. So, I can text you?

Participant: Yes.

Staff Member: Okay, thanks. What phone number should I use when I text you?

Participant: My number, 439–345–1733.

Staff Member:	I am programming that into my phone as we speak—thanks. I have it. Now, let me send you a text message just to be sure I got your number correct. There, I just sent you a message that says, "Welcome to the study." Did you receive it?
Participant:	Yes, it just came in.
Staff Member:	Great! Now, did you say that I can also reach you by phone if we ever needed to actually talk?
Participant:	Well, I guess that would be OK, but please text me first if you wouldn't mind.
Staff member:	Happy to do so. Any particular time of day that is best for you to talk?
Participant:	Any weekday before I go to work—I go to work at 3:00 every afternoon.
Staff member:	OK, so usually early afternoons then?
Participant:	Yes, fine with me.
Staff member:	If I ever needed to mail something to you, how would I do that?
Participant:	Let me give you my PO box address, I check that about twice each week.

As you can readily see from this vignette, the staff member was quite wise in programming the mobile phone number into his or her own mobile phone "on the spot"—this ensures that the participant gave the correct number and that they are now electronically connected. The staff member was also smart to subtly assume that he or she could call the person and talk by voice and then present the question as one of simply asking when the best times are in a given week. Once the rhythm of exchange was established, the staff member used that momentum to collect the mailing address.

Collecting contact information and making contact are, of course, two very different things. When making phone contact with a participant, it is important to converse extemporaneously rather than read through a scripted agenda. The staff member should have and show a genuine interest in the person. This interest may elicit potentially important information. For example, the staff member might ask, "When we talked last, you were living in an apartment that you hated; have you had any luck getting a better one?" This question may yield a new address (information that may also be critical to keeping the retention rate high).

Mail Contacts

Birthday cards, holiday cards, and postcards can all be efficient ways to keep the study and the staff member relatively fresh in the minds of participants. Sending cards requires thoughtful use of the time between when participants complete the baseline assessment and when they are given their promised incentive. If the birth date was not collected in the assessment, then it can be requested during this time. Honesty is important—simply tell participants that you want to send them a birthday card! Similarly, it is easy enough to think about upcoming holidays and then to ask participants whether or not they celebrate these.

Although sending birthday and holiday cards may be hit or miss, every participant should be sent a postcard if possible. Postcards are an informal way of keeping in touch with someone, and their use can be casual—almost anonymous. The word "anonymous" is important because it may be that the study involves a sensitive topic (sex, drugs, disease) and the participant does not want his or her involvement disclosed. Thus the postcard should be from a place rather than a person, and the place should be generic rather than specific. For example, it may come from the Greater Chicago Board of Human Resources rather than from the Substance Abuse Prevention Center of Greater Chicago. To promote later recognition of this communication, the staff member could actually show a blank postcard to the respondent and say, "I would like to send one of these to you before we meet again—if that is okay with you, then what address should I use?" The postcard should only be a greeting—it should not be personalized to the point where participants' involvement in the study is disclosed in any way. Postage for this card should include Return Service Requested. This is an important way for a staff member to know that someone in the cohort has moved without leaving a forwarding address. This event necessitates immediate attempts to make phone contact.

In promoting retention, it is critical to assign one staff member as a retention coordinator whose primary role is to track the participants. This should be the same staff member who performs the baseline assessment and, more important, interfaces with the participant to collect

> **IN A NUTSHELL**
>
> In promoting retention, it is critical to assign one staff member as a retention coordinator whose primary role is to track the participants.

contact information (phone and address) and provides the incentive payment. Regardless of other roles this person takes on during the course of the research, the most important thing is her personality. Key attributes to enhance retention include being personable, amiable, and outgoing—the retention coordinator should be someone who is considered a "people person." Once this person is in place, it should be made clear that she will be the only person maintaining contact with each participant and that the purpose of each contact is to ensure that there are no barriers for the participant to complete the follow-up assessment on the day and time planned. Naturally, planning this day and time should be a very deliberate process, guided by the needs of the participant only (research staff *should not* be under the illusion that data collection must occur between 9 A.M. and 5 P.M., Monday through Friday). Once the day and time are planned, this information should be provided to the participant on a brightly colored appointment card that also clearly indicates how the participant can contact the staff member. If time allows, then the staff member should run the card through a lamination machine to give it some durability and to make it stand out. As the appointment nears, participants should get a reminder by phone, e-mail, or text message, as they prefer.

Attrition bias is naturally a prime concern. If, for example, people who drop out do so for a variety of practical reasons (for example, change of residence, employment schedule conflicts with appointment times, lack of transportation to the appointment), then the odds of developing a biased final sample are relatively low. But if people drop out based on lack of interest in the study or personal conflicts with the nature of the research questions, then the odds of developing a biased final sample go up substantially. Indeed, the final sample might comprise only people who really like the study topic and who are not in conflict with the topic in any way. In health promotion research, this skewed sample may rarely reflect reality. Here are just a few of many possible examples of topics that may create this problem:

IN A NUTSHELL

If people drop out based on lack of interest in the study or personal conflicts with the nature of the research questions, then the odds of developing a biased final sample go up substantially

- Sex and sexuality research
- Research on eating disorders
- Vaccine-acceptance research
- Substance-abuse prevention research
- Drunk-driving prevention research
- Cancer prevention research
- Research on compliance with exercise and diets to improve cardiovascular health

Summary

Although observational research is often a forerunner to experimental research, it may also constitute the terminal point of evidence in the research chain. Either way, rigor in observational research is essential. This chapter has described some of the key concepts that ensure this rigor. An initial concern is gaining access to the desired population, followed by the creation and implementation of a successful recruitment protocol. Assessment—the main activity in observational research—is important in its own right and is also related to whether volunteers return for scheduled follow-up interview sessions. Given the importance of using prospective designs in health promotion research, multiple steps can and should be taken to ensure an optimally high retention rate. Ultimately, constant attention to the everyday operation of observational research is vital to ensuring a high degree of rigor. This attention includes careful record-keeping, thorough training of research staff, and periodic monitoring of all recruitment and retention procedures. The successful study will be one that is planned in great detail and implemented with fidelity.

KEY TERMS

Active recruiting	Quality assurance
Attrition	Respondent fatigue
Gatekeepers	Response bias
Incentives	Retention
Participation bias	Social desirability
Passive recruiting	

For Practice and Discussion

1. This chapter emphasized the importance of recruitment that is both systematic and effective. Write a one-paragraph summary of what each of these terms means, then use that as a guide to do the following:
   a. Locate a journal article that is somewhat flawed with respect to systematic recruiting (we, the authors, assure you that plenty of examples can be found).
   b. Locate a journal article that is somewhat flawed with respect to effective recruiting (we, the authors, assure you that thousands of examples can be found).

c. For each example, determine how you would have avoided the problem had you been the principal investigator of the study.

2. Again using existing journal articles, locate at least 6 different studies that report dollar amounts provided to research participants as incentives (compensation for their time). Cite each article and next to each citation list the incentive schedule for the study, including dollar amounts. Then annotate this list with your opinion on whether the amount was too high (being coercive), too low (possibly hurting the participation rate), or just right. Explain and defend each opinion.

3. Often recruiting volunteers is more of an art than a science—creativity carries the day! Imagine that you are conducting a study that requires volunteers to donate blood and urine specimens on a monthly basis and asks them to complete weekly electronic diaries using their own smartphones. Unfortunately for you, the topic is a sensitive one—substance abuse (including alcohol)—and your population is somewhat paranoid about disclosure because they are teenagers. Getting these teens to enroll has proven to be a difficult challenge. Your task is to create a recruitment protocol that will meet this challenge. Once you have this protocol on paper, label each strategy as "passive" or "active" and explain your answers. Note, a reasonable protocol for this challenge will involve at least five different strategies, so plan carefully—the study depends on you!

4. Respondent fatigue is a common issue when long questionnaires are used. One of the best ways to truly learn about this problem is to experience it! Go online and locate a codebook (another term for a questionnaire) from a public use dataset and pretend to take the questionnaire as if you were a study participant. (Be sure to find a challenging dataset such as the CDC's Behavioral Risk Factor Surveillance System—BRFSS). Time yourself as you go through the questions; be sure that you read each question carefully and that you respond thoughtfully and accurately to each item. If your attitude to completing the questionnaire changes at any point, note the time, the question you've reached, and what changed for you. Once you are done, answer the following questions:

a. Was there a breaking point at which you wanted to quit? If so, when did that happen?

b. Was there a point when you became less thoughtful in your responses and simply answered the remaining questions in a hurry? If so, when?

c. Was there a point when you found yourself being basically annoyed by the questions? If so, when?

d. Given your answers to a, b, and c, what are your recommendations for a time (or length) limit on this questionnaire when it is next revised for use with study volunteers?

References

Crosby, R. A., Charnigo, R., Weathers, C., Caliendo, A. M., and Shrier, L. A. (2012). Condom effectiveness against non-viral sexually transmitted infections: A prospective study using electronic daily diaries. *Sexually Transmitted Infections*, *88*, 484–488.

Crosby, R. A., and DiClemente, R. J. (2004). Use of recreational Viagra among men having sex with men. *Sexually Transmitted Infections, 80*, 466–468.

Huck, S. W., and Cormier, W. H. (1996). *Reading statistics and research*. New York: Longman.

Shi, L. (1997). *Health services research*. Albany, NY: Delmar Publishers.

Sim, J., and Wright, C. (2000). *Research in health care: Concepts, designs, and methods*. Salisbury, Wiltshire, UK: Stanley Thrones (Publishers) Ltd.

Tucker, J. D., Peng, H., Wang, K., Chang, H., Zhang, S.-M., Yang, L. G., and Yang, B. (2011). Female sex worker social networks and STI/HIV prevention in South China. *PLoS ONE, 6*(9), e24816. doi:10.1371/journal.pone.0024816

Webster, G., Teschke, K., and Janssen, P. A. (2012). Recruitment of healthy first-trimester pregnant women: Lessons from the Chemicals, Health & Pregnancy Study (CHirP). *Maternal and Child Health Journal, 16*(2), 430–438.

CHAPTER 10

METHODOLOGICAL CONSIDERATIONS IN THE DESIGN, IMPLEMENTATION, AND REPORTING OF RANDOMIZED CONTROLLED TRIALS IN HEALTH PROMOTION RESEARCH

Ralph J. DiClemente
Laura F. Salazar
Richard A. Crosby

The randomized controlled trial (RCT) represents an advanced and rigorous true experimental research design used to assess the effectiveness of health promotion programs. Implementing a randomized controlled trial to evaluate a health promotion program differs distinctly from traditional drug trials and requires a high degree of attention to seven key steps. These steps describe a range of approaches to address pertinent methodological issues in the design and implementation of randomized controlled trials.

Much of the research in health promotion has been observational in nature, as noted in Chapters Four and Nine. However, the very definition of—and indeed the identity of—the discipline of health promotion is predicated on the premise of designing programs that promote health. As such, a mainstay of health promotion is the development, implementation, evaluation, and publication of programs whose express purpose is to enhance the health of human populations.

The term "health promotion program" (HPP) can be ambiguous. Broadly defined, an HPP can be any intervention that is intended to change health. Such interventions

LEARNING OBJECTIVES

- Understand the advantages and strengths of using a randomized controlled trial for evaluation of health promotion programs.

- Learn the different categories of variables often used in randomized controlled trials for health promotion programs.

- Learn the nine steps in the process of conducting a randomized controlled trial.

- Become familiar with the standardized format for reporting the results of randomized controlled trials.

may include, for example, a new school smoking-cessation curriculum, a new exercise-enhancement class at a community-based organization, a program to enhance use of a medication (for example, the Nicoderm patch to reduce cigarette smoking), changing diet to reduce low-density lipoproteins (LDLs), or an HIV-prevention program designed to promote using condom protection in sexual intercourse.

To determine whether or not an HPP is effective, we use experimental research. Experimental research is used in many fields; in health promotion we focus mainly on evaluating whether HPPs are efficacious in enhancing biological indicators of health, health-protective behaviors, and health-protective attitudes, beliefs, knowledge, and intentions. There are many different types of research designs applicable for these assessments (see Chapter Five). Experimental designs, like ice cream, come in a wide variety of flavors. Among the diverse array of choices, we have chosen to focus in this chapter on one specific type of experimental research design—the randomized controlled trial.

randomized controlled trial (RCT)

a specific type of scientific experiment; its key distinguishing feature is that subjects, after assessment of eligibility and recruitment but before the intervention to be studied begins, are randomly allocated to receive one or another of the alternative treatments under study

The randomized controlled design is referred to as a mixed design in that there is a both a between-group factor and a within-group factor. The between-group factor allows the observed outcomes to be compared between two or more groups who receive different interventions; the within-subjects factor allows the observed outcomes to be compared within groups over time. Mixed designs are commonly used in health promotion research. The **randomized controlled trial (RCT)** is one type of mixed design that is a "true" experimental design; it can also be described as a **parallel group design,** meaning there are two treatments implemented: one (the HPP) to the treatment group and one (an placebo-attention or standard of care) to the control group. In the RCT, participants are randomly assigned (that is, by chance) to either receive or not receive the HPP.

parallel group design

a design that involves a comparison between two groups

extraneous variables

variables that may affect the study outcomes but are not of interest to the research question, but may threaten the trial's validity

The RCT is considered the optimal design for isolating and quantifying the effects of an HPP because it controls for **extraneous variables** that threaten to compromise the validity of the HPP evaluation. Recall from Chapter Five that extraneous variables are those variables that may affect the study outcomes but are not of interest to the research question. Indeed, whether the field of scientific inquiry is medicine, psychology, or public health (specifically, health promotion), the RCT is the cornerstone of research and is widely considered the gold standard for evaluating programs in any discipline involving human populations. Because of the importance of the RCT to health promotion research, this chapter provides an in-depth description of how to design and implement an RCT. We describe key concepts in designing, implementing, and reporting randomized controlled trials in health promotion research. Though it is not an exhaustive treatment of this methodology, we describe the essential concepts that form the foundation of randomized trial design and discuss the importance of these concepts in enhancing the validity of health promotion research.

What Is an Experiment in Health Promotion Research?

As stated in Chapter Five, one experiment in health promotion research involves the manipulation of an **independent variable** and control of extraneous variables; the independent variable (IV) is intentionally changed, modified, or altered by the research team. In terms of the RCT, the IV is the "treatment" that is given to the participants and can assume multiple levels. In its simplest form, the IV would have two levels or arms: the HPP arm and a comparison/control arm. Because this is an RCT, participants must be randomized to one arm or the other.

The effects of the IV can be measured by assessing the prespecified outcome variables. In the parlance of experimental research, the outcome measures are what you are trying to affect with your HPP; these are designated as **dependent variables** (DV) and can include such health-related outcomes as weight, BMI, blood pressure, depressive symptoms, C-reactive protein, blood glucose levels, and LDLs, to give a few examples. These assessments are administered over time; depending on the research question, they can take months or years and include multiple follow-ups.

To illustrate these somewhat abstract concepts more clearly, we will explore a hypothetical case. Let's say you have developed an innovative approach designed to motivate older adults to increase their consumption of fruits and vegetables. You have developed this innovative program based on evidence derived during the explanatory stage of research from numerous observational epidemiologic studies, which observed significantly fewer adverse health outcomes (such as heart disease) for older adults reporting greater fruit and vegetable consumption. The innovative HPP comprises five group sessions, designed to: (1) enhance older adults' awareness of the risk of heart disease and cancer, (2) describe the health benefits associated with greater fruit and vegetable consumption, (3) provide an opportunity to learn heart-healthy cooking techniques (such as substituting olive oil for palm oil), and (4) mobilize group support to motivate adults to change their dietary behavior. This is not an easy task, as modifying dietary behaviors is a formidable undertaking that often necessitates changing individuals' eating habits acquired over their lifetime. However, you are undaunted. You feel strongly that your heart-healthy HPP, based on a solid foundation of health promotion theory and utilizing new motivational techniques and strategies, will be effective in changing dietary behaviors. The next step is to evaluate your program.

independent variable
the variable that is manipulated by the investigator

dependent variables
the trial's outcome measures or endpoints

You recruit about two hundred older adults from local senior citizen homes. You describe the study, answer any questions individuals may have, request written informed consent, and collect the forms. Next, you ask participants to: (1) complete a baseline questionnaire that assesses their consumption of fruits and vegetables and measures hypothesized key **mediators** of behavior change, such as knowledge, attitudes, and perceived norms, and (2) provide a blood specimen. In this context, mediators are the variables that the HPP expects to affect or change through its activities; they are, in turn, related to your DVs. The blood specimen will be assessed for LDL, the putative etiological factor associated with heart disease that you are hoping to change (reduced LDL levels in the blood) as a function of participation in your HPP. Subsequently, you randomly assign participants to either your innovative heart-healthy HPP or a group of participants who do not receive any health promotion intervention (this could be some other program that does not include a focus on enhancing fruit and vegetable intake). Next, you present the five-session program and then ask participants (from both groups) to return, let's say 12 months after completing the intervention, to complete the same questionnaire administered at baseline so that significant changes in the DV can be determined. At this point, you hypothesize (and hope) that participants in the heart-healthy HPP report consuming more fruits and vegetables over the past 12 months relative to participants in the comparison group. Let's say you observe differences between the two groups in the quantity and frequency of fruit and vegetable consumption, with greater fruit and vegetable consumption in the heart-healthy HPP. This would be a clear indication that the program worked. Congratulations—you have just conducted an experimental research study! The final step is to disseminate the findings through publication in a peer-reviewed journal (see Chapter Seventeen for details on the publication process). This is a simplified illustration of how to conduct an RCT; of course, there will be many design nuances that need to be considered in your study. But we have described the basic structure of the RCT.

mediators

variables through which the intervention causes changes in the trial's outcomes or end points

Advantages of an Experimental Research Design

The major advantage of experimental research over observational research is the strength of **causal inference** it offers. Causal inference implies that a valid conclusion can be made regarding the effect of an independent variable on a dependent variable (that is, a change in x will create a corresponding change in y). As stated in Chapter Five, experimental designs are powerful research designs for controlling potential confounding influences. As our fruits-and-vegetables HPP RCT example illustrates, the causal inference is

causal inference

the process of drawing a conclusion about a causal connection based on the conditions of the occurrence of an effect

based on comparing the DVs (outcomes) observed among the older adults in the heart-healthy HPP relative to the older adults not receiving the HPP. Because randomization controls for multiple extraneous variables, by randomizing participants into groups and then observing differences in outcomes for those exposed to the HPP and those who were not exposed to the HPP, we can say with confidence that the HPP caused the positive changes in behavior.

There are, of course, many variations of the RCT design. In this chapter, we restrict our discussion to describing the basic research structure of the RCT. Readers interested in more detailed presentations are referred to Piantadosi (1997) and Pocock (1993). We have adapted the basic structure of the RCT design as described by Schulz, Altman, and Moher (2010) and Moher et al. (2012) to enhance its relevance for health promotion research. For more information about RCTs, we recommend visiting the **CONSORT** website at www.consort-statement.org. CONSORT stands for Consolidated Standards of Reporting Trials. The standards were developed by the CONSORT group, a dynamic group comprising experts in clinical trial methodology, experts in guideline development, biomedical journal editors, and research funders.

CONSORT
broadly accepted standards for reporting trials

Conceptualizing a Randomized Controlled Trial Design

An RCT is graphically depicted in Figure 10.1. Although the research design may appear to be basic, you should not underestimate its strength: this is a powerful evaluation design. Also, do not be overwhelmed by the number or sequencing of steps needed to effectively implement an RCT. Although there are a number of key steps that necessitate careful decision-making on the part of the investigator, in Table 10.1 we provide a step-by-step approach to designing and implementing an RCT that may facilitate an understanding of the design and its component parts so you can feel confident when you conduct your first RCT.

Step 1. Conduct a Power Analysis—This Is Essential!

Before you evaluate your HPP, you must first conduct a power analysis to determine the sample size needed to help show, using quantitative statistical techniques, whether or not your HPP was effective. A **power analysis** is a mathematical procedure for determining, before you start your experiment, how large a sample size is needed to adequately ensure that your statistical tests are accurate and valid and also the likelihood that your statistical tests will detect effects of your HPP for a given **effect size**. The effect size is the magnitude of the difference between two groups.

power analysis
a priori statistical analysis to determine the appropriate number of subjects needed in the trail in order to detect a meaningful statistical effect

effect size
the magnitude, or size, of the effect of an intervention

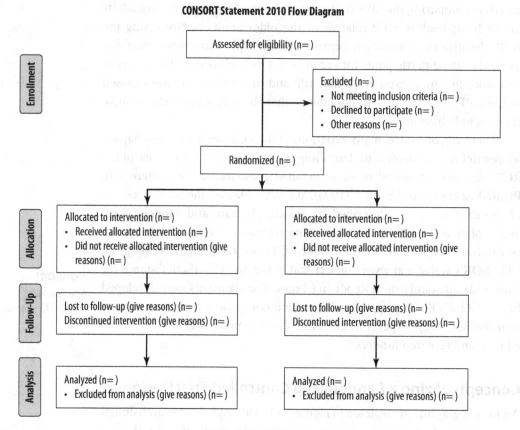

Figure 10.1   A Schematic Illustration of a Randomized Controlled Trial (RCT)

Table 10.1   The Basic Steps in Designing and Implementing an RCT

Step	Objective at This Step
1. Conduct a power analysis	Power analysis will provide the size of the sample that must be used to detect effects of the HPP and ensure validity of the RCT.
2. Register the trial	See clinicaltrials.gov for detailed instructions on how to register the trial.
3. Enrollment	Select and define the study sample.
4. Baseline assessment	Measure dependent and mediating variables (for example, knowledge, perceived norms, attitudes, behavioral intentions, changes in dietary behaviors, blood levels of low-density lipoprotein) prior to participating in the trial.
5. Allocation	Randomize participants to study groups ("trial arms").
6. Implement study conditions	Implement the HPP and control/comparison groups as prescribed in the research protocol and manual of operations.
7. Follow-up	Follow participants post-HPP to monitor changes in the independent variables and the outcomes.
8. Analysis	Compare the changes in outcomes observed among participants in the HPP condition with those observed among participants in the comparison condition.
9. Reporting the trial findings	Prepare a report that describes the entire process as well as the trial findings—use the CONSORT checklist.

RCTs necessitate large resources to implement in terms of both time and money, so you want to make sure that you have enough power statistically to show an effect if one is truly there. If your sample size is too small, the trial will lack precision and will have been all for naught. Conversely, if your sample size is too large, time and resources will have been wasted. You should consult with the statistician on your project beforehand to help with this procedure; there are many online sample size power calculators that can assist.

Step 2. Register the Trial—This Is Critical!

Registering the RCT creates a formal record of your design, hypotheses, planned analyses, and dependent variables. Registering the trial makes public and explicit the objectives and goals of the trial. Moreover, trial registration is a requirement for publication in many journals and must occur prior to the implementation of the trial.

Step 3: Enrollment—Select and Define the Study Sample

The third step is to select and define the study sample. The key decision is who will be in the study and how best to recruit them to participate. It is important when defining the study sample to establish a set of **inclusion and exclusion criteria** that specify the target population and are appropriate to the research question. These criteria, sometimes referred to as eligibility criteria, establish the parameters for determining who is able to participate (inclusion) and who is not able to participate in the study (exclusion). Referring back to our illustration earlier in this chapter, a researcher might decide that only adults over 60 will be eligible for trial enrollment. Another hypothetical inclusion criterion could be adults over 60 who have clinically documented high levels of LDL. An exclusion criterion may be older adults who are not able to understand or complete the psychosocial assessment. In any event, it is critical to carefully document the inclusion and exclusion criteria and the rationale for these criteria. There is no magic formula for defining the inclusion and exclusion criteria. It is based on understanding the HPP that is to be evaluated: understanding the key outcomes of interest as well as weighing the competing concerns of **internal validity** (the extent to which the study evaluates the hypotheses) and **external validity** (the extent to which the results of the study can be extended beyond the sample in the study to a broader population).

Numerous strategies can be used to recruit a target sample (see Chapter Six). Referring back to our example, we could send study recruiters to

inclusion and exclusion criteria
criteria that define the characteristics used for determining whether or not a subject is appropriate to participate in the trial

internal validity
the confidence that we can place in the cause-and-effect relationship identified in the trial

external validity
degree to which the study findings can be generalized to other study populations with different characteristics

senior assisted-living facilities to solicit participation, essentially generating a convenience sample. Alternatively, we could enhance the generalizability of our findings by recruiting a random sample of seniors. For instance, we could use a variety of random sampling methods to determine who would be approached at a medical facility and asked to participate. The sampling strategy should be based on the purpose of the study. Once the sampling strategy is defined, then sample selection, recruitment, and informed consent procedures can begin.

Step 4: Baseline Assessment—Measure Dependent and Mediating Variables Prior to Participation in the Trial

Variable selection is a critical step that requires investigators to first articulate the short-term and long-term objectives of the HPP. The short-term objectives are typically conceptualized as the theory-driven mediating variables of the HPP, meaning that the activities of the HPP will affect these variables and, in turn, affect the long-term objectives (such as behavior or biological outcomes). We recommend conducting a thorough review of the empirical literature and conceptually "mapping" the mediating variables to the underlying psychosocial or health promotion theory that was used to develop the HPP. Formative research with the targeted population is also helpful to ensure that all key and relevant variables are assessed. Once the variables have been selected, focus on choosing the appropriate instrument, scale, or metric (see Chapter Seven for a more detailed discussion). Without good metrics for your study variables, the internal validity of your RCT may be jeopardized.

logic model
a depiction, usually graphical, of the logical relationships between the resources, activities, outputs, and outcomes of an intervention

Critical at this juncture is the creation of a logic model for identifying the primary and secondary outcomes. A **logic model** is a formalized schematic to describe the hypothesized linkage between sets of variables and the trial's outcomes (also referred to by epidemiologists as "trial endpoints"). We provide a basic description of logic models and how they can be useful for an RCT. Let's think back to our central example of developing an HPP to change the dietary behaviors of older adults to reduce LDL as a way of lowering the risk of heart disease. A simple logic model can be developed; it is presented in Figure 10.2. Some logic models can become extremely complex; what we propose in Figure 10.2 is a heuristic to illustrate a point about variable selection.

As shown, this HPP is designed to target those factors identified theoretically or empirically as being associated with dietary behavior. This model assumes that the HPP will affect older adults' personal cognitions, social networks, attitudes, norms, and knowledge, which in turn will result

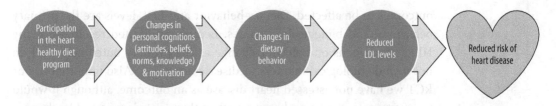

Figure 10.2 Logic Model Depicting the Hypothesized Pathway between Exposure to the Health Promotion Program and Changes in Mediators, Behavior, and Biological Markers

in changes in dietary behavior. As a consequence of older adults changing dietary behavior, they will have lower LDL levels. Continuing with the logic model, observed changes in LDL levels will positively impact on older adults' health (that is, they will result in lower risk for heart disease). Thus one implicit assumption in the logic model of HPPs is that there is a direct, linear relationship between exposure to the HPP and its effect on theory-driven mediators, which in turn should result in corresponding changes in the health-promoting behavior (that is, dietary behaviors) and outcome (that is, reduced risk of heart disease). This is the plausible causal chain stemming from participation in the HPP and ultimately better heart health.

Now that we understand the underlying logic of the trial, let's review the four categories of variables used in an RCT: (1) the independent variable, (2) theory-driven mediators, (3) the behavioral dependent variable, and (4) biological dependent variables (in this example, LDL levels). The independent variable is the treatment administered to the older adults; adults are randomly assigned either to receive the HPP or to a control arm (no exposure to the HPP). The theory-driven mediators are those psychosocial variables derived from the underlying theoretical framework and empirical literature—such as readiness to change dietary behaviors, attitudes toward healthy eating, knowledge about the connection between poor dietary behavior and high LDL levels, beliefs that healthy eating will lower LDL levels, and self-efficacy to eat healthy—that are expected to change as a function of exposure to the HPP. The behavioral dependent variable in this instance is dietary behavior, and it should be affected by changes in the theory-driven mediators. The biological dependent variable is the LDL level, and it should in turn be affected by changes in dietary behaviors.

From an HPP perspective, this RCT has multiple dependent variables or outcomes. The theory-driven mediators are considered **intermediary outcomes** because of the temporal order in which they are affected by the HPP relative to the primary outcomes. In other words, the intermediary outcomes must be influenced or affected by the HPP in order for the primary

intermediary outcomes
common preliminary outcomes, typically on the causal pathway to the final outcome

outcomes to be affected. Dietary behavior and LDL levels are the primary behavioral and biological outcomes. Because of limited resources, many HPPs often focus on behavior change as the primary outcome(s) and do not include biological markers or disease outcomes. Also note that in our RCT we have not assessed heart disease as an outcome, although it would be of utmost interest to know whether there are demonstrable changes in incidence of heart disease. As health promotion researchers, it is the actual health outcomes that we are ultimately trying to affect through development of and participation in our HPPs. Although tracking disease reduction is, ultimately, the most desirable outcome for evaluating the efficacy of the intervention, most HPP RCTs do not include actual disease as an outcome because some diseases manifest over long periods of time (for example, heart disease, lung cancer) or because the incidence of some diseases is too low to detect change in the population targeted (such as HIV infection). Including disease outcomes in the RCT would require suitably large sample sizes followed over extended time periods to ascertain whether HPP participation resulted in a lower incidence of disease. As an alternative, it is more realistic and appropriate to assess whether the HPP produced a clinically meaningful decline in a biologically assessed risk factor for heart disease, such as LDL.

For these reasons, few RCTs of HPPs include assessment of disease outcomes. However, we maintain that in the past decade there has been a **"biological revolution."** New biomedical technologies enable meaningful and noninvasive measurement of biological risk indicators for disease (for example, C-reactive protein as a risk factor for heart disease). This has created the opportunity to select surrogate biological endpoints in the absence of *actual* disease endpoints. There has been great interest recently in using surrogate endpoints—laboratory measurements or physical signs used as a substitute for a clinically meaningful disease endpoint, such as LDL—or other laboratory measures to reduce the cost and duration of HPP RCTs.

biological revolution

marked changes in the capacity to measure changes in people's health status using less invasive technology

Step 5: Allocation—Randomize Participants to Trial Groups (or "Trial Arms")

Once you have decided on all the variables for inclusion and how they will be measured, the baseline assessment can be administered. The next step is to randomize participants to either receive the HPP or not. Randomization, one of the most critical aspects of the RCT, has a number of advantages in experimental research. Foremost, randomization comparably distributes participant characteristics that were assessed at baseline across groups. Moreover, randomization provides an efficient strategy for also distributing characteristics that were not measured. Often, for a variety of reasons (for example, prohibitive cost, time, participant burden), the baseline assessment cannot reasonably measure all variables that could affect the relationship between exposure to the HPP and key outcomes. For example, people who are stressed may tend to

IN A NUTSHELL

Randomization comparably distributes participant characteristics that were assessed at baseline across groups. Moreover, randomization provides an efficient strategy for also distributing characteristics that were not measured.

overeat as their coping mechanism. For an HPP designed to increase healthy food consumption, stress levels may not be a variable of primary interest but could affect study outcomes. To address this, randomization would theoretically ensure that the two groups have comparable stress levels. A word of caution to the aspiring researcher: although randomization is a powerful procedure to guard against systematic bias in allocating participants to the trial arms and controls for numerous threats to validity, randomization does not mean that the participants in the arms are equivalent (in fact, rarely will they be equivalent).

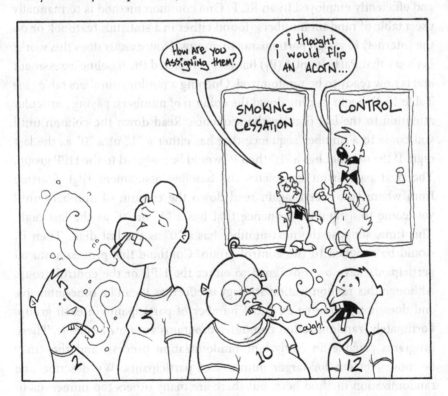

Dincus's Simple Randomization Procedure

How to Randomize Participants

IN A NUTSHELL

There are two main features to consider when randomizing participants to study conditions: first, implementing a valid randomization procedure, and second, establishing procedures to safeguard the integrity of the randomization procedure so that unintentional or intentional biases do not influence the participant allocation process.

Because randomization is the major strength of the RCT, it is important that it be conducted properly. In general, there are two main features to consider when randomizing participants to study conditions: first, implementing a valid randomization procedure, and second, establishing procedures to safeguard the integrity of the randomization procedure so that unintentional or intentional biases do not influence the participant allocation process.

Implementing randomization requires reliable procedures that create comparability between or among groups. As with many other aspects of research, there are many randomization procedures that could be effectively and efficiently employed in an RCT. One common method is to manually use a table of random numbers (found either in a statistics textbook or on the Internet) to assign participants to groups. How exactly does this work? Let's say that Participant 1 (P_1) has just completed the baseline assessment and is now ready to be randomized. Opening a random numbers table (see Table 10.2), begin reading down the column of numbers, paying particular attention to the last digit in the sequence. Read down the column until you come to a number sequence that has either a "1" or a "0" as the last digit. If the number has a "1," then P_1 would be assigned to the HPP group. The next participant completes the baseline assessment (P_2). Starting from where you ended, again read down the column of numbers until you come to a number sequence that has a "1" or "0" as the last digit. This time, suppose the next number has a "0" as the last digit. Then P_2 would be assigned to the control group. Continue this process until all participants have been assigned to either the HPP or the control group. Although this randomization strategy is effective, it can be time-intensive and does not guarantee an equal number of participants in each group. Fortunately, randomization computer programs are now available. These programs provide an equivalent randomization process, and they may be more efficient for larger numbers of participants. We describe one randomization method here, but there are many others too numerous to describe individually. For a more thorough description of randomization procedures, we refer you to Piantadosi (1997) and Pocock (1993).

Table 10.2 Random Numbers Table

52384	4797	71955	11581	46419	89706	27721	39561
3646	8192	51970	23053	71287	12341	91304	29056
81473	44938	95355	91376	20566	16977	95272	36178
37552	73865	75287	37734	45424	85909	35327	98437
27951	30078	71621	95589	40610	69232	2384	17280
2721	91473	59494	47777	46710	80923	88878	69497
20211	95941	39068	54813	25633	73888	18195	43099
55923	1652	94599	11664	58284	26631	93212	69249
31904	83060	47985	85095	30247	41983	42294	18602
31510	65211	46309	23609	76682	23982	32035	46802
21216	67487	97093	5064	5656	31258	49538	77893
35031	20469	89136	50750	87218	81376	94599	72280
89666	13674	50360	58074	73321	74676	95244	59061
25152	65990	69179	30796	74746	66360	44085	43055
73531	21813	28708	51741	50630	8293	92192	36329
51576	98453	47390	35442	77039	77748	70011	26273
89214	83822	84019	90247	86499	49943	29698	51413
48108	77480	85897	23054	64364	9162	69159	6005
21909	2832	59466	85099	76470	57675	26711	80801
37131	96487	7593	80233	99944	61103	4420	52266
93670	59536	38295	25539	88393	91356	32083	95808
57626	12006	14110	47864	86510	2420	65409	46010
48414	87287	66007	86323	44922	53889	4434	85588
91408	19449	50286	15538	789	3361	90186	33638
83151	55246	81281	55926	70076	26986	86926	69987
76281	44729	32869	19716	71425	86214	12260	12236
39241	86436	43377	335	67171	21099	15746	12030
39535	24879	14977	5117	42049	93843	89091	27236

Safeguarding the Integrity of the Randomization Procedure

The second concern is to safeguard the integrity of the randomization procedure to avoid unintentional or intentional biases. This is essential to reduce potential confounding effects associated with bias. In terms of health promotion research, this means designing randomization procedures so that members of the research team who have contact with participants cannot influence the allocation of the participant to the HPP or the control group. Sometimes, given the nature of the HPP, a team member involved in the randomization procedure may tacitly decide that a particular participant could benefit from being in the HPP group. This person may assign that participant to the HPP group without adhering to the established randomization procedure. In this instance, the participant did not have an equal chance of being in either the HPP or control group. In effect, the randomization procedure has been subverted.

To avoid subverting the randomization procedure, participants could be assigned to study conditions using well-established **concealment of allocation** procedures. (See Schulz, 1995; Schulz and Grimes, 2002; and Schulz, Chalmers, Hayes, and Altman, 1995, for a thoughtful discussion of concealment of allocation in randomized controlled trials and for a more detailed account of subverting randomization.) Essentially, this entails developing procedures, prior to beginning study enrollment, in which an investigator generates the allocation sequence, using a random numbers table. This pregenerated sequence must be adhered to when randomizing all participants. In practice, this procedure would operate as follows: the randomization sequence, 0 (control group) or 1 (HPP group), is written on a piece of paper and placed in sealed, opaque envelopes. As participants are ready to be randomized, they are either given or asked to draw the envelope from the top of the stack of envelopes containing the randomization sequence. The investigator (or the participant, if she drew the envelope) opens the envelope and displays the group allocation. Although this is an effective procedure to protect the randomization process, it is critical that the randomization sequence is determined beforehand and that only the principal investigator or the project statistician is involved in constructing the stack of envelopes. Minimizing the involvement of other staff, and having a predetermined randomization sequence that is concealed from other research team members, will help safeguard the integrity of the randomization procedure.

concealment of allocation
strategies designed to mask participants' knowledge about their group assignment

IN A NUTSHELL

Although concealment of allocation techniques is effective in protecting the randomization process, it is critical that the randomization sequence is determined beforehand and that only the principal investigator or the project statistician is involved in constructing the stack of envelopes.

Step 6: Implementing the Study Conditions—Implement the HPP and Comparison Groups as Prescribed in the Research Protocol and Manual of Operations

Implementing an RCT requires particular attention to a number of methodological issues concerning the HPP. Four key issues to consider are: (1) blinding, (2) designing the control/comparison condition, (3) ensuring fidelity of HPP implementation, and (4) enhancing participation in the HPP.

Blinding may be used with study participants, study investigators and staff, and study statisticians. With respect to participants, blinding is a research procedure that prevents them from knowing whether they have been assigned to the experimental or control condition. This procedure reduces problems known collectively as **demand characteristics**. These manifest when participants behave differently as a consequence of knowing they are being studied or because of social desirability; in essence, participants may *selectively change their behaviors or distort their reports of behaviors upon assessment.*

> **IN A NUTSHELL**
>
> Demand characteristics manifest when participants behave differently as a consequence of knowing they are being studied or because of social desirability; in essence, they may selectively change their behaviors or distort their reports of behaviors upon assessment.

blinding
strategies to reduce participants' knowledge of the group to which they have been assigned

demand characteristics
experimental artifacts wherein participants form an interpretation of the experiment's purpose and may alter their behavior or responses

Blinding also has applicability for study staff. For example, if the research staff is aware of the study hypothesis, their behavior could affect study outcomes if they differentially evaluate individuals in each of the trial arms. This phenomenon is called **experimenter bias**. To control for this bias, a double-blind procedure can be implemented. For example, in medical trials, particularly studies designed to evaluate the differential effectiveness of medication, double-blind trials are often implemented. In a **double-blind trial**, neither the investigator nor the participant is aware of whether the participant is allocated to the experimental (experimental drug) arm or the control (placebo medication) arm.

experimenter bias
a process in which the investigators performing the trial may influence the results

double-blind trial
an experimental method used to ensure impartiality and avoid errors arising from bias

Finally, the staff member conducting data analysis (the study statistician) could be biased by knowing what condition participants were assigned. Here another form of blinding applies, in that the study statistician may need to be blinded as well. When this occurs, a study is deemed triple-blinded. In this case, participants, investigators, and statistician are all unaware of whether the assigned condition is experimental or control.

Although an effective procedure, blinding is difficult to implement in the context of an HPP RCT. In other words, it may be impossible to keep participants from knowing to which condition they are randomized. Typically, due to the nature of HPP research, participants and group facilitators are aware of participants' group assignments. For example, in our illustration of the HPP with older adults to change dietary behavior, it would be difficult if not impossible to effectively blind participants and group facilitators who are, respectively, being exposed to the HPP and administering it. Indeed, the facilitators are often involved in developing the HPP and thus blinding on this level would be impractical. Likewise, blinding participants is difficult, because they have to be informed of the study intent and procedures and sign a written informed consent form prior to participation in the study. Participants would be aware that they would be assigned to one of (at least) two groups and would know what each group would receive as part of the RCT. Once the HPP begins, they will fully understand to which group they have been assigned. Therefore, for many HPP RCTs, blinding is not a viable way to control for these types of biases. In fact, one type of demand characteristic that is particularly difficult to control in HPP RCTs is social desirability. This occurs when participants underreport or overreport their behaviors to conform to the established social norms created by the group and the group facilitator. For example, an abstinence-based program for teen pregnancy prevention may create a norm suggesting that engaging in sex is wrong, thereby leading participants to *underreport* their true sexual behavior because they do not want to appear to be having sex. This would suggest an intervention effect (that is, that the HPP was effective in reducing sexual behavior) that is spurious.

Hawthorne effect
phenomenon that affects many research experiments in social sciences; a process in which subjects participating in an experiment may change their behavior simply because they are enrolled in a trial

Another common demand characteristic is known as the **Hawthorne effect**. The Hawthorne effect is a form of reactivity whereby subjects improve or modify an aspect of their behavior in response to being studied (McCarney, Warner, Iliffe, van Haselen, Griffin, and Fisher, 2007) rather than in response to any particular experimental manipulation. The term was coined in 1950 by Henry A. Landsberger when analyzing older experiments from 1924 to 1932 at the Hawthorne Works (a Western Electric factory outside Chicago) that found that employee productivity varied with changes in lighting. The study produced surprising results. As might be expected, productivity increased when lights were made brighter. However, unexpectedly, productivity also increased when the lights were dimmed! Landsberger drew the conclusion that simply knowing they were being observed caused employees to increase their productivity. This form of bias can be minimized by the use of a structurally comparable comparison group. In other words, a group that does not receive the HPP, but receives an **placebo-attention program**. A placebo-attention comparison group would

placebo-attention program
program to control for attentional bias

be similar to the HPP with respect to time, frequency of meetings, intensity of activities, and enjoyment of intervention activities. In the illustration used earlier, the HPP consisted of five group sessions focused on healthy diet. A comparable placebo-attention comparison group would therefore mirror the number of group sessions (also known as the intervention dose), the frequency with which the sessions are offered, the duration of sessions, and the level of interactivity within each session. The use of an placebo-attention comparison program provides a suitable remedy to the Hawthorne effect, although this increases the cost of conducting the study as additional staff is needed to develop and implement the comparison group.

Designing the Comparison Condition

There are three types of comparison groups. For one type, the comparison group receives no health promotion intervention or additional attention from study staff other than what is required to collect participant assessments. This is referred to as a **true control group**. Essentially, participants who are assigned to the control group would return to complete follow-up assessments on the same schedule as participants randomized to the HPP group. Typically, if the study is conducted in a clinical setting that routinely offers treatment and counseling, the comparison group receive the "usual care or standard-of-care treatment or counseling" typically offered. In the second type, the **wait-list control group**, participants assigned to the comparison group enter the HPP *after* their final assessment. This is an ethically appropriate design that ensures that all participants receive the HPP. The third type has been discussed; it involves constructing a structurally similar "placebo-attention comparison group," which does not receive information, education, or skills hypothesized to affect dependent variables to prevent potentially compromising the validity of the RCT and producing null findings. Yet a structurally similar placebo-attention comparison condition should also be relevant and beneficial to participants.

true control group
group that receives no intervention, but only usual care

wait-list control group
a group that receives no intervention until participants have completed their final assessment

IN A NUTSHELL

Be careful that the comparison HPP program does not provide information, education, or skills relevant to the goals of the HPP.

Ensuring Fidelity of HPP Implementation

In any RCT it is imperative that implementation of the HPP be monitored regularly to safeguard against **drift** (that is, deviation from the established

drift
deviation from the established protocol

protocol). Drift is typically not an issue when the HPP is a web-based or a computer-based program, but it is an issue when a facilitator(s) or health educator(s) deliver the intervention. Drift happens when program facilitators unintentionally or intentionally deviate from the established intervention protocol. At times they may interject personal experiences or anecdotes into a given HPP that clearly deviate from the HPP curriculum. In addition, they may perceive that the situation or circumstances necessitate presenting information that is not included in the scripted curriculum.

Implementation drift can affect the internal validity of the RCT and reduce the ability to detect effects of the HPP on study outcomes. Internal validity may be compromised because the intervention is delivered differentially by staff members or by the same staff member throughout the course of the study. Thus evaluation of the "HPP" is problematic because it may have assumed several forms throughout the trial.

To minimize drift, it is critical to develop an implementation monitoring or quality assurance protocol. This protocol governs what can and cannot be done. The protocol should be sufficiently detailed, including: (1) specification of each activity, (2) the goal and objectives for each activity, (3) who will implement the activity, and (4) the time allocated to each activity. Investigators and research staff need to be acutely aware of all aspects of the protocol and taught to adhere to it diligently. Although a detailed training program can be useful, continual monitoring of HPP implementation is also needed to ensure that drift is avoided. That way, if drift does occur, it can be promptly detected and rectified.

Detecting drift requires ongoing monitoring of HPP implementation staff. To this end, a number of procedures have proven useful. In our own research, we use a dual-method quality assurance methodology. First, participants are asked to anonymously complete a rating form that lists all the HPP session activities. Participants "check off" whether the health educators or program facilitators implemented each session activity (yes/no). The health educators and program facilitators are blind to the participants' ratings, as these are placed in unmarked envelopes and collected by staff other than health educators or program facilitators. Thus the investigators have an objective determination of the HPP activities that participants report being exposed to during the group session. This record is then checked against the implementation manual. Inconsistencies can then be addressed in meetings with the health educators.

The second method for assessing fidelity of implementation is to have a rater assigned to each HPP intervention group session and comparison group session if possible. If not feasible, then at a minimum, a rater can be assigned to a percentage of intervention and comparison group sessions. In addition, an alternative approach could be to audio-record the HPP sessions and then have a rater independently review the recording. In fact, audio-recording may be the only way to assess quality assurance for HPPs that are one-on-one (facilitator and participant), because having a rater in the room would significantly alter the intervention. No matter how the quality assurance is implemented, the rater completes a checklist much like the participants' rating form; however, the rater's checklist is significantly more detailed. The rater assesses whether particular HPP activities were implemented, the amount of time allocated to each activity and whether the planned intervention activities were implemented correctly according to the intervention manual. These quality assurance methods can be used to quickly identify a health educator or program facilitator who is not compliant with the HPP manual and to help minimize the adverse effects of poor implementation fidelity.

Enhancing Participation and Retention in the HPP

In any multisession HPP there is the potential that some participants will not complete the full HPP program, so they do not receive the full dose of the intervention. It is critical to develop strategies designed to maximize participant completion of all HPP sessions. For example, consider a study designed to test whether yoga exercises conducted during one-hour sessions for 30 consecutive days help reduce blood pressure. Unfortunately, nearly 36 percent of the participants in the HPP (yoga) group do not attend all 30 sessions, so they have not received the "full dose" of the HPP.

Not completing the full HPP can reduce the likelihood that HPP effects will be detected. To remedy the situation, it may be tempting to discard or eliminate data from participants who do not complete the full intervention. However, to do so would be inappropriate. Once participants have been randomized to their respective treatment groups, they must be analyzed within those groups, regardless of whether or not they complete all required procedures. A common phrase that captures this rule is "once randomized, always analyzed." This is referred to as an **intent-to-treat** analysis and is critically important to complying with the rules. An intent-to-treat analysis involves analyzing everyone who was enrolled and randomized, regardless of whether they completed all of the

IN A NUTSHELL

Once participants have been randomized to their respective treatment groups, they are analyzed within those groups, regardless of whether or not they complete all required procedures. A common phrase that captures this rule is "once randomized, always analyzed."

intent-to-treat
inclusion of all participants in the summative analysis, whether they were treated or not

HPP sessions or assessments. This is important because those who do not attend all sessions may differ from those who are "completers" on other characteristics relevant to the dependent variables. If "non-completers" are deleted from analyses, this introduces bias to the sample. In essence, eliminating those with incomplete attendance in the HPP changes what had initially been a randomized group. The second rule of the intent-to-treat analysis is that it should be applied when issues arise relative to missing follow-up assessments or missing data within assessments. Again, the initial temptation may be to delete participants' data from the analysis. Again, this would introduce bias into the findings. Many statistical techniques have been devised to address missing data; these should be used when appropriate. For a discussion of these techniques, consult Graham, Hofer, Donaldson, MacKinnon, and Schafer (1997) or Schafer (1999).

Because statistical solutions to missing data are not as desirable as design-based solutions, it is important to consider how best to ensure full participation in the HPP and follow-up assessments. A number of strategies have been designed to reduce HPP attendance barriers. First, compensation may be offered to participants for attending the HPP and for completing assessments. Typically, assessments are administered at baseline and subsequent follow-up time points after the completion of the HPP activities. Some funding agencies, however, may not permit the use of monetary (or other) compensation for simply being a participant. They might, however, approve of providing compensation for completing assessments, so it may be helpful to build in brief assessments that coincide with the HPP intervention sessions. One example would be to compensate participants for completing the quality assurance rating form. Another example would be to provide compensation for childcare, if necessary. Also, providing compensation in the form of stipends for transportation to and from the HPP sessions and for completion of assessments can be effective in reducing barriers to, and enhancing participation in, the HPP. Finally, designing an HPP that is perceived by participants as valuable, enjoyable, and engaging, and having health educators (program facilitators) who are perceived as caring, knowledgeable, and dedicated are critical features of any HPP and may enhance retention.

Step 7: Follow-Up—Follow Participants Post-HPP to Monitor Changes in Outcomes

Maintaining the study cohort over protracted periods of time may be one of the most formidable challenges in conducting an RCT. Several problems can easily arise. We describe here some of the problems that are unique to RCTs; Chapter Nine provides more detail about procedures that can be used to retain study cohorts over time.

Conducting the Follow-Up Assessment. Follow-up is critical to capturing data that measure the effectiveness of the HPP. After participants complete an HPP, you will need to follow them over time and ask them to return for another assessment so that you can measure changes in attitudes, beliefs, intentions, behaviors, or health indices. This presents a number of issues.

One question associated with the follow-up assessment is, who will collect the follow-up data? Anyone involved in program implementation of the HPP or of the placebo-attention comparison condition should not be involved in conducting the follow-up assessments. Health educators or facilitators typically establish relationships with participants, which may influence participants' responses to questions and result in social desirability bias. Likewise, health educators could knowingly or unknowingly influence participants' responses. Using a staff member not known to the participants may reduce this form of bias. The most effective strategy is to maintain a strict distinction between HPP implementation staff (for example, health educators, program facilitators, program interveners) and the data collection staff (assessors).

IN A NUTSHELL

Health educators or facilitators typically establish relationships with participants, which may influence the way participants respond to questions and result in social desirability bias.

A related issue involves the mode of administration of the assessment instrument. Interview-administered assessments may create greater potential for bias, as participants may respond in socially desirable ways (that is, providing answers they think the assessor wants to hear). This potential for bias from interviewer administered assessments may be

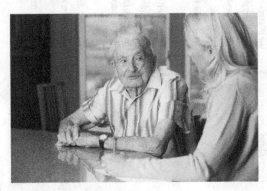
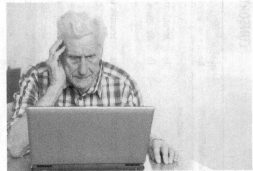

Figure 10.3 Comparison of Assessment Modes

CONSORT 2010 checklist of information to include when reporting a randomized trial*

Section/Topic	Item No	Checklist item	Reported on page No
Title and abstract			
	1a	Identification as a randomized trial in the title	
	1b	Structured summary of trial design, methods, results, and conclusions (for specific guidance see CONSORT for abstracts)	
Introduction			
Background and objectives	2a	Scientific background and explanation of rationale	
	2b	Specific objectives or hypotheses	
Methods			
Trial design	3a	Description of trial design (such as parallel, factorial) including allocation ratio	
	3b	Important changes to methods after trial commencement (such as eligibility criteria), with reasons	
Participants	4a	Eligibility criteria for participants	
	4b	Settings and locations where the data were collected	
Interventions	5	The interventions for each group with sufficient details to allow replication, including how and when they were actually administered	
Outcomes	6a	Completely defined pre-specified primary and secondary outcome measures, including how and when they were assessed	
	6b	Any changes to trial outcomes after the trial commenced, with reasons	
Sample size	7a	How sample size was determined	
	7b	When applicable, explanation of any interim analyses and stopping guidelines	
Randomization:			
Sequence generation	8a	Method used to generate the random allocation sequence	
	8b	Type of randomization; details of any restriction (such as blocking and block size)	
Allocation concealment mechanism	9	Mechanism used to implement the random allocation sequence (such as sequentially numbered containers), describing any steps taken to conceal the sequence until interventions were assigned	
Implementation	10	Who generated the random allocation sequence, who enrolled participants, and who assigned participants to interventions	
Blinding	11a	If done, who was blinded after assignment to interventions (for example, participants, care providers, those assessing outcomes) and how	
	11b	If relevant, description of the similarity of interventions	

Section/Topic	Item No	Checklist item
Statistical methods	12a	Statistical methods used to compare groups for primary and secondary outcomes
	12b	Methods for additional analyses, such as subgroup analyses and adjusted analyses
Results		
Participant flow (a diagram is strongly recommended)	13a	For each group, the numbers of participants who were randomly assigned, received intended treatment, and were analyzed for the primary outcome
	13b	For each group, losses and exclusions after randomization, together with reasons
Recruitment	14a	Dates defining the periods of recruitment and follow-up
	14b	Why the trial ended or was stopped
Baseline data	15	A table showing baseline demographic and clinical characteristics for each group
Numbers analyzed	16	For each group, number of participants (denominator) included in each analysis and whether the analysis was by original assigned groups
Outcomes and estimation	17a	For each primary and secondary outcome, results for each group, and the estimated effect size and its precision (such as 95% confidence interval)
	17b	For binary outcomes, presentation of both absolute and relative effect sizes is recommended
Ancillary analyses	18	Results of any other analyses performed, including subgroup analyses and adjusted analyses, distinguishing pre-specified from exploratory
Harms	19	All important harms or unintended effects in each group (for specific guidance see CONSORT for harms)
Discussion		
Limitations	20	Trial limitations, addressing sources of potential bias, imprecision, and, if relevant, multiplicity of analyses
Generalizability	21	Generalizability (external validity, applicability) of the trial findings
Interpretation	22	Interpretation consistent with results, balancing benefits and harms, and considering other relevant evidence
Other information		
Registration	23	Registration number and name of trial registry
Protocol	24	Where the full trial protocol can be accessed, if available
Funding	25	Sources of funding and other support (such as supply of drugs), role of funders

*We strongly recommend reading this statement in conjunction with the CONSORT 2010 Explanation and Elaboration for important clarifications on all the items. If relevant, we also recommend reading CONSORT extensions for cluster randomized trials, non-inferiority and equivalence trials, non-pharmacological treatments, herbal interventions, and pragmatic trials. Additional extensions are forthcoming: for those and for up to date references relevant to this checklist, see www.consort-statement.org.

Figure 10.4 Consolidated Standards of Reporting Trials (CONSORT) Checklist

minimized, although not entirely eliminated, with self-administered modes such as using computer-assisted technology to administer the assessments (Turner, Ku, Rogers, Lindberg, Pleck, and Sonenstein, 1998). Figure 10.3 illustrates these two modes.

Step 8: Perform Analysis

The objective of the RCT is to compare changes in outcomes observed among participants in the HPP with those observed among participants in the comparison arm(s). In the current example, you would determine whether participation in the HPP resulted in significant, observed, and measurable changes in the three classes of outcomes: (1) theory-driven mediators associated with dietary behavior; (2) dietary behaviors, and (3) blood LDL levels. Although seemingly straightforward, analysis of an RCT can be complex. The description of the statistical approaches—and there are many—is beyond the scope of this chapter; however, Chapter Fifteen describes analytic approaches for RCTs in more detail. Further, we recommend strongly that anyone undertaking an RCT consult with a statistician.

Step 9. Reporting the Trial Findings—Conduct Structured Reporting of RCTs

Methodologically rigorous research warrants dissemination of the findings to stakeholders, interested participants, or, in the case of funded evaluations, the funding agency. In certain instances, the findings may also be communicated to policy makers. Indeed, this step may enhance the likelihood that the HPP's benefits will extend beyond just those who participated in the study. If the HPP is found to be effective and the results are disseminated, other agencies and organizations could adopt the program, thereby improving public health.

In the event that the findings are not supportive of the HPP, the results can provide empirical evidence that may be useful in guiding the direction of future research. Far too often HPPs are implemented without adequate evaluation. This is to the detriment of the participants in these programs, society, or organizations that bear the costs of these programs, and also to the science of health promotion.

To assist in reporting of RCTs, a well-articulated, structured format (a checklist) has been developed by the CONSORT group. The checklist is considered *de rigueur* in high-impact journals. Figure 10.4 shows this structured reporting format in considerable detail.

Summary

The aim of this chapter was to provide fundamental information to help guide the design of randomized controlled trials assessing the effectiveness of HPPs. Two limitations of this chapter are that it could not cover all aspects of RCT design—most prominently, statistical analysis—nor could it provide an in-depth discussion of the issues presented. Notwithstanding these limitations, the chapter provides a broad overview of key issues to be considered in designing and implementing an RCT. In addition, we emphasize how these issues affect the validity of the study and the interpretation of the findings. Finally, we propose practical solutions. Given the importance of HPPs and the cost and time associated with designing and implementing these programs, it is critical that we also consider how best to evaluate their effectiveness. The RCT, carefully designed and implemented, represents a rigorous methodological approach to assessing the effectiveness of health promotion interventions.

KEY TERMS

Biological revolution	Inclusion and exclusion criteria
Blinding	Independent variable
Causal inference	Intent-to-treat
Concealment of allocation	Intermediary outcomes
CONSORT	Internal validity
Demand characteristics	Logic model
Dependent variables	Mediators
Double-blind trial	Parallel group design
Drift	Placebo-attention program
Effect size	Power analysis
Experimenter bias	Randomized controlled trial
External validity	True control group
Extraneous variables	Wait-list control group
Hawthorne effect	

For Practice and Discussion

1. Imagine that you accessed a population of low-income Hispanic women who are at high risk of cervical cancer. Your intent is to develop

a randomized controlled trial (RCT) to test an HPP that you have developed that is designed to promote regular Pap testing. The HPP is a 9-hour program delivered in three sessions. Women will be paid $50 to complete a baseline assessment and another $50 to complete a follow-up assessment. All women will be asked to provide permission for study investigators to track their medical records for the next 5 years. Because these women would not otherwise have any education designed to promote Pap testing, you decide to use a do-nothing control group for your RCT. Please provide justification for your choice of a "true" control group. Then assume that the justification is not sufficient and provide an alternative plan that can be defended on the basis of rigor alone (excluding ethical concerns from your argument).

2. This chapter emphasized the importance of using an intent-to-treat analysis for RCTs. Unfortunately, quite a few articles reporting RCTs have been published that do not employ the intent-to-treat principle. Consider a hypothetical scenario in which 140 women were randomized to the HPP condition and 110 women were randomized to an attention control condition. Baseline measures were collected on all 250 women. In the ensuing 6 weeks, women were expected to attend a two-hour intervention on each Saturday afternoon. By the end of the sixth week, 90 percent of the women in the HPP condition remained in the study (that is, they attended the sessions as required). By contrast, only 50 percent of the women in the control group remained in the study. How might failure to use an intent-to-treat analysis influence the study findings? Keep in mind that the influence is a form of bias that can affect the validity of the findings. Discuss the intent-to-treat principle, why it is important, and how it could affect this study's findings and the interpretation of the findings.

3. Earthshaking new research suggests that too much television viewing results in increased risk for obesity. These newspaper reports are based on an observational study. Now you would like to test this hypothesis in an RCT. You decide to randomize a group of college freshmen during the incoming orientation to two conditions (arms): (1) the intervention arm—they are not permitted TV use during the semester or (2) the control arm—they are permitted as much TV viewing as they would like. You assess their weight and height at baseline during orientation; this will yield a measure of body mass index (BMI), TV exposure in the prior 4 months, and other potential confounding factors, such as alcohol and drug use, exercise, and diet. Working in a group, complete the experiment (you supply the data). Calculate effect sizes for TV exposure on obesity as determined by BMI. Interpret your findings and make recommendations based on the results.

4. Read a journal article that examined a randomized trial of a dietary enhancement intervention in the field of health promotion and discuss how the authors designed the study. Pay particular attention to the selection and recruitment of the sample, the allocation of subjects to the study conditions, the follow-up or retention rates, whether intent-to-treat analyses were conducted, and how the investigators conducted their analysis to determine if the intervention was efficacious. Also, what measures of effect do the investigators report to demonstrate the efficacy of the intervention?

References

Graham, J. W., Hofer, S. M., Donaldson, S. I., MacKinnon, D. P., and Schafer, J. L. (1997). Analysis with missing data in prevention research. In K. Bryant, M. Windle, and S. West (Eds.), *The science of prevention: Methodological advances from alcohol and substance abuse research* (pp. 325–366). Washington, DC: American Psychological Association.

McCarney, R., Warner, J., Iliffe, S., van Haselen, R., Griffin, M., and Fisher, P. (2007). The Hawthorne Effect: a randomised, controlled trial. *BMC Medical Research Methodology, 7*, 30. doi:10.1186/1471–2288–7–30. PMC 1936999. PMID 17608932.

Moher, D., Hopewell, S., Schulz, K., Montori, V., Gotzsche, P. C., . . . CONSORT. (2012). CONSORT 2010 Explanation and elaboration: Updated guidelines for reporting parallel group randomized trials. *International Journal of Surgery, 10*(1),28–55.

Piantadosi, S. (1997). *Clinical trials: A methodologic perspective.* New York: Wiley.

Pocock, S. J. (1993). *Clinical trials.* New York: Wiley.

Schafer, J. L. (1999). Multiple imputation: A primer. *Statistical Methods in Medical Research, 8,* 3–15.

Schulz, K. F. (1995). Subverting randomization in controlled trials. *Journal of the American Medical Association, 274,* 1456–1458.

Schulz, K. F., Altman, D. G., and Moher, D., for the CONSORT Group. (2010). CONSORT 2010 Statement: Updated guidelines for reporting parallel group randomized trials. *BMJ, 340,* c332. doi:10.1136/bmj.c332

Schulz, K. F., Chalmers, I., Hayes, R. J., and Altman, D. G. (1995). Empirical evidence of bias: Dimensions of methodological quality associated with treatment effects in controlled trials. *Journal of the American Medical Association, 273,* 408–412.

Schulz, K. F., and Grimes, D. A. (2002). Blinding in randomized trials: Hiding who got what. *Lancet, 359,* 696–700.

Turner, C. F., Ku, L., Rogers, S. M., Lindberg, L. D., Pleck, J. H., and Sonenstein, F. L. (1998). Adolescent sexual behavior, drug use and violence: Increased reporting with computer survey technology. *Science, 280,* 867–873.

CHAPTER 11

COMMUNITY-BASED PARTICIPATORY RESEARCH IN THE CONTEXT OF HEALTH PROMOTION

Ralph J. DiClemente
Laura F. Salazar
Richard A. Crosby

To address the significant public health challenges of the twenty-first century, including addressing a wide range of health disparities experienced by many people globally, traditional community-based research methods have evolved and have been augmented with a new methodological paradigm. This paradigm encompasses new research models that place community partners on equal standing with academic researchers. Community-based participatory research (CBPR) is considered one of these models. CBPR embraces an equal and collaborative partnership between community and academia that enhances the likelihood that adoption, integration, and sustainability of public health innovations will be achieved.

Although substantial progress has been made in public health on several fronts since the first edition of this book, the need to further accelerate health promotion efforts to reduce risk behaviors and associated diseases means that new research paradigms may be required. Many academic researchers conduct studies in communities deemed "high-risk" in that they are characterized by high unemployment, low social capital, high poverty, and low educational attainment; thus these communities also experience significant disparities in health-related outcomes. Indeed, if public health is to effectively confront risk and disease in these most adversely impacted communities, it may require engaging the community

LEARNING OBJECTIVES

- Distinguish between traditional community research models and community-engagement models.

- Learn the motivation for newer and more equitable community-engagement models.

- Understand the underlying principles of the community-based participatory research model.

- Learn about ways to navigate the potential challenges of partnering with communities.

as a partner in the research enterprise rather than as a "recipient of research" as in traditional research models (Blumenthal, DiClemente, Braithwaite, and Smith, 2013a). A number of community engagement models have been developed to facilitate this work, including participatory action research (PAR), participatory learning and action (PLA), community-based participatory research (CBPR), feminist participatory action research (FPAR), and empowerment evaluation (EE). These models require community involvement in research projects, but the roles of the researcher(s) and the community members vary. For example, in PAR the researchers are more heavily involved and are responsible for coordinating the project and community action. On the opposite end of this continuum, EE does not *require* a researcher unless the community decides that they would like outside help with their project, though most communities choose to work with a professional evaluator or researcher. The remaining models fall somewhere in the middle in terms of degree of researcher input and level of community control. To some degree these models grew out of communities' concerns over being exploited, lack of input into the research process, lack of trust, who owned the data, and sustainability of efforts. These models address these concerns by first and foremost establishing a partnership as the basis for conducting all project activities. In this way, these newer paradigms are much like a square dance—that is, multiple partnerships are a requisite, and each participating partner must listen to the caller and work together as they perform a rather complex sequence of steps. If each partnership and the sets of partnerships are all in sync, then the square dance will be orchestrated beautifully and will result in an enjoyable time and productive research that benefits the community.

Typically, the traditional community research model involves the community providing the context in which the research is conducted and, in turn, researchers engage community representatives to serve on their **community advisory boards** (CAB), providing periodic input on project implementation issues such as recruitment and retention. A CAB is defined as a board made up of community representatives who serve as a source of leadership and provide direction and input on project design, implementation, evaluation, and dissemination of the findings. Establishing a CAB typically begins with a well-publicized informational meeting (we recommend providing refreshments to enhance turnout) to discuss the purpose of the CAB, opportunities for involvement, and terms for participation. Establishing this partnership may begin with this first meeting; however, sustaining a CAB can be a time- and labor-intensive process involves building relationships over time and making a long-term commitment. Having a CAB is certainly necessary, but may not be sufficient,

community advisory boards

a type of advisory board consisting of representatives of the general public or key stakeholders who meet with representatives of the study to ensure that the community has equal voice, power, and decision-making capability with academic partners in all facets of the research enterprise.

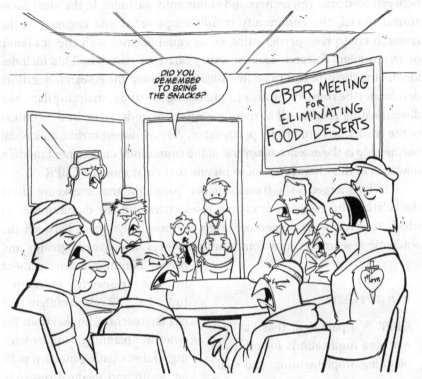

Mincus and Dincus Conflict Arises at First Community Advisory Board Meeting

The need to identify a more cohesive and equitable community research alignment has inspired a new form of researcher-community relationship. In addition to some of the community concerns already highlighted, this new "evolution of alignment" can also be attributed to a practical concern over an increasing emphasis on community-based and translational research by government and private funders. This changing emphasis reflects the realization that medical and public health innovations—be they medical devices, pharmaceutical therapies, or health promotion programs—are unlikely to achieve their full promise and potential to reduce risk behaviors and disease without their adoption, integration, and sustainment in highly affected communities. Consequently, a more close-knit and collaborative model between academia and the community that fosters greater adoption, integration, and sustainability of medical and public health innovations now exists.

The emerging **zeitgeist** (the literal translation is "spirit of the times") for community-based research avoids conducting research *on* a community,

zeitgeist
the spirit of the time; general trend of thought or feeling characteristic of a particular time period

or even *in* a community, but rather conducts research *with* a community. This contemporary perspective is indicative of an equitable partnership between academic researchers and community partners. In the ideal operational model, the community is fully empowered and engaged in the research enterprise, participating as an equal partner with the academic or government research team in every phase of research. This includes identifying the problem to be investigated, defining the research question, developing the research protocol, conducting the study, analyzing data, and disseminating results. All of these activities are undertaken in the context of the academic-community partnership. As mentioned earlier, this equal partnership is the essence of several of the community engagement models; however, in this chapter we focus on one particular model—CBPR.

CBPR emerged as a transformative paradigm that markedly alters the relationship between academic researchers and the communities in which research is implemented, levels the power dynamics between the academic researchers and community partners, and fosters greater and deeper community engagement in the research enterprise. Indeed, CBPR is a paradigm that has far-reaching implications for ethically planning, implementing, and evaluating modern public health and medical research. CBPR is increasingly gaining traction in the cognate fields of public health and medicine.

IN A NUTSHELL

CBPR is a paradigm that has far-reaching implications for ethically planning, implementing, and evaluating modern public health and medical research.

In this chapter we define CBPR, identify the impetus and rationale for CBPR, and describe its underlying principles. We also describe the advantages and potential challenges of utilizing CBPR and offer potential solutions to overcome these challenges. Finally, we describe the application of CBPR in community-based research.

Impetus for CBPR

Recent advances in public health and medicine have resulted in significant reductions in disease morbidity, and as a consequence, major gains in life expectancy have been achieved. However, it has become increasingly clear that medicine and public health, in their present incarnation, may not be optimally effective in furthering gains in health. Over the past few decades, medical expenditures have increased consistently and substantially, although improvement in health indicators has been more modest and gradual; essentially, gains in health are not commensurate with expenditures (Fineberg, 2013). Indeed, there is a growing awareness of the need to actively engage the community as a research partner to advance scientific knowledge at the community level. Furthermore, even though there are rapid innovations in medicine and public health, these innovations are unlikely to achieve their full promise and potential to reduce risk behaviors and the resultant morbidity and mortality without the adoption, integration, and sustainment of these innovations in highly affected communities. CBPR as a research paradigm may improve public health and enhance potential solutions for reducing and/or eliminating racial and ethnic health disparities at the community level. This paradigm stands in stark contrast to pre-CBPR research that was oriented primarily to the interests and desires of academic researchers, who were often not integrally involved in the communities in which they implemented research and thus had little personal investment in the future of these communities. As a consequence, when pre-CBPR research ended, often when government or private sector foundation funding expired, this created a gap in community-based services. Often communities could not replicate or reconstitute these services, resulting in feelings of abandonment, resentment, and anger.

Before describing the core principles of CBPR, it is important to note that CBPR is not a research methodology per se nor is it a research design. CBPR is a paradigm for how community research should be planned, developed, implemented, evaluated, and disseminated. CBPR provides the overarching contextual framework that guides the research enterprise. It does not alter the

IN A NUTSHELL

CBPR is not a research methodology per se nor is it a research design. CBPR is a paradigm for how community research should be planned, developed, implemented, evaluated, and disseminated.

methodological rigor or processes inherent when undertaking the research process; rather, CBPR utilizes the same scientific methods and principles as other types of research endeavors, as well as similar processes by which hypotheses are developed and tested and considerations of study design are decided. There are, however, important considerations that apply uniquely to CBPR. These include principles that govern relationships between academic researchers and community partners to develop equitable academic-community partnerships. These equitable partnerships are integral to the successful implementation of CBPR and ultimately the research enterprise. Recall the square dance analogy and how important partnerships are to an enjoyable and successful experience.

Defining Community-Based Participatory Research

A formal definition of community-based participatory research (CBPR) can be found in a review of the topic commissioned by the federal Agency for Healthcare Research and Quality (AHRQ) (Viswanathan et al., 2004). In this definition CBPR is a collaborative research approach designed to ensure and establish structure for participation by communities affected by the issue being studied, representatives of organizations, and researchers in all aspects of the research process to improve health and well-being through taking action, including social change.

Within the CBPR paradigm all types of research designs, whether qualitative, observational, or experimental, are appropriate. Importantly, CBPR may enhance the research enterprise by engaging the community as active and equal partners, thus providing a unique and valuable perspective that may promote and enhance the research planning process by facilitating research implementation, assisting in contextualizing the evaluation, and promoting dissemination of the study findings. Of particular note, CBPR transcends what has become broadly known as "community engagement" or community-based research. Within the CBPR paradigm the community is actively engaged in the research enterprise; however, the community can be engaged without developing a fully functional, equitable, and operational partnership, whereby a power imbalance would remain typically favoring academic researchers. Rather than simply engaging the community, CBPR is distinguished by a core set of principles that, first and foremost, intrinsically value an equal, shared, and reciprocal relationship between community partners and academic researchers. Figure 11.1 provides a brief summary of the key features inherent in a CBPR approach in contrast to more traditional approaches.

IN A NUTSHELL

CBPR is distinguished by a core set of principles that, first and foremost, intrinsically values an equal, shared, and reciprocal relationship between community partners and academic researchers.

With any emerging paradigm, a taxonomy and consensus regarding terminology is established over time. This is true for CBPR. A number of authors and programs have developed sets of principles for guiding CBPR. Rather than describe each of these, we refer the interested reader to Blumenthal et al. (2013a, b) as well as a widely cited articulation of CBPR principles developed by Israel and colleagues (Israel, Schultz, Parker, and Becker, 1998). We articulate these underlying CBPR principles as follows:

1. *Recognizes community as a unit of identity.* This principle acknowledges that a community may be a geographic entity, but alternatively a

Traditional Community Research Models	Community-based Participatory Research Model
• Role of community is passive	• Role of community is one of "dynamic and equitable engagement"
• Project leadership is mainly under control of academic researchers	• Project leadership is jointly controlled by community partners and academic researchers
• Identification of the research problem is governed by academic researchers	• Identification of the research problem is governed by community partners in close collaboration with academic researchers
• Research planning, implementation and evaluation is the purview of academic researchers	• Research planning, implementation, and evaluation is the purview of the community partners and academic researchers
• Dissemination is governed by academic researchers usually through publication of results in medical and public health journals	• Dissemination is governed by community partners and academic researchers. This may include publication of results in medical and public health journals, but goes well beyond academic dissemination vehicles to focus on providing feedback to the community thereby gaining increased "buy in" for future planning or actions
• Sustainability of the project or innovative program is not part of the academic research agenda	• Sustainability of the project or innovative program is a priority that provides direct and immediate benefit to the community; avoids lapses in program/service implementation that may be deleterious to community members

Figure 11.1 Differentiating Traditional Community Research Models from CBPR

community may be defined by other commonality among members, such as ethnicity or occupation.

2. *Builds on strengths and resources within the community.* This principle recognizes that public health workers and researchers have often described communities according to their needs and problems, but a more appropriate approach to community health needs assessment calls for an inventory of the community's assets as well (Sharpe, Greaney, Lee, and Royce, 2000). Assets may include businesses, churches, schools, organizations, and agencies.

3. *Facilitates collaborative partnerships in all phases of the research.* This principle reaffirms that communities should share control over all phases of the research process. Indeed, this is the virtual *de facto* definition of CBPR.

4. *Integrates knowledge and action for mutual benefit of all partners.* This principle asserts that the results of community-based research should not be simply an academic enterprise that adds to the knowledge base of

community health, but should also be used as a platform to promote local efforts directed at action-oriented community change.

5. *Promotes co-learning and an empowering process that attends to social inequalities.* This principle suggests that researchers and community members learn from each other. Moreover, researchers recognize the inherent inequality between themselves and community members and attempt to address this factor by sharing information, decision-making power, resources, and support.

6. *Involves a cyclical and iterative process.* This principle is indicative of a cycle that proceeds from partnership development and maintenance through community assessment, problem definition, development of research methodology, data collection, analysis, and interpretation, through dissemination of results, determination of action and policy implications, taking action, and establishing mechanisms for sustainability. By implication, the process would then start over once this cycle is complete.

7. *Addresses health from both positive perspectives (such as wellness) and ecological perspectives.* This principle asserts that the former is the more limited model of health that emphasizes physical, mental, and social well-being. The latter recognizes the role of economic, cultural, historical, and political factors.

8. *Disseminates findings and knowledge gained to all partners.* This principle emphasizes sharing the results of the research with community partners in easy-to-understand language and includes the need to consult with participants prior to submission of manuscripts for publication, acknowledging the contributions of participants and developing coauthored publications, when appropriate.

9. *Involves a long-term commitment by all partners.* This principle asserts that a true partnership does not dissolve because a three-year grant has come to an end. The partnership continues even in the absence of funding; the partners may search for new funding while continuing unfunded activities.

Distillation of the Core Principles of CBPR

ethical engagement
a partnership that yields benefits for the community partner

Although CBPR has several underlying principles, essentially CBPR can be distilled to two overarching or anchoring principles from which all others are derived and tethered (Blumenthal, 2011). The first overarching principle is that of **ethical engagement**. Ethical engagement refers to active partnering with communities so that the community derives benefit from the research. This principle is critical, as it addresses a history of exploitation by academics and public health researchers—especially in minority and low-income communities—whereby research participants and their communities received scant benefit. Unfortunately, there are also some instances in which community members were harmed by research (for example, the Tuskegee Syphilis Study). The second overarching principle is that of **community empowerment.** Community empowerment refers to a process in which communities are enabled to gain control over their lives and the decisions affecting their community. This principle has domestic roots that are manifest in the concept of maximum feasible community participation (Blumenthal, 2011). This principle acknowledges that low-income communities rarely have had control over the programs that have an impact on their lives. Programs that affect a community's schools, medical facilities, or public housing, to name but a few examples, rarely reside under community purview—including the design, management, or control of such programs. As community participation expands, deepens, and becomes inextricably woven into the research enterprise, community residents acquire an increased sense of empowerment and, as a consequence, control and decision-making capability over programs that impact their health and well-being and the future of the community.

community empowerment
community exertion of control

Sustainability of Innovative Health Promotion Programs

Sustainability, in the context of CBPR, refers to the endurance of the research, programs, outcomes, or evaluation monitoring plans that were implemented. Sustainability is a critical and constant challenge in health promotion research. Unless environmental and social conditions associated with risk behaviors and diseases are changed, the potential for durable and meaningful health improvements is limited. Mindful of its direct impact on health, a major focus of CBPR is to be a driver of community change. CBPR strives to influence public policies and the strategic stimulation of private, entrepreneurial investment in adversely impacted communities.

sustainability
persistence or durability

To further enhance and support sustainability, a key challenge in health promotion research is creating readily translatable programs. With the increasing emphasis on translational research (Noonan and Emshoff, 2013), transferring medical and public health innovations to community venues is important. There has been a concomitant emphasis on the role CBPR can play to facilitate the translational research agenda as CBPR focuses on thinking systemically and contextually so that evidence-based programs can be embraced by the community and fully integrated into the community infrastructure. Sustainability therefore is more likely when conditions foster the growth of community capacity and empowerment to choose, adopt, adapt, and sustain effective health promotion programs.

Another key issue in translational HPP research has been the question of how to create an infrastructure to sustain health promotion programs following termination of government or private-sector grant funding. The academic-community partnership must therefore always be attentive to the need for identifying and securing resources that enhance the capacity for program continuation after government and private-sector grant funding concludes. Ultimately, it is critical that effective health promotion programs be broadly disseminated and integrally embedded as self-sustaining programs in communities. Without creating community capacity, *ceteris paribus*, health promotion programs are less likely to be sustainable and, as a consequence, also less likely to be able to provide services beneficial for the health and well-being of community members (that is, less likely to reduce disease-associated risk behaviors, disease morbidity, and disease mortality). Thus a question often arises: How are these goals achieved? Answers to this quandary are complex; however, a few observations may provide some clarification. The CBPR process must include a focus on enhancing the community's capability to strategically analyze, plan, and initiate political action designed to help leverage resources and gain political power. Although this is a difficult task to achieve, the synergy of academic-community partnership optimizes the odds for success.

IN A NUTSHELL

The CBPR process must include a focus on enhancing the community's capability to strategically analyze, plan, and initiate political action designed to help leverage resources and gain political power.

CBPR is increasingly recognized and utilized as a vital component to expand access to quality care, prevent disease, and achieve equity in health care. Researchers recognize the value of involving community constituents in the process of identifying appropriate research questions and creating meaningful, testable hypotheses that reflect the interests and priorities of the community. This movement of promoting active and full partnership between communities and academic researchers in participatory research may involve youth, parents, educators, government officials, faith-based community leaders, and other sector groups (Blumenthal, Hopkins, and Yancey, 2013b).

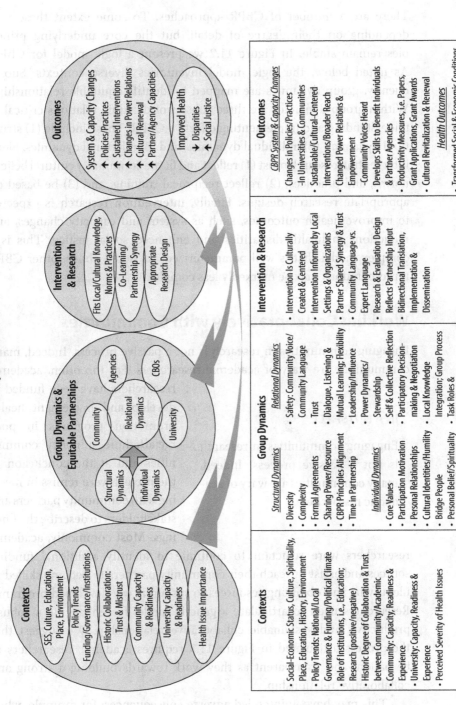

Figure 11.2 CBPR Conceptual Logic Model

Source: Adapted from Wallerstein and Duran (2010) and Wallerstein, Oetzel, Duran, Tafoya, Belone, and Rae (2008).

Logic Model for CBPR

There are a number of CBPR approaches. To some extent these vary depending on their degree of detail, but the core underlying principles remain stable. In Figure 11.2 we present a logic model for CBPR. As noted below, the logic model inventories diverse contexts. Subsequently, group dynamics are mapped to identify equitable relationships. Within group dynamics are three subsets of dynamic relations critical to understanding and implementing effective CBPR. These include (1) structural dynamics, (2) individual dynamics, and (3) relational dynamics. Next, intervention research must (1) reflect and fit the community cultural beliefs, norms, and practices, (2) reflect reciprocal training, and (3) be based on appropriate research designs. Finally, intervention research is expected to improve health outcomes, such as system and capacity changes, and reductions in health disparities and enhanced social justice. This is a complex model that is well parameterized. As noted above, other CBPR representations may be markedly less complex.

Working Collaboratively with Communities

Engaging communities in research is not a passive process. Indeed, many communities are wary of academic researchers. Far too often, academic researchers have been funded to develop and implement health promotion programs in poor racial/ethnic minority communities and at the conclusion of the project were remiss in meeting with community partners and stakeholders to describe the findings. Most commonly, academic researchers were reluctant to continue to identify additional funding sources and assist or teach their community partners to become skilled in identifying and obtaining resources to sustain newly developed programs. Researchers need to articulate a generic model for enhancing a robust, productive, and sustainable collaborative relationship. We suggest that the process articulated in Figure 11.3 requires academic researchers to be patient and transparent as they work towards building a strong and collaborative relationship.

This may have unintended adverse consequences; for example, when academic researchers are under time constraints to respond to a Funding

IN A NUTSHELL

Engaging communities in research is not a passive process. Indeed, many communities are wary of academic researchers.

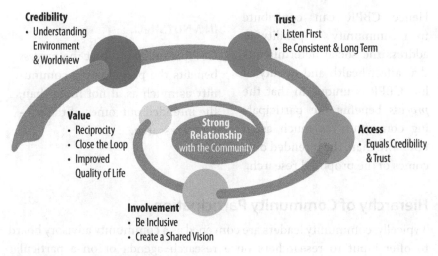

Credibility
- Understanding Environment & Worldview

Trust
- Listen First
- Be Consistent & Long Term

Value
- Reciprocity
- Close the Loop
- Improved Quality of Life

Strong Relationship with the Community

Access
- Equals Credibility & Trust

Involvement
- Be Inclusive
- Create a Shared Vision

Figure 11.3 Keys to the Community

Source: "Engaging and Mobilizing the Grassroots Community," *MEE's UrbanTrends Newsletter, 20*(1).

Opportunity Announcement (FOA) from NIH, CDC, or another public or private funding source. We address some barriers in translating CBPR principles into action in the following section.

Community-Based Research and Level of Community Involvement

As we noted earlier in this chapter, CBPR is often implemented in minority and other disadvantaged communities, and this is likely to become even more frequent in the future as researchers address marked racial and ethnic health disparities. These are often powerless communities that are accustomed to being the purported beneficiaries of health and social programs over which they have no control. CBPR and its principles also work to organize community members to partner with public health workers and researchers in seeking better ways to improve their health through the building of skills for conducting research, advocacy, and lobbying; through training and educational opportunities as community health workers; and through the building of new partnerships and collaborations. As a result, the community is empowered to initiate action on other issues such as education for the poor, unemployment, environmental justice, inadequate transportation or housing, violence, and drug use. These are also public health issues; in fact, these social determinants of health may have a greater impact on community health than access to medical care (Marmot, 2011).

Hence CBPR can contribute to a community's capability to address the social determinants that affect health and quality of life. CBPR is unique in that the *process* benefits the participating community as much as, if not more than, the intended outcomes of the proposed research.

IN A NUTSHELL

CBPR is unique in that the *process* benefits the participating community as much as, if not more than, the intended outcomes of the proposed research.

Hierarchy of Community Participation

Typically, community leaders are convened as a community advisory board to offer input to researchers on a research agenda or on a particular project. While valuable, this type of relationship is not reflective of CBPR in that it still represents an imbalanced power relationship: the researcher is still considered the expert asking the advisory board members for input, but the advisory board has no real authority. Hatch, Moss, Saran, Presley-Cantrell, and Mallory (1993) described a gradient or hierarchy of community participation that includes the typical academic-advisory board relationship and moves upward to greater engagement and equity (see Figure 11.4).

At the lowest level of the hierarchy, persons consulted by researchers are at the periphery of the community, often working for human service

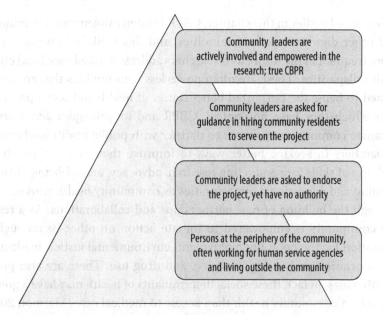

Figure 11.4 Hierarchy of Community Participation in Research

agencies and living outside the community. In this model, community residents are unaware of the purpose of the research and have no influence on its design. Moreover, the disconnect between program development and assisting community partners in identifying sources of funding to sustain programs has led to distrust of academic researchers.

At the second level, the project's advisors are leaders drawn from organizations and churches in the community; however, there is no equitable sharing of power or authority, as the researchers retain total control of the project. In this model, there is community involvement, but it is passive.

At the third level, community leaders are asked not only for endorsement of the project but also for active participation and guidance in hiring community residents to serve as interviewers, outreach workers, and the like. This model is "community-based but not community-involved, because community members do not contribute to the design of the research nor do they have a significant role in interpreting findings" (Hatch et al., 1993). This model may also offer potential for manipulation of the community, because those hired may essentially become patronage workers, which means positions may be awarded to some as political favors with strings attached.

The fourth level both involves and empowers the community. Here community representatives are "first among equals" in defining the research agenda, identifying the problem to be studied, analyzing its contributory factors, and proposing possible solutions. The community "negotiates as a collaborator the goals of the study, the conduct of the study, and analysis and use of study findings" (Hatch et al., 1993). At the fourth level, there are likely to be conflicts and differences between researchers and the community. The challenge to the researchers is to negotiate these differences and build a trusting relationship with the community rather than to search for another, more compliant venue in which to implement their project. This level of relationship between community and researcher is the most difficult to attain but the one that is most conducive to conducting effective and ethically responsible community-based participatory research.

Advantages of CBPR

Advantages of CBPR can be identified in the three stages of research: (stage 1) development, (stage 2) implementation, and (stage 3) dissemination. Advantages of CBPR in the developmental stage of research include the generation of questions that are meaningful and important to a community and the merging of academic theory with lay knowledge that provides a richer and more textured understanding of health problems and their determinants within the community context. CBPR also can lead

IN A NUTSHELL

CBPR also can lead to improved cultural sensitivity and relevance of research methods and intervention strategies, increased reliability and validity of measures, and a better fit of research activities into local realities.

to improved cultural sensitivity and relevance of research methods and intervention strategies, increased reliability and validity of measures, and a better fit of research activities into local realities (Minkler, 2005; Cargo and Mercer, 2008). While research is in the active implementation stage, CBPR can help to increase recruitment and retention of study participants, build community ownership and trust, and contribute to higher response rates (Jagosh et al., 2012; Cargo and Mercer, 2008). Lastly, in the later stages of research, CBPR contributes to a richer interpretation of findings, can accelerate the translation of research into practice, and increases the likelihood that research findings will be acted on (Jagosh et al., 2012; Cargo and Mercer, 2008).

Translating CBPR Principles into Practice: The Devil Is in the Details

While the guiding principles of CBPR specify that the relationship between the community partners and academic researchers and CBPR is a more equitable and ethical community research paradigm, there are substantial challenges in translating CBPR principles into practice. Some of these challenges are highlighted in Table 11.1 along with a description of their place in the CBPR process.

The transition from principles to practice can be fraught with many challenges. These challenges need to be resolved in an equitable manner so participants do not feel alienated or isolated. The "goodness of fit" between the academic researchers and the community partners in terms of the disease or disease-specific determinant to be targeted in the grant application, the methodology employed in the study, and other operational and logistic issues are key factors affecting the effectiveness of CBPR collaborations. Conflict resolution strategies may be useful in identifying the root of some of the aforementioned conflicts and beginning to address them in a manner that not only solves the current problem but also, in the process, strengthens the community partnership.

Growth of CBPR Fueled by Increased Investment

Within the United States, CBPR has garnered increasing support as a research paradigm, and this is reflected in the rapidly growing fiscal support for CBPR. The Centers for Disease Control and Prevention (CDC) and

Table 11.1 Challenges in Translating CBPR Principles into Practice

Challenge	Description	Potential Solution
1. Time constraints	Time constraints often focus on the near horizon in developing a response to an FOA. Thus academic researchers need to move quickly to secure support from stakeholders and community agencies and develop budgets that adequately reflect their level of involvement in the research enterprise. In CBPR there is a slow trajectory through which academic researchers engage the community partners. This period of building a relationship, while critical, may be lengthy, thereby impeding the timely submission of a grant application.	Commitment to the CBPR process involves building a strong relationship well before submitting an application in response to a specific FOA. One cannot begin this process if an FOA is posted with a 6-week turnaround; this is anathema to the principles of CBPR. Building an authentic relationship is a time-intensive endeavor. Once forged, the academic–community partnership will be in an advantageous position to respond when an FOA is posted.
2. Willingness to equitably share power and decision-making authority	Although in principle the academic researcher should be equitable with the community in terms of decision-making authority, in reality either the academic researchers or the community partners may hold a greater share. This is particularly likely to be problematic when deciding how to allocate scarce resources involved in conducting the research. Community members may want to use the funds for items not allowable. Who is ultimately responsible for fiscal oversight?	Typically, academic researchers submit the grant application, which includes a budget and budget justification; once funded, the academic institution oversees the administration of the budget. To avoid this particular conflict, provide education and training to community partners on how the grant process works, what items can be included in a budget, what cannot be included in the budget, and the administration of the funds. The academic researcher should work together with the community partners in developing the budget prior to the grant submission.
3. Shared involvement in the process of disseminating the research findings	Issues may arise when there is conflict over who owns the data and how the findings will be disseminated to the community and to the public via publications and professional presentations.	As part of the CBPR process, the community is involved in partnership with the researchers in collecting the data, analyzing and interpreting the data, and disseminating findings back to the community. As such, key community members need to have adequate research training and skill building. Yet an important part of this process is also education of community members in how the publication process works and who can be listed as an author on publications, based on level of involvement, and the federal guidelines pertaining to data ownership and sharing.
4. Human subjects and the need for institutional review board (IRB) approval	Implementing CBPR activities by community partners that relate specifically to human subjects research, whether it is conducting interviews or focus groups, could potentially result in violations of federal guidelines overseeing human subjects research or, at worst, could result in an adverse event. The academic researcher and her academic institution are responsible for oversight of the research activities and ensuring that the research is implemented correctly and ethically.	First and foremost, all community members participating in research activities involving human subjects must be listed on the institutional review board protocol along with their role. This requires that the academic researcher ensure that each community member undergo training and certification in conducting human subjects research. Additionally, education and training about implementing the research protocols, which emphasize the importance of adhering to the research protocols to avoid IRB violations, should also be conducted.

(continued)

Table 11.1 (*Continued*)

Challenge	Description	Potential Solution
5. Conflict arises between community partners and academic researchers in targeting a particular disease or disease-specific determinant	Academic researchers typically have skill sets to intervene on specific public health issues (such as HIV or obesity) and thus will target a particular disease for intervention or a disease-specific determinant. These diseases or determinants are based on a researcher's capacity to construct a "winnable" grant application and obtain funding for the project. A conflict emerges when the academic researchers cannot reach agreement with community partners on which disease or disease-specific determinants should be targeted. While the academic researchers have one skill set and disease competency, the community partners may decide that another disease or disease-specific determinant is a greater priority. This conflict creates inertia and must be resolved amicably in order for the academic–community partnership to move forward.	CBPR involves a time commitment to establishing an authentic relationship and ultimately improving the health of the community through joint research projects and implementation of interventions. At times, if the skill set of the academic partner does not match the research priority of the community, instead of abandoning the project, one solution is to bring in additional researchers or seek out new resources to expand the collective expertise of the academic–community partnership.
6. Conflict arises between community partners and academic researchers in meeting the specified requirements of the FOA	Similar to #5, but different, this challenge involves overcoming conflict when the community research priority differs from the requirements of the FOA. Both community partners and academic researchers may each strongly feel that the funding mechanism can be used to support their priority research project even though it is expressly not supported by the FOA. Thus there is a mismatch between the interest of the investigative team and the requirements of the FOA. Extending this to its logical conclusion, submitting an application that is off-target would result in its being considered "nonresponsive" and not being funded.	When a funding opportunity announcement (FOA) is posted, the academic researcher can bring the FOA to a community meeting for discussion. The FOA should be reviewed by relevant community partners rather than having the academic researcher present to the community what she would like to submit in response. Consequently, familiarizing the community with the parameters of the FOA allows for better understanding and consensus regarding which relevant research priorities will be targeted.
7. Development of a consensus for a research design	In submitting a response to an FOA, even when academic researchers and community partners agree on the research priority to be targeted in the grant application, there remain other barriers to developing an effective grant application. One key hurdle is the methodological design. For instance, if the FOA is requiring interventions to reduce determinants of diabetes, and both the academic researchers and community partners reach consensus on this focus, there may be less agreement on the use of randomized controlled trial (RCT) design to evaluate innovative diabetes prevention intervention. Although in most cases RCTs are considered the optimal design to evaluate new health promotion intervention programs, community partners may feel that it is unethical to withhold the HPP from half the sample. Thus conflict arises over the issue of randomization to study conditions. Certainly, other research designs can be proposed; however, they may be perceived by the Scientific Review Group (the researchers who review the grant application at NIH) as less rigorous and consequently may receive a poorer score that results in the application not being funded. This is particularly relevant in the constrained fiscal climate at NIH, CDC, and other funding agencies.	The academic research partner has a responsibility to provide information and enhance community members' understanding of the grant process prior to the start of a proposal, educating them in how grants are reviewed and scored and the requirements of the specific funding mechanism. This process can be viewed as an opportunity to increase community members' awareness of research designs, including the advantages and disadvantages of different designs. The PI has a responsibility to share his expertise with the community and must be willing to explain one design's superiority. Also, if community members are particularly against an RCT because of the absence of benefit to the control group, the academic research partner must be prepared to describe the advantages of a wait-list control condition (Chapter Five) or having a control group that receives a placebo-attention equivalent of known value (Chapter Twelve).
8. Navigating uncharted waters	If this is the initial foray of academic researchers into a community, they may be unaware of the community culture or of interpersonal conflicts between community partners. Thus the community partners may be in disagreement on some issues.	Community research requires engaging communities long before the need to respond to an FOA. It is recommended that researchers interested in community research begin the engagement process now so they can begin to appreciate the community culture. This process is time intensive, entailing, for example, meeting with key stakeholders, attending neighborhood meetings and community forums, talking to community members, and holding meet-and-greets.

the National Institutes of Health (NIH) have been leaders in promoting the application of CBPR to health issues by creating funding initiatives that require CBPR. The Agency for Healthcare Research and Quality (AHRQ) has also invested in a participatory approach to research. Foundations and non-profit organizations, such as the W.K. Kellogg Foundation and Community Campus Partnerships for Health, have similarly marshaled resources to further the adoption of CBPR as a research paradigm. International resources also exist, with the World Health Organization advocating community-engaged approaches to health promotion.

Sources of Guidance and Tools for Conducting CBPR

As interest in CBPR grows, there is a growing need and demand for educational resources that help build the knowledge and skills that investigators and community partners need in order to develop and sustain effective CBPR partnerships. Many materials have been developed and are readily available online. Overall, these materials are designed to assist investigators and community partners in acquiring the knowledge base and skill base needed to develop and sustain community-based participatory research partnerships. Much of the material available is also designed to foster critical thinking and action on issues affecting CBPR and community-institution partnerships. Many are developed using a combination of experiential and didactic approaches to teaching and learning. The learning objectives are manifold: (1) provide a deeper understanding of the basic principles of CBPR and strategies for applying them, (2) understand the key steps involved in developing and sustaining CBPR partnerships, (3) identify common challenges faced by CBPR partnerships and suggested strategies for overcoming them, and (4) develop and enhance skills for all partners that will enhance their capacity for supporting and sustaining authentic CBPR partnerships.

Five categories of tools and resources have been identified to assist with the CBPR process (Kegler, Fletcher, Honeycutt, and Wyatt, 2013):

1. *Planning for CBPR*: These tools provide information about the infrastructure required to conduct CBPR and other issues that community and research partners may wish to consider before initiating a CBPR project.

2. *Building CBPR partnerships*: These tools provide resources for partners to come to a shared understanding about their project and each partner's role, and to strengthen trust in the partnership. These tools also provide specific examples of partnership agreement documents, such as sample Memoranda of Understanding (MOUs) and publication guidelines.

3. *Evaluating CBPR partnerships*: These tools can be used to assess various aspects of CBPR partnerships, including partnership functioning, satisfaction, accomplishments, and areas for improvement.

4. *Seeking funding*: These tools may assist partnerships with developing strong CBPR research proposals; they include examples of successful CBPR proposals.

5. *Conducting ethical research*: These tools highlight ethical considerations specific to CBPR.

Policy through CBPR

Case studies may be particularly useful for partnerships seeking to influence policy (Minkler and Wallerstein, 2008). These case studies describe the CBPR projects' policy efforts, and several organizations have developed guides or how-to manuals on conducting CBPR with specific populations. For example, the *Community-Based Participatory Research (CBPR) Toolkit* developed by the Association of Asian Pacific Community Health Organizations and the National Association of Community Health Centers offers resources to support research partnerships with Asian Americans, Native Hawaiians, and other Pacific Islanders.

Partners engaged in CBPR may benefit from reviewing case studies or examples of other CBPR partnerships and projects, particularly those that include recommendations or practical implications. For example, *Promoting Healthy Public* describes outcomes and summarizes lessons learned, successes, and challenges in conducting CBPR projects. In addition, it lists sample policy and related outcomes in which the CBPR partnerships played a role. The *Clinical and Translational Science Awards* (CTSA) provides examples of successful CBPR projects and includes a description of how each one applies the principles of community engagement (Clinical and Translational Service Awards, 2013). Several collections of CBPR case studies or project examples are authored by community members who have partnered with researchers on CBPR projects. For example, *Achieving the Promise of Authentic Community-Higher Education Partnerships: Community Case Stories* describes nine CBPR projects, each written by community partners involved in the research (Community-Campus Partnerships for Health, 2007). This collection of case studies gives community partners a voice to document their CBPR experiences, while also creating a useful resource to inform and strengthen community-academic partnerships.

Summary

It is becoming apparent that more traditional research models, although useful, are not sufficient to reduce disease morbidity and mortality in the most adversely impacted communities. In terms of effective health promotion, CBPR represents a new paradigm for interfacing with communities and developing effective and sustainable community-academic partnerships. It is through these partnerships that communities find a voice in the research enterprise, a voice that has long been neglected or missing. It is through CBPR that communities, particularly those that have been disproportionately affected by the burden of disease, can become intimately engaged, as equal partners, in each of the nine steps of the research process—from identifying the problem to developing more effective solutions, implementing them, and determining whether or not they work. Although the process of developing academic-community partnerships is often labor- and time-intensive, relative to other traditional community-based research models, there is enhanced potential for these partnerships to develop, implement, and evaluate socially meaningful, culturally relevant, and ethically responsible community research.

KEY TERMS

Community advisory boards (CAB)	Sustainability
Community empowerment	Zeitgeist
Ethical engagement	

For Practice and Discussion

1. CBPR is sensitive to issues of social justice. Please discuss how CBPR addresses social justice issues in community-based health promotion research (HPP) research.

2. Describe four challenges in adopting CBPR to design, implement, and evaluate HPP in high-risk communities.

3. You, as an HPP expert, have been asked by the mayor and city council to help in reducing the prevalence of substance use among youth. Please design a randomized controlled trial of a drug prevention program in a low-income, drug-impacted community. How would CBPR be applicable to developing, implementing, evaluating, interpreting, and disseminating the results of this program?

4. Please select an HPP article that describes an application of CBPR. Please review the article carefully and discuss how CBPR was applied to the following: (a) selection of the research question, (b) development of the HPP, (c) selection of the target sample, (d) sample recruitment, (e) maintenance of the study sample (reducing attrition over time), and (f) the data analysis. In this article, did the investigators acknowledge the community input and did the investigators provide suitable feedback to the community at the conclusion of the study? Were next steps explicitly articulated between the investigators and community with respect to seeking additional funding or policy recommendations/changes as a result of the study? Discuss some of the potential barriers to maintaining a cohesive and functional academic-community partnership, even after conducting an HPP study.

References

Blumenthal, D. S. (2011). Is community-based participatory research possible? *American Journal of Preventive Medicine* (*40*), 386–389.

Blumenthal, D. S., DiClemente, R. J., Braithwaite, R. L., and Smith, S. A. (Eds). (2013a). *Community-based participatory health research: Issues, methods and translation to practice*. New York: Springer.

Blumenthal, D. S., Hopkins III, E., and Yancey, E. (2013b). Community-based research: An introduction. In D. S. Blumenthal, R. J. DiClemente, R. L. Braithwaite, and S. A. Smith (Eds.), *Community-based participatory health research: Issues, methods and translation to practice* (1–18). New York: Springer.

Cargo, M., and Mercer, S. (2008). The value and challenges of participatory research: Strengthening its practice. *Annual Review of Public Health*, *29*, 325–350.

Clinical and Translational Service Awards (CTSA). (2013). National Center for Advancing Translational Sciences. Bethesda, MD: National Institutes of Health.

Community-Campus Partnerships for Health (CCPH). (2007). Celebrating a Decade of Impact. Toronto, ON: Community-Campus Partnerships for Health.

Fineberg, H. V. (2013). The state of health in the United States. *Journal of American Medicine*. doi:10.1001/jama.2013.13809

Hatch, J., Moss, N., Saran, A., Presley-Cantrell, L., and Mallory, C. (1993). Community research: Partnership in black communities. *American Journal of Preventive Medicine*, *9*(6 Suppl), 27–31; 2001.

Israel, B. A., Schulz, A. J., Parker, E. A., and Becker, A. B. (1998). Review of community based research: Assessing partnership approaches to improve public health. *Annual Review of Public Health*, *19*, 173–202.

Jagosh, J., Cacaulay, A. C., Pluye, P., Salsberg, J., Bush, P. L., Henderson, J . . . . Greenhalgh, T. (2012). Uncovering the benefits of participatory research: Implications of a realist review for health research and practice. *Milbank Quarterly*, *90*(2), 311–346.

Kegler, M. C., Fletcher, D., Honeycutt, S., and Wyatt, A. (2013). Public and private investments and resources for community-based participatory research. In D. S. Blumenthal, R. J. DiClemente, R. L. Braithwaite, and S. A. Smith (Eds.), *Community-based participatory health research: Issues, methods and translation to practice* (79–110). New York: Springer.

Marmot, M. (2011, October 1). Global action on social determinants of health. *Bulletin of the World Health Organization, 89*(10), 702.

Minkler, M. (2005). Community-based research partnerships: Challenges and opportunities. *Journal of Urban Health, 82*(2 Suppl 2), ii3–ii12.

Minkler, M., and Wallerstein, N. (Eds.). (2008). *Community based participatory research for health: From process to outcomes.* San Francisco: Jossey-Bass.

Noonan, R., and Emshoff, J. (2013). Translating research to practice: Putting "what works" to work. In R. J DiClemente, L. F. Salazar, and R. A. Crosby (Eds.), *Health behavior theory for public health* (pp. 309–332). Burlington, MA: Jones & Bartlett Learning.

Sharpe, P. A., Greaney, M. L., Lee, P. R., and Royce, S. W. (2000, March-June). Assets-oriented community assessment. *Public Health Rep, 115*(2–3), 205–211.

Viswanathan, M., Ammerman, A., Eng, E., et al. (2004). Community-based participatory research: Assessing the evidence. Evidence Report/Technology Assessment No. 99 (Prepared by RTI—University of North Carolina Evidence-based Practice Center under Contract No. 290–02–0016). AHRQ Publication 04-E022–2. Rockville, MD: Agency for Healthcare Research and Quality.

Wallerstein, N., and Duran, B. (2010). CBPR contributions to intervention research: The intersection of science and practice to improve health equity. *American Journal of Public Health, S1*(100), S40–S46.

Wallerstein, N., Oetzel, J., Duran, B., Tafoya, G., Belone, L., and Rae, R. (2008). "What predicts outcomes in CBPR." In Minkler and Wallerstein (Eds.), *CBPR for health: From process to outcomes.* San Francisco: Jossey-Bass.

CHAPTER 12

PROGRAM EVALUATION

Nancy J. Thompson
Michelle C. Kegler

Evaluation of health promotion programs is critical to furthering our understanding of whether the programs we implement work, how well they work and for whom, whether there are unintended consequences, and whether or not they make sense in terms of cost. Although program evaluation by definition is not considered research, because the knowledge gleaned is relevant only to the specific program, program evaluation still utilizes rigorous research methods and strategies to obtain the information. Moreover, program evaluation is typically mandated by the agency that funds the program and thus must be fulfilled as a routine part of program implementation.

Program evaluation uses social science research methods to determine whether programs or parts of programs are sufficient, appropriate, effective, and efficient. Evaluation also generates information about how to improve programs that do not meet these criteria. If a program has unexpected benefits or creates unforeseen problems, evaluation will let us know about these as well (Deniston and Rosenstock, 1970; Thompson and McClintock, 1998). In short, evaluation provides information to serve a variety of purposes, as shown in Box 12.1.

LEARNING OBJECTIVES

- List the purposes of program evaluation.

- Discuss why timing, integration into the program, and budgeting are important to evaluation planning.

- Enumerate key elements needed to describe an evaluation.

- Describe formative, process, and outcome evaluation.

- Name and describe five types of economic evaluation.

- Discuss objectives of an evaluation report.

The authors would like to thank David Holtgrave for his contributions to this chapter. This publication was partially supported by Cooperative Agreement Number # 5U48DP001909 from the Centers for Disease Control and Prevention. The content does not necessarily represent the official position of the Centers for Disease Control and Prevention.

BOX 12.1. REASONS TO EVALUATE

Why do we evaluate? So we can:

- Learn whether the program plans can work before we start using them
- Find out if the materials are a fit for the people who will get them
- Be sure that a program is being delivered the way it was designed to
- Monitor whether a program or activity is getting the desired results
- Get an early warning about problems that could become serious if not addressed
- Find out if a program has any unexpected benefits or problems
- Give program managers the information they need to improve services
- Keep track of progress toward the program's goals
- Produce data on which to base future programs
- Show the program's effectiveness to the target population, the public, those who want to run similar programs, and those who are providing the funds

Source: Adapted from Thompson and McClintock (1998) and Tobacco Technical Assistance Consortium (2005).

There are also indirect benefits that may result from formally evaluating a program. First, program staff have the opportunity to hear from the people they are trying to serve; this in turn lets the program participants know that they have a voice in the running of the program and that the program personnel respect what they have to say. It conveys the message that the program is not being imposed on them. Evaluation can also improve staff morale by providing evidence that either their efforts have been fruitful or leadership is aware of problems and is taking appropriate steps. Staff also get to hear the good news about the program in the words of the people served. A third indirect benefit is that the results of an evaluation can demonstrate an effect or impact, such that the media may develop an interest, further promoting the program (Thompson and McClintock, 1998).

effectiveness

measure of the ability to achieve a desired result in actual practice, not in a controlled or laboratory setting

Evaluation differs from research in that its primary purpose is to provide information to decision makers to help them make judgments about the **effectiveness** of a program and to improve it. In this context, effectiveness refers to a measure of the ability of a program to achieve a desired result in actual practice, not in a controlled or laboratory setting. Evaluations are typically guided by the needs of key stakeholder groups and should be designed in a way that is sensitive to the dynamic and political organizational settings in which programs exist. More so than with pure research, evaluation methods must balance scientific rigor with the need to produce meaningful findings in a timely manner with minimal disruption of program operations.

Many full texts have been written on evaluation (Rossi, Lipsey, and Freeman, 2004; Patton, 2008; Smith, 2010; Weiss, 1997). This chapter draws from these sources as well as from commonly accepted wisdom in the field, to highlight some of the major concepts and issues in evaluation. Topics covered include planning for evaluation, stakeholders, description of the program, target population, logic models, formative evaluation, process evaluation, outcome evaluation, economic evaluation, and evaluation reports.

Evaluation Planning

A frequent error made in developing a program is to add on evaluation after the fact. Evaluation should begin while the program is being created—indeed, as soon as someone has the idea for a program. Once begun, it should continue through the duration of the program, ending only once a final assessment has measured the extent to which the program met its intended goals. The following scenario describes why it is important to start the evaluation process so early.

Suppose a health worker creates a program to reduce motorcycle-related injuries by providing reduced-cost motorcycle helmets to motorcycle drivers in Uganda (see Figure 12.1). To initiate the program, program staff place posters in petrol stations and markets throughout the districts they hoped to reach. The posters invite drivers to come to the program location for a reduced-cost motorcycle helmet. Some

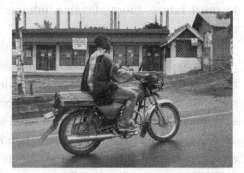

Figure 12.1 Ugandan Motorcyclist without a Helmet
Source: "Bota Bota" by Nazareth College licensed under BY-NC-SA Attribution 2.0 Generic Creative Commons license.
https://creativecommons.org/licenses/by/2.0/.

drivers respond, but not as many as expected. To determine why the numbers were low, the health worker decides to evaluate. The staff may learn that drivers in the area are at work during the hours the program is open. They may learn that drivers are concerned about the weight of the helmet, the smell associated with wearing it, or that the helmets still cost too much, even at a reduced price. They may learn that the location is too far for most drivers to travel. As a result, the staff now needs to rewrite the posters and flyers, change the hours, or move the location. Had the health worker assessed drivers' interest, access to the location, and typical financial resources before the program began, it would have saved time, money, and the disappointment and frustration of the program staff.

A public health program that is well designed incorporates methods to assess progress in achieving its goals and objectives and should produce most of the information needed to evaluate its effectiveness in the course of running the program. Thus evaluation can and should be integrated into the design and operation of the program. If this happens, evaluation may require little more than analyzing the information collected throughout the operation of the program.

IN A NUTSHELL

Evaluation can and should be integrated into the design and operation of the program.

Failure to evaluate a public health program can be considered irresponsible and perhaps even unethical. It is evaluation that allows us to determine whether a program benefits or harms the people it is designed to serve. We do not use medications that are untested, and we should not use educational, behavioral, or social interventions that have not been tested, either. Ineffective programs can discourage people from behavior change, and insensitive programs can build public resentment, causing people to resist future, more effective, interventions (Thompson and McClintock, 1998).

Let's look at an example. Suppose the staff of an injury prevention program were to invite a 55-year-old with a spinal cord injury to talk to students about the hazards of driving above the speed limit. The staff hope that this person's story about speeding at age 16 and the subsequent health effects he has suffered will discourage the students from driving above the speed limit. Evaluation might show, however, that many teenagers do not relate to the problems of people over age 30 and are not influenced by what they have to say. Evaluation could also show what type of people the students *would* listen to—perhaps sports stars or other young people (their peers) who have had difficulty finding a job because of their driving history. It can be nonproductive, and even counterproductive, when the wrong person delivers a message, no matter how good the message is.

Budgeting for evaluation is an important part of the planning stage. The **cost** of evaluation varies. Operating a program with a design that includes a **comparison group** or multiple repeated assessments over time is more expensive than operating a service program, but evaluation is built into the program design, so it is included in the cost of the program (Thompson and McClintock, 1998). What is more, programs with comparison groups or repeated measures will most clearly demonstrate whether or not the program is producing the intended result. Though they may be more costly, such programs may have the greatest likelihood of receiving funding. Box 12.2 lists some of the costs commonly encountered when conducting an evaluation.

cost
what is sacrificed or exchanged to achieve an outcome. Potential costs can include money, time, labor, difficulty, emotions, stamina, or energy, among others

comparison group
a group of participants used in an evaluation study who are similar to participants in the group who received the treatment or program in order to assess effects

---

BOX 12.2. COMMON EVALUATION-RELATED COSTS

The following costs are commonly encountered in an evaluation:

- Flyers, press releases, or other recruitment materials
- Meeting or interview space
- Telephone costs for scheduling and/or conducting interviews or focus groups
- Purchasing, copying, or printing of data collection instruments or questionnaires
- Recording devices
- Audiotapes or videotapes
- Participant or interviewer transportation
- Mailing
- Incentives for participants
- Transcriptionists for taped material
- Computer(s)
- Data entry personnel
- Statistical consultant
- Printing or copying of final report

Source: Adapted from Tobacco Technical Assistance Consortium (2005).

Stakeholders

One of the first steps in conducting an evaluation is to identify and engage stakeholders in the planning process (Centers for Disease Control and Prevention, 1999). Stakeholders include all persons who have an interest in the program being evaluated, the conduct of the evaluation, and the evaluation findings. Stakeholders include program participants; program staff and volunteers; those providing funding to the program or the evaluation; those providing other resources, such as space, for the program; and evaluation personnel. Depending on the program, the stakeholders may also include parents or family members of participants, or all community members, whether or not they participated in the program. Involving major stakeholders in the process of evaluation planning, execution, and analysis ensures that the evaluation results will have value. It also helps to ensure that the results of the evaluation will be used to improve the program.

IN A NUTSHELL

Involving major stakeholders in the process of evaluation planning, execution, and analysis ensures that the evaluation results will have value.

Describing the Program

Another early step in the evaluation process is to develop a thorough understanding of the program to be evaluated (Centers for Disease Control and Prevention, 1999). Key elements that should be carefully considered include the target population, need for the program, goals and objectives, program components and activities, underlying logic, resources, the stage of development of the program (such as the program planning stage, pilot stage, or implementation), and the program context (Centers for Disease Control and Prevention, 1999).

Target Population

The target population is the group the program is intended to serve. The more clearly this population has been defined, the easier it will be to determine whether the population has been reached and whether the program was effective for these people. As a part of evaluation planning, it is important to determine whether the program intends to reach all people in the county, for example, or only those individuals who currently use the services of the county health department, or only males between the ages of 18 and 50 who use the services of the county health department. The method by which you can best reach each of these groups will vary.

Logic Models

An important part of describing a program is understanding its underlying logic. The evaluation should identify the program's ultimate goal(s) and enumerate clearly the program's activities and how they are expected to lead to the goal. Putting this information together with sufficient detail to be of value can be difficult. A logic model is a tool designed to help you with this process. It provides a picture of the relationships among the various aspects related to a program and its evaluation.

The five components of a logic model are inputs, activities, outputs, outcomes, and impact (goals). Figure 12.2 shows the sequence of actions that describe what the program is and what it will do and the linkages to results. *Inputs* (resources, contributions, investments that go into the program) are the resources that the program must have in order to conduct the program's activities. These include funding, personnel (staff as well as volunteers), equipment, supplies, and space. They may also include collaborations with other organizations and people whose interests are consistent with those of the program. Planning, too, is an input required in order to conduct program activities.

Activities (tasks, services, events, and products that reach people who participate or who are targeted) are the actual events that take place when the program is occurring (Tobacco Technical Assistance Consortium, 2005). These may include events such as conducting an education program, distributing condoms or smoke alarms, or holding support groups. But activities can also include inviting collaborators to a meeting, sending letters to supporters, building relationships with the communities to be served, gathering materials for a resource center, maintaining an inventory of resources, responding to telephone inquiries, and disseminating information to interested parties.

Outputs are measures that can be used to demonstrate that the program was conducted. These include indicators like the number of training sessions held or the number of collaborators in attendance at a meeting. In contrast, **outcomes** are measures that can be used to demonstrate that program participants *received* what you put out there. Outcomes would include indicators like an increase in knowledge or changes in attitudes or

outputs
indicators to show that the program was implemented, with whom it was implemented, and how many received it

outcomes
indicators to show the short-term or medium-term effects of the program

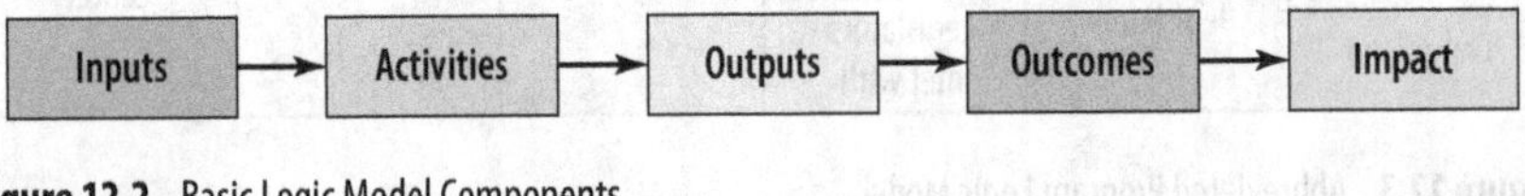

Inputs → Activities → Outputs → Outcomes → Impact

Figure 12.2 Basic Logic Model Components

behavior. In the case of tobacco use prevention programs, outcomes could include an increase in the belief that smoking is dangerous, and a decrease in the rate of smoking.

impact
the long-term effect of a program

The **impact** of a program is the measure of whether or not the overall program goal was achieved and, usually, whether or not the effects are long-term. For health programs, this is typically a measure of decreases in morbidity and mortality. In our smoking example, the program's impact could be a decrease in new cases of lung cancer or deaths from this disease. It could also be a decrease in overall smoking-related mortality, including both cancer and heart disease.

A logic model can be developed for an entire program or for one of its parts, such as a particular activity. Figure 12.3 presents an example of an abbreviated logic model for a program to reduce tobacco-related cancer. Figure 12.4 presents an example of a more detailed logic model for the process portion of a cardiovascular disease prevention program designed to reduce disparities in physical activity.

summative evaluation
type of evaluation that determines whether a program met its goals or objectives in terms of outcomes and/or impact

Types of Evaluation

There are several typologies for the different kinds of evaluations that can be done. A common distinction is made between summative and formative evaluation. Rossi and colleagues (2004) define **summative evaluation** as "evaluation activities undertaken to render a summary judgment on certain critical aspects of the program's performance, for instance, to determine if specific goals and objectives were met" (p. 65). They define **formative evaluation** as "evaluative activities undertaken to furnish information that will guide program improvement" (p. 63). In public health and health promotion, four types of evaluation are widely recognized: formative, process, outcome, and economic. Each of these is described here.

formative evaluation
type of evaluation that takes place before or during a project's implementation with the aim of improving the project's design and performance

Formative Evaluation

The purpose of formative evaluation is to determine that an element of the program (for example, materials, message, or location) is **feasible**,

feasible
having the capability to be implemented with the targeted population

Inputs	Activities	Outputs	Outcomes		Impact
			Short-term	**Long-term**	
Staff	Coalition meetings	Groups attending	Policies adopted	Decrease in smoking	Decrease in tobacco-related cancer
Volunteers	Meetings with legislators	Meetings attended			
Computers		Legislators met with			

Figure 12.3 Abbreviated Program Logic Model

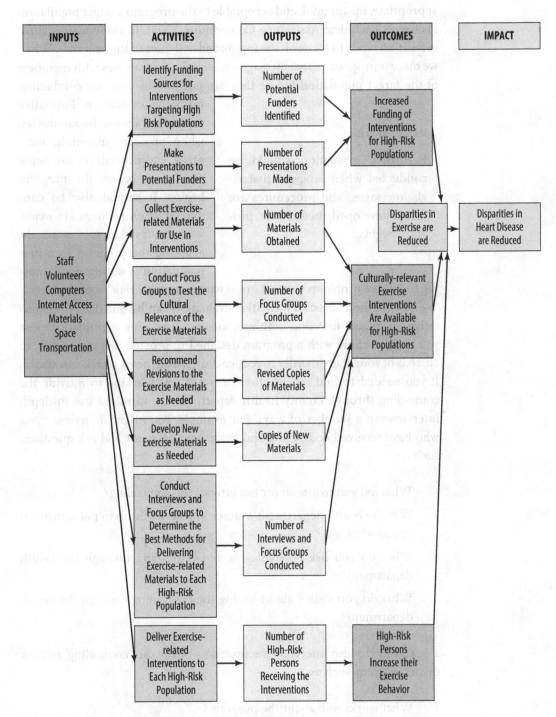

INPUTS   **ACTIVITIES**   **OUTPUTS**   **OUTCOMES**   **IMPACT**

Figure 12.4   Logic Model with Detailed Inputs, Activities, and Outputs

appropriate, meaningful, and acceptable to the program's target population (Tobacco Technical Assistance Consortium, 2005). In essence, formative evaluation tends to focus on the inputs and activities of the program. When we discuss program plans, messages, materials, or strategies with members of the target population before they are put into use, we are conducting formative evaluation. Formative evaluation should be conducted when program materials, messages, and procedures are being developed, before the program begins. It should also be conducted when changes are made, such as revising the materials, adapting the program to a new population or setting, or attempting to resolve problems that occurred with prior materials or procedures.

IN A NUTSHELL

Formative evaluation should be conducted when program materials, messages, and procedures are being developed, before the program begins.

The methods used in formative evaluation can be qualitative, quantitative, or mixed, meaning both methods are used. For example, suppose you were working with a program designed to provide diet counseling to citizens of your state in order to reduce deaths from heart attack and stroke. If you needed to find out whether or not it was working to provide the counseling through county health departments, you might use in-depth interviews in a number of ways. For example, you might interview those who have received counseling and those who have not and ask questions such as:

- What led you to attend (or not attend) the counseling?
- Was the health department a factor in your decision to participate? If yes, in what way?
- What do you like about having the counseling through the health department?
- What do you dislike about having the counseling through the health department?

You might also interview the providers of the diet counseling and ask them questions such as:

- What works well about the program?
- What does not work well?
- What are the benefits of providing the counseling through the health department?

- What are the problems with providing the counseling through the health department?
- What are some better ways to provide the counseling?

You might interview program administrators and ask:

- Why was the health department chosen as the means of providing the counseling?
- What were the perceived benefits of using the health department? *Probe*: Have these benefits been realized?
- What were the perceived drawbacks of using the health department? *Probe*: Have these drawbacks occurred?

You might also interview administrators of the health department and ask:

- What do you know about the diet counseling program?
- What are the benefits to the health department associated with this program?
- What are the costs to the health department associated with this program?

Many of these same questions could also be addressed by conducting focus groups with each of these types of program affiliates.

Naturalistic observation (as described in more detail in Chapters Four and Eight) is another qualitative method that can be used for formative evaluation. Suppose you were working with a program designed to provide hypertension screening in rural areas of your state through churches and civic groups and you wanted to determine whether the civic group screenings were working. An observer at the screening locations could note:

- How the facilities are laid out and whether the physical setup works
- What problems participants appear to encounter
- Whether participants appear to know where to go
- How much participants and program personnel interact
- Whether any of the participants complain as they leave

In observing program personnel, the observer could note:

- How they set up for the screening
- Who is responsible for what tasks

- How they approach participants
- What steps they take to ensure privacy
- Whether they take time to explain each step
- What feedback they provide to those who were screened

In observing participants, the observer could note:

- Do they tend to be of similar ages or social backgrounds?
- Do any people approach and choose not to participate? If so, are their characteristics similar to those of the people who choose to participate?
- How do people respond when approached by program personnel?
- Do they ask questions? What kind of questions do they ask?

Quantitative methods, such as cross-sectional surveys (as described in more detail in Chapter Four), can also be used to conduct formative evaluation. Suppose, for example, you wanted to assess the effectiveness of your advertising for a screening program such as the one just described. You could survey people who did and did not participate in the screening, using questions similar to those shown in Table 12.1. Combined with demographic information, the responses to questions like these could be used to determine for whom the advertising is and is not appropriate and effective.

Process Evaluation

Process evaluation assesses the way the program is being delivered, rather than the program's effectiveness. It documents what is actually being provided by the program and compares that to what was supposed to

Table 12.1   Sample Survey

Please indicate the extent to which you agree or disagree with each of the following statements	Strongly Agree	Agree	Neither Agree nor Disagree	Disagree	Strongly Disagree
There was enough advertising.	SA	A	N	D	SD
The location of the advertising was good.	SA	A	N	D	SD
The ads were easy to understand.	SA	A	N	D	SD
Overall, I liked the ads.	SA	A	N	D	SD

be provided to determine whether there are any gaps. In other words, process evaluation functions as a form of quality control. It also serves many other purposes, such as providing managers with feedback on the quality of delivery, documenting the **fidelity** and variability of program delivery across sites and personnel, providing information to assess which components of the program are likely to be responsible for particular outcomes, and providing data that can be used to demonstrate what the program is doing to funders, sponsors, participants, and the public. To serve these purposes, process evaluation focuses on the activities and outputs of the program; for example, what is done in each screening, and how many screenings are held. Program context, reach of the program, dose delivered and received, fidelity to the original program plan, implementation, and recruitment are some of the typical components of process evaluation (Linnan and Steckler, 2002).

fidelity
strict observance to or conformity to an agreement, guidelines, or protocol

> **IN A NUTSHELL**
>
> Program context, reach of the program, dose delivered and received, fidelity to the original program plan, implementation, and recruitment are some of the typical components of process evaluation.

Common process evaluation questions (adapted from Patton, 2008) include:

- What are the program's main characteristics as perceived by major stakeholder groups?
- Who participates in the program, and how do they compare to the intended target population for the program?
- Which components of the program are working as expected? What is not working well? What challenges and barriers have been encountered?
- What do participants and staff like and dislike?
- What has changed from the original implementation design and why?
- What are the startup costs of the program? What are the ongoing costs of implementation?
- What has been learned about the program that might inform efforts elsewhere?

As in formative evaluation, the methods used in process evaluation can be qualitative or quantitative. For example, suppose you were working with a program designed to provide child safety seat checks and education to caregivers who transport children under the age of 7 years in their vehicles. If you wanted to find out how the checks were being conducted, you could use observation. The observer could note whether or not the program technician checked both the installation of the seat and the placement of the child in the seat. The observer could also note whether the technician involved the caregiver in the seat check, whether or not she discussed any problems that were identified with the caregiver, and whether or not she provided instruction to the caregiver about how to correct the problem.

Quantitative methods can also be used for process evaluation. For example, counts of number of vehicles checked, number of seats checked, and number of caregivers educated could be used to verify the program's output. If the program was advertised through a radio campaign, counts of radio spots developed and taped, stations contacted and stations accepting spots, number of spots aired, frequency of airing per spot, and minutes of air time would also be elements of process evaluation. Other common data collection methods in process evaluation include interviews, diaries or logs, document review, record abstraction, and monitoring or tracking systems.

Outcome Evaluation

experimental
a research design where participants are assigned to receive the treatment (program) or an alternative by a random process

Outcome evaluation is linked to the outcomes in the program's logic model, and almost always uses **experimental** or quasi-experimental study designs, along with quantitative methods (as described in more detail in Chapter Five). Short-term outcome evaluation can measure the short-term effects of the program on a participant immediately after participation. Consequently, it measures outcomes that can change rapidly as a result of an intervention, such as knowledge, attitudes, and intended behavior. Changes in these outcomes are typically assessed with pretest-posttest designs, administering the measures before and after the participant takes part in the program. Short-term outcome evaluation provides evidence of the degree to which a program is meeting its short-term or intermediate goals, such as increasing participants' awareness of the hazards of radon gas, or changing their knowledge, attitudes, and beliefs about radon gas. Surveys, interviews, and observation are common data collection methods in these kinds of evaluations.

IN A NUTSHELL

Short-term outcome evaluation provides evidence of the degree to which a program is meeting its short-term or intermediate goals, such as increasing participants' awareness of the hazards of radon gas, or changing their knowledge, attitudes, and beliefs about radon gas.

Changes in outcomes like actual behavior, such as getting one's home radon tested, usually take longer to manifest themselves. As a consequence, they are usually assessed with pretest-posttest follow-up designs, or with observational follow-up, also known as cohort designs. Control or comparison groups are often used to aid in attributing the observed effects to the program. See Chapters Four and Five for more detailed discussion of experimental and observational research designs.

The value of outcome evaluation is that it provides an indicator of both program effectiveness and the extent to which a program's objectives are being met. When combined with process evaluation, outcome evaluation can indicate which activities and outputs appear to have the greatest influence and can allow program managers to shift resources from less effective to more effective elements of the program. Demonstrating a program's ultimate impact on morbidity and mortality, however, can be challenging due to the long-term nature of these outcomes and the multiple influences on them. Program evaluations in public health and health promotion therefore often focus on intermediate outcomes rather than on morbidity and mortality.

Economic Evaluation

Part of evaluating a program is determining whether or not the effects it produces are worth the program's costs. In other words, we must determine whether the outcomes and impact achieved through the program were worth the inputs and time that went into the program. Economic evaluation methods are a family of techniques that can answer questions about the program's **affordability** (that is, being within one's economic or other means) and **efficiency** (that is, its ability to achieve an outcome with the least expenditure), and the standards the program must achieve to be considered cost-saving or **cost-effective**. In the context of program evaluation, cost-effectiveness means a degree of desired outcome that is worthwhile in relation to its costs. Five cost-related evaluation questions are of real interest to decision makers: (1) affordability; (2) assessing costs of **unmet needs** (that is, the deficit in services that has not been adequately addressed); (3) performance standard setting; (4) comparing programs in one disease area to each other; and (5) comparing programs in one area to health-related services in other disease areas.

Cost Analysis (Determining Affordability)

Consider the following question. "There is a highly effective risk-reduction program that was developed in another community—can we afford to offer

affordability
being within one's economic or other means

efficiency
ability to achieve an outcome with the least expenditure

cost-effective
having a degree of desired outcome that is worthwhile in relation to the cost

unmet needs
the deficit in services that has not been adequately addressed

the service in my home town?" To answer this "affordability" question, we need to know the cost of delivering the program activities. This might mean knowing the dollar cost of conducting each activity per participant served, or it might mean simply knowing, in detail, what types of human resources and materials are needed to conduct the activity.

The economic evaluation technique of cost analysis is perfectly suited to answering the affordability question. In a cost analysis of a prevention program, a table is constructed with the categories of resources consumed by the program as the rows (for example, staff time, incentives given to participants, materials distributed, staff travel time) and inputs as the columns of the table. These inputs include (1) a definition of each resource category, (2) a definition of the unit of each resource category, (3) the number of units of each resource category consumed, (4) the dollar value of each resource category, and (5) the product of the number of resource units consumed and the dollar value of each unit for each resource category. Summing these products across all resource categories gives the total cost of the program. Dividing the total cost by the number of clients yields the per-client cost of the program.

Overall, there are seven basic steps in a cost analysis:

- Choose a time period for the cost-analysis.
- Count the clients served during this time period.
- Inventory the resources, in specific units, required for all program activities.
- Calculate the cost per unit of each resource used.
- Count the number of units of each resource used in the time period specified.
- Calculate the total costs of the program.
- Calculate the expected cost per client served.

IN A NUTSHELL

Cost analysis can determine the price of delivering a program, and it can provide detailed information about the exact types (and quantities) of resources consumed by the program.

If a decision maker is interested in questions of the affordability of particular programs, the economic evaluation technique of cost analysis is perfectly suited to providing answers. Cost analysis can determine the price of delivering a program, and it can provide detailed information about the exact types (and quantities) of resources consumed by the program.

Cost of Unmet Needs Analysis (Assessing Costs of Unmet Needs)

Consider another question: "How much would it cost to run a program that really addresses the unmet prevention service delivery needs of a population?" From time to time, decision makers may need to know how much it would cost to address the unmet needs of a particular population or populations. Cost of unmet needs analysis is a technique that is perfectly suited to this need. A cost of unmet needs analysis has just a few basic steps:

- The number of people in need of a particular activity or service is estimated (for example, using epidemiologic and behavioral information).

- The most effective activities or services for this population are identified (for example, using the published literature or local evaluation information).

- The per-client cost of these activities or services for this population is identified (for example, using the published literature or local cost analyses).

The per-client costs of the programs are multiplied by the number of people needing the programs; this yields the cost of unmet needs for this particular population. Cost of unmet needs analysis can answer cost of unmet needs questions for decision makers, *and* it can also equip decision makers to answer questions from media, state legislators, federal agencies, and others interested in the real cost of unmet needs in a particular locale.

Threshold Analysis (Performance Standard Setting)

Another important question might be, "The state legislature wants to know if it is saving money by preventing disease and averting medical costs. How much disease would this program have to prevent in order to be cost-saving?"

In a threshold analysis, we start by taking the cost of a particular program. Then we divide it by the **present value** of the lifetime medical care cost of treating one case of the disease the program is designed to prevent. (Present value is a technical term meaning, roughly, that we use a 3-percent annual discount rate to bring future health care costs into present value.) The result tells us how many cases of disease would have to be permanently prevented by this program in order for it to be considered cost-saving. Note that we do not have to know anything about how much disease is actually prevented by this program in order to calculate the cost-saving threshold.

present value
current value of some future sum of money

These simple calculations constitute a threshold analysis in its entirety. However, we can go one step further and ask whether the approximate number of cases of disease that might be prevented by a particular program is likely to be above or below the threshold. For instance, if a state does a threshold analysis on its HIV counseling and testing program and finds that only 5 HIV infections would have to be prevented for the program to be cost-saving, it can try to identify whether there is evidence to suggest that the actual number of infections prevented is above or below 5 (even if the precise number is unknown). Often there will be sufficient evidence to determine whether or not it is likely that a threshold is being met, even when the exact level of effectiveness is not known. Identifying whether the number of infections prevented is above or below a threshold can be a much more practical evaluation question to answer, rather than trying to estimate the exact number of infections prevented.

IN A NUTSHELL

Identifying whether the number of infections prevented is above or below a threshold can be a much more practical evaluation question to answer, rather than trying to estimate the exact number of infections prevented.

Cost-Effectiveness Analysis (Comparing Programs in One Disease Area to Each Other)

Consider another question: "We would like to prevent as much disease as possible given the level of resources that our county has available—how can we do this?" People working in disease prevention all desire to avert as many cases of illness as possible—indeed, that is the very nature of their work. Consequently, they want to give priority to prevention programs that will prevent as much disease as possible. Of course, a real limitation is the amount of resources available, so public health personnel have to maximize the amount of disease prevented within those resource constraints.

The technique of cost-effectiveness can help with this decision. As applied here, cost-effectiveness analysis would provide the cost-per-case of disease prevented by a given program in a given population. Theoretically, cost-effectiveness would provide the cost per case of disease prevented for any program for any population. Then one would start funding the specific program or population combinations with the lowest cost per disease averted until resources were exhausted.

Figure 12.5 presents selected data from a cost-effectiveness analysis of the United States president's fiscal year 2007 initiative to expand HIV counseling and testing (Holtgrave, 2007). These selected data are presented

Input

Parameter	Value
Budget	$93 million
Technical assistance, targeting, and evaluation	$9.3 million
HIV– client counseling and testing (societal)	$59.13
HIV+ client couseling and testing (society)	$169.31
Percentage of clients HIV+	1.5%
HIV+ annual transmission rate (unaware of seropositivity)	8.8%
HIV+ annual transmission (unaware of seropositivity)	2.4%

Analysis

	Payor
Total no. clients reached	1,377,147
HIV+ persons newly reached	13,014
Transmissions averted from HIV+ clients	833
Gross cost per transmission/infection averted from HIV+ clients	$111,645
Discounted lifetime medical care costs of one case of HIV disease	$200,000
Cost-effectiveness (cost–cost saved)	<$0 (cost saving)

Figure 12.5 Cost-Effectiveness of HIV Counseling and Testing Expansion

Source: *Journal of Public Health Management and Practice* by Lippincott Williams & Wilkins. Reproduced with permission of Lippincott Williams & Wilkins in the format reuse in a book/textbook via Copyright Clearance Center.

from the societal perspective; that is, counting all costs that accrue to the payer, the client, or others. Some of the inputs (left side of the figure) include parameters such as the cost of counseling an HIV negative (HIV–) client ($59.13) versus an HIV positive (HIV+) client ($169.31), as well as the percentage of clients expected to be HIV+. The analysis (right side of the figure) includes a determination of the number of HIV+ clients newly reached; this is a product of clients reached times the proportion who are HIV+ times the proportion who are not already aware of their seropositivity (0.63, not shown in figure). By making the newly reached HIV+ clients aware of their seropositivity, their likelihood of transmitting their HIV is reduced from 8.8 percent to 2.4 percent, a reduction of 6.4 percentage points. Applied to the total of 13,014 people newly reached, this results in 833 transmissions averted. While the original paper investigated additional infections averted, these 833 transmissions averted from HIV+ clients, alone, produce a cost per transmission averted of $93,000,000/833, or $111,645, far less than the discounted lifetime medical care costs of one case of HIV disease ($200,000).

Cost-Utility Analysis (Comparing Programs in One Area to Health-Related Services in Other Disease Areas)

Consider a question posed at the national level. "The Office of Management and Budget in the White House is wondering whether investment in HIV prevention is better than investments in diabetes, or cancer, or heart disease. How can we even begin to answer a question like that?"

Many public health policymakers must set priorities across disease areas. For instance, appropriations committees in the U.S. Congress must work to make funding decisions across many areas of expenditure, including making health service funding decisions that must choose among cancer programs, heart disease programs, HIV prevention programs, diabetes control programs, and so on. The Office of Management and Budget in the White House has endorsed cost-benefit and cost-utility analysis as important forms of input into such decision making. (We'll focus here on the more broadly useful cost-utility analysis rather than cost-benefit analysis.)

Cost-utility analysis evaluates a program in terms of the cost per **quality-adjusted life-year (QALY)** saved (or cost per QALY saved, for short). QALY refers to both the quality and the quantity of a life that is affected by health-related interventions. It is the arithmetic product of life expectancy and the quality of the remaining life years. A value of 1 = one year in perfect health; anything less than perfect health gets a score of <1.

quality-adjusted life-year (QALY)
an indicator of disease burden that equates with the years of life affected by the program and considers quality as well as quantity

Note that in the cost-effectiveness analysis discussed earlier, the cost-effectiveness outcomes were in the form of cost per case of a disease prevented; that outcome form is useful for comparing different prevention programs that target the same disease, but is not useful for comparing prevention programs for one disease to those in other disease areas. The cost-utility analysis outcome of cost per QALY saved can be used across disease areas, because a quality-adjusted life year saved in one year is (at least theoretically) the same as a QALY saved in another disease area.

Simply put, a cost-utility analysis can show that a program is cost-saving, cost-effective, or not cost-effective. If a cost-utility analysis shows that the costs prevented (usually health care costs prevented) by a program are greater than the cost of delivering the program itself, then the program is said to be cost-saving. Clearly, if a program saves more money than it costs to deliver, it can justifiably be labeled "cost-saving."

However, a program may cost more to deliver than it saves, yet still be quite worthwhile. For instance, kidney dialysis, many forms of surgery, and many medical screening programs cost more than they save but as a society we readily accept them and invest in them. Although there is no magic cutoff value, very commonly it is cited that programs that are not cost saving but cost less than $50,000 per QALY saved should be labeled as cost-effective. (Note that some researchers would place the cutoff at $80,000, $100,000, or even $120,000 rather than $50,000.) Programs that cost more than the cutoff value (say, $50,000 per QALY saved) cannot be justifiably labeled as cost-effective.

The Evaluation Report

No matter what type of evaluation is conducted, the results have to be shared with major stakeholders. Generally, the main function of an evaluation report is to provide answers to the questions posed at the beginning of the evaluation and discuss what these answers mean. In evaluation, meaning is often derived through some form of comparison. Patton (2008) discusses comparing program outcomes to outcomes from a similar program, to stated program objectives, to outcomes from the same program in a prior time period, or to external standards of desirability. Other objectives of an evaluation report include providing management with a basis for decisions regarding program changes, soliciting continued funding, providing staff with feedback, making others aware of the program and its contributions, and making recommendations for future action.

The reporting of results is especially important in evaluation as it becomes the basis for future action. Without an adequate report of the findings, the evaluation is largely worthless. In formulating the report, consider each of the categories of stakeholders, their needs, and their interests. Also consider what actions they might want to take as a result of the report. This will ensure that you provide them with sufficient information to inform their action as fully as possible.

There are numerous additional issues to consider in reporting evaluation findings. For example, should the report be written or oral? If it is written, options include an executive summary followed by a full report, an executive summary only, press releases, newsletters, or a traditional academic research monograph (Patton, 2008). Other issues to consider include authorship and contributors to the report, as well as whose perspectives are represented. Options range from including only the evaluator's perspective to the evaluator writing the report on behalf of a particular stakeholder group.

Applying Some Key Evaluation Concepts: A Case Example

An example of a program evaluation was conducted by Glanz, Geller, Shigaki, Maddock, and Isnec (2002). The program, called "Pool Cool," was a sun safety program initially implemented in Hawaii and Massachusetts and subsequently disseminated nationwide. Because of its comprehensive evaluation, we will use the Pool Cool program to illustrate many of the key concepts covered in this chapter. Designed as an intervention research study, the project included formative, process, and outcome evaluation. (For a more detailed description of the program and related evaluation findings, please see Glanz, Geller, Shigaki, Maddock, Isnec, 2002; and Glanz, Isnec, Geller, Spangler, 2002.)

Stakeholders

Stakeholders are those who have a stake or a vested interest in evaluation findings; they include individuals who make decisions about a program or those who simply desire information about the program or its evaluation. For Pool Cool, major stakeholders included the Pool Cool staff (behavioral scientists, health educators, research assistants, and data managers), the aquatics and recreation staff, parents of young children, and children taking swimming lessons at the participating pools. The funding agency is also considered a stakeholder; for the initial evaluation of Pool Cool, this was the Centers for Disease Control and Prevention. Patton (2008) advised evaluators to go beyond identification of stakeholders and to develop a strong relationship with at least one primary intended user. This required evaluators to find strategically located people who were enthusiastic about an evaluation and committed to using the results. For Pool Cool, the project team both designed and evaluated the program. This integration facilitated use of the evaluation findings in making decisions about the program.

Defining the Program

A critical step in designing an evaluation for Pool Cool or any other program is to develop a thorough understanding of the program. The Pool Cool program uses both behavioral and environmental strategies to prevent skin cancer by improving sun protection behaviors, reducing sunburns, and promoting sun safety policies and environments at swimming pools (Glanz, Geller, Shigaki, et al., 2002). The *target audience* for the Pool Cool program is children who take swimming lessons and their parents, as well as aquatics instructors at the participating pools (Glanz, Isnec, Geller, and Spangler, 2002; Glanz, Geller, Shigaki, et al., 2002). *Educational strategies* include lifeguard and aquatic instructor training, sun safety lessons to be implemented as part of swimming lessons, a series of interactive activities, and incentives. *Environmental strategies* include informal consultation on policy change and provision of sunscreen pump bottles, a shade structure (such as a tent, a canvas cover or tarp, or an umbrella), and signage with sun-safe messages.

The Pool Cool program is based on the social cognitive theory, which asserts that behaviors are influenced by the social and physical environment and that people, their behaviors, and the environment have a reciprocal relationship, with each influencing the other (Glanz, Geller, Shigaki et al., 2002; Bandura, 1986). The *logic* underlying the Pool Cool program is relatively straightforward. If knowledge and skills, health beliefs, and social and physical environments can be altered to support sun safety, the prevalence of preventive behaviors will increase among children taking swimming lessons, their parents, and aquatics instructors. An increase in these behaviors will lead to reductions in sun exposure and sunburns among program participants, and in the long term, reductions in skin cancer. Thus short-term outcomes include changes in knowledge and skills, health beliefs, social norms, social acceptability, and physical environments. Specific environmental and policy-related outcomes include existence of shade structures and sun safety signage and availability of sunscreen at the participating swimming pools. Intermediate behavioral outcomes include use of sunscreen, wearing protective clothing, seeking shade during peak sun hours, and wearing sunglasses. The longer-term outcomes that would, in theory, result from an increase in these preventive behaviors include reduced sun exposure, reduced sunburns, and, ultimately, a lower incidence of skin cancer.

Types of Evaluation

Formative evaluation, usually conducted in the developmental phase of a program, provides input that can be used to modify a program and document the feasibility of program implementation. Data from formative evaluations are useful in crafting and tailoring intervention strategies and messages that effectively reach the target population, resonate with selected audiences, and are culturally appropriate. Formative evaluation was valuable in the program development phase of the Pool Cool program.

Planning a successful program requires a solid understanding of the knowledge, attitudes, behaviors, and culture of the target audience (Green and Kreuter, 2005). In Pool Cool, this required learning the culture of the swimming pool environment and

IN A NUTSHELL

Planning a successful program requires a solid understanding of the knowledge, attitudes, behaviors, and culture of the target audience.

learning about the sun safety practices and views of lifeguards, aquatics instructors, and pool managers. It also required developing an understanding of sun safety beliefs and practices of parents and children.

The Pool Cool formative evaluation used multiple data collection methods (Glanz, Carbone, and Song, 1999; Glanz, Isnec, Geller, and Spangler, 2002). Qualitative evaluation methods included focus groups, discussion groups, and interviews with children, parents, recreation staff, pool managers, aquatics instructors, and lifeguards. Site visits to swimming pools were also completed. Quantitative data were collected through self-administered written surveys. Several issues affecting program design emerged from the formative component of the evaluation.

The *process evaluation* component of Pool Cool was multifaceted and served several purposes (Glanz, Isnec, Geller, and Spangler, 2002). For example, it assessed the extent of implementation of the educational and environmental program components, how much time was spent delivering the program, exposure to program components, program reach, and how the target audience—lifeguards and children—rated the various aspects of the program. It was also designed to catch any unintended consequences or unexpected circumstances that might influence either program implementation or outcomes.

Three types of data collection were employed in the process evaluation: monitoring forms, observation records, and select items from posttest surveys. The monitoring forms were completed by lifeguards and aquatics instructors and were designed to assess delivery of the eight sun safety lessons. They were also used to assess the presence of parents at the pools, how well lessons were received, and which components were taught.

Staff logs were used for quality assurance purposes and were completed on site visits to the participating pools. Staff logs helped to document that participation and implementation were affected by the weather. Relevant survey items asked parents about participation, their reactions to the program, and incentives they had received. Overall, the process evaluation findings enabled the project team to feel comfortable that the program was being implemented as planned. Good documentation of the implementation process also shed light on how the program outcomes were achieved.

The *outcome evaluation* design for the Pool Cool program was a randomized controlled trial with swimming pools as the unit of randomization and analysis (Glanz, Geller, Shigaki, et al., 2002). Pools were randomized into either the intervention arm (n=15) or the control arm (n=13), with the latter receiving an attention-matched injury prevention program. Primary outcome data were collected through self-administered written surveys completed by two cross-sectional samples of parents at the beginning of the summer and 8 weeks later. These were parents of children ages 5 to 10 who were taking swimming lessons. Major measures included demographic factors, knowledge about skin cancer and sun protection guidelines, attitudes, policies for sun protection at the pool, parent and child's sun protection practices, and child's sunburn experiences for the previous summer and the summer when the program took place. Environmental outcomes were assessed through observation at three points in time: the beginning, middle, and end of the summer. Two independent observers completed observations forms to assess availability of sunscreen, shaded areas, sun-safety signage, and lifeguard sun-safety practices.

Results showed significant intervention effects in children's use of sunscreen, staying in shade, and sun protection habits. Use of sunscreen, wearing a hat, and sun protection habits also increased among parents. Further, pool sun protection policies increased in the intervention pools. Environmental results documented greater improvements in avail-

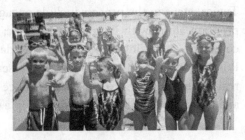

Figure 12.6 Pool Cool Kids
Source: Photo courtesy of Pool Cool.
http://www.med.upenn.edu/poolcool/.

ability of sunscreen, posting of sun-safety signs, and lifeguard shirt use in intervention pools relative to control pools. Overall, outcome evaluation results showed a modest but significant program effect. Evaluation results have been disseminated through publication in peer-reviewed journals. The program was subsequently disseminated nationwide. This second phase of the project also included process and outcome evaluations (Escoffery, Glanz, Hall, and Elliott, 2009; Rabin, Nehl, Elliot, Deshpande, Brownson, and Glanz, 2010).

Summary

Evaluation involves the systematic collection of information to answer questions about a program. These questions can be classified into four types of evaluation: formative, process, outcome, and economic. Formative evaluation is conducted during the developmental phase of a program to determine whether specific components such as materials, message, and learning activities are feasible and acceptable to the program's target population. Both qualitative and quantitative methods are common in formative evaluation. Process evaluation focuses on the internal operations of a program and attempts to provide information that can lead to program improvement. It also uses both qualitative and quantitative methods. In contrast, outcome evaluation usually employs quantitative methods to determine the effectiveness of a program—in other words, it asks, is the program achieving the desired outcomes? As described in this chapter, numerous types of economic analysis can be conducted under the rubric of program evaluation. These include cost analysis, cost of unmet needs analysis, cost effectiveness, threshold analysis, and cost-utility analysis.

Evaluation is similar to applied research and draws heavily on social science research methods. It differs from research in its emphasis on stakeholder involvement and its focus on providing information to decision makers to aid them in making judgments about a particular program. Typical steps in the process include engaging stakeholders; describing the program along with its underlying logic; focusing the evaluation design; collecting, analyzing, and interpreting data; and reporting study results. Program evaluation exemplifies how research methods can be applied to real-world situations to make a difference both in how we approach social and public health problems and in people's day-to-day lives.

KEY TERMS

Affordability	Formative evaluation
Comparison group	Impact
Cost	Outcomes
Cost-effective	Outputs
Effectiveness	Present value
Efficiency	Quality-adjusted-life-year (QALY)
Experimental	Summative evaluation
Feasible	Unmet needs
Fidelity	

For Practice and Discussion

1. You are an evaluator in the State Health Department, and your supervisor approaches you about a new project. It seems that a coalition in one of the cities of your state has received some new funding for its two-year-old program to increase exercise among people with arthritis. The pain associated with arthritis can cause arthritis sufferers to not use their muscles, and, as a result, their muscles can atrophy. The goal

of the arthritis exercise program has been to increase participants' joint flexibility and aerobic fitness while preventing the loss of their muscle condition. So far, they have served 225 people with arthritis.

The program planners are excited about the additional funding and the potential to reach more people. The staff has just learned, however, that before the funds will be released, the program must submit a complete evaluation plan to their funder. You are assigned to develop their evaluation plan. How would you begin? Since the program has already been running for two years, what problems might that create in developing the plan? What parts of the plan might be easier to write for an existing program?

2. You have been asked by the director of a local hospital's cardiac rehabilitation department to evaluate a program conducted through the department. In this program, women with a history of myocardial infarction or of coronary artery bypass surgery who exercise regularly are asked to make telephone calls to other women with a similar history who do not regularly exercise. The purpose of the calls is to encourage the nonexercisers to participate in group exercise as a means of providing social support, since studies have found that women who persist in exercising after cardiac rehabilitation are more likely to have social support.

Although program evaluations can produce positive findings as well as negative findings, the personnel in charge of the program are not enthusiastic about the evaluation. Specifically, they express fear that it will not show all the good things their program is doing. As the evaluator, what can you do to help the program personnel become invested in your evaluation plan?

3. You have been conducting an evaluation of a state program designed to encourage African Americans to consider becoming organ donors. As a part of the evaluation, television stations in the state aired television spots about the need for organs in the African-American community. African Americans in the state were later surveyed, and their knowledge and attitudes about organ donation were compared to those of African Americans in a neighboring state.

After completing the evaluation, you are invited to present your findings at a national meeting. A hepatologist (liver doctor) in the audience complains about your results, saying that you did not randomly assign people to receive the program or not. How would you respond to this person?

4. Read a journal article that highlights a cost analysis of a health promotion program. Did the authors follow the seven steps outlined in

this chapter in conducting their cost analysis? Provide the information for the seven steps from the article. What specific type of cost analysis did they perform? Describe the resources that went into implementing the program. How did the authors arrive at the associated costs for these resources? Do you think their dollar value was accurate? Did the authors discuss QALY? Discuss the results and provide your opinion on whether or not the program should be implemented widely.

References

Bandura, A. (1986). *Social foundations of thought and action: A social cognitive theory*. Englewood Cliffs, NJ: Prentice-Hall.

Centers for Disease Control and Prevention. (1999). Recommended framework for program evaluation in public health practice. *MMWR Recommendations and Reports*. Atlanta, GA: Centers for Disease Control and Prevention.

Deniston, O. L., and Rosenstock, I. M. (1970). Evaluating health programs. *Public Health Reports, 85*(9), 835–840.

Escoffery, C., Glanz, K., Hall, D., and Elliott, T. (2009). A multi-method process evaluation for a skin cancer prevention diffusion trial. *Evaluation and the Health Professions, 32*(2)184–203.

Glanz, K., Carbone, E., and Song, V. (1999). Formative research for developing targeted skin cancer prevention programs for children in multiethnic Hawaii. *Health Education Research, 14*(2), 155–166.

Glanz, K., Geller, A., Shigaki, D., Maddock, J., and Isnec, M. (2002). A randomized trial of skin cancer prevention in aquatics settings: The Pool Cool program. *Health Psychology, 21*(6), 579–587.

Glanz, K., Isnec, M., Geller, A., and Spangler, K. (2002). Process evaluation of implementation and dissemination of a sun safety program at swimming pools. In A. Steckler and L. Linnan (Eds.), *Process evaluation for public health interventions and research*. San Francisco: Jossey-Bass, pp. 58–82.

Green, L., and Kreuter, M. (2005). *Health promotion planning: An educational and ecological approach* (4th ed.). New York: McGraw-Hill.

Holtgrave, D. R. (2007). The president's fiscal year 2007 Initiative for Human Immunodeficiency Virus counseling and testing expansion in the United States: A scenario analysis of its coverage, impact, and cost-effectiveness. *Journal of Public Health Management Practice, 13*(3), 239–243.

Linnan, L., and Steckler, A. (2002). *Process evaluation for public health interventions and research*. San Francisco: Jossey-Bass.

Patton, M. Q. (2008). *Utilization-focused evaluation* (4th ed.). Thousand Oaks, CA: Sage.

Rabin, B., Nehl, E., Elliot, T., Deshpande, A., Brownson, R., and Glanz, K. (2010, May 31). Individual and setting level predictors of the implementation of a skin cancer prevention program: A multi-level analysis. *Implementation Science, 5*, 40.

Rossi, P. H., Lipsey, M. W., and Freeman, H. E. (2004). *Evaluation: A systematic approach* (7th ed.). Thousand Oaks, CA: Sage.

Smith, M. (2010). *Handbook of program evaluation for social work and health professionals.* New York: Oxford University Press.

Thompson, N. J., and McClintock, H. O. (1998). *Demonstrating your program's worth: A primer on evaluation for programs to prevent unintentional injury.* Atlanta: Centers for Disease Control and Prevention, National Center for Injury Prevention and Control.

Tobacco Technical Assistance Consortium. (2005, January). The power of proof: An evaluation primer. http://www.ttac.org/power-of-proof/index.html

Weiss, C. (1997). *Evaluation: Methods for studying programs and policies.* Englewood Cliffs, NJ: Prentice-Hall.

CHAPTER 13

SURVEY RESEARCH FOR HEALTH PROMOTION

Richard A. Crosby
Laura F. Salazar
Ralph J. DiClemente

Survey research is a type of health promotion research with a distinct purpose. Specifically, survey research is used to describe key aspects of a population through statistical estimates thought to represent the true parameters of that population. Rather than testing prespecified hypotheses or testing health programs, survey research is generally descriptive. Because the results from this type of research are typically generalized to an entire population (such as a state or an entire country), they may be used to inform the allocation of health promotion programs or even health promotion policy. As such, survey research is typically characterized by the use of probability sampling and rather large samples. This type of research carries its own set of challenges and issues, all of which are important.

In nations with a representative government, the tradition of electing a leader is most often preceded by several months (or years) of seemingly endless media reports that predict who will win the election. These predictions are the result of **survey research**, a specific type of health promotion research that is extremely important to the field, as results are often used to inform decisions and policies. Just as survey research can predict who will win a political contest, it can also describe other national phenomena such as trends in obesity, the incidence of diabetes, or whether teen pregnancy is rising, falling, or staying at a constant level. For example, a global United Nations report on food and agriculture showed that according to survey research, Mexico's obesity rate (32.8 percent) has exceeded

LEARNING OBJECTIVES

- Understand how survey research differs from research that tests hypotheses.

- Distinguish between various forms of survey modalities in the larger context of self-administered versus interviewer-administered options.

- Describe how the chosen sampling method limits and defines the choice of survey modality.

- Explain various methods of conducting survey research.

- Describe the construction of a manual of operations and the principles that guide the development of a survey instrument.

- Calculate the standard error and the margin of error and distinguish between the two in the context of survey research.

survey research
research describing health behaviors in very large, often nationally representative, samples

that of the United States (31.8 percent) and that now 70 percent of Mexican adults are overweight compared with 69 percent of U.S. adults (Food and Agriculture Organization of the United Nations, 2013). Given this example, you can quickly understand that the primary difference between survey research and other types of health promotion research described in the rest of this textbook is that survey research may focus on a single variable (such as body mass index) rather then testing the association between variables. This is a key difference that will become more apparent to you as you read this chapter.

probability sampling
use of chance to select a study sample

By necessity, all survey research uses **probability sampling**, involving the implementation of some form of random selection procedure to generate the sample, as doing so allows the findings to be widely generalized. Thus many of the key concepts of probability sampling will become very important to you as you read this chapter and prepare to someday conduct survey research. Many of the skills you acquired from reading the chapter on measurement (Chapter Seven) will prove vital to planning survey research. However, beyond using what you have already learned from the previous chapters, this chapter will provide you with skills in five additional domains that are unique to survey research:

sampling frame
a list of all possible sampling elements

1. It is vital to determine the **sampling frame,** an exhaustive list of all possible sampling elements that includes every member of the targeted population.

2. You must decide on the *modality* that will be used to administer the survey (computer-administered, interviewer-administered, or self-administered).

3. You need to determine the *sample size* (as this estimate will become critical to budgeting) as well as the time allocated to the survey, staff needs, and your ability to make accurate statistical inferences.

4. You must create a *manual of operating procedures* (MOP) describing all protocols that apply to the modality of data collection that you select. For example, the manual will specify the number of contact attempts to be made before giving up on a potential survey respondent. Additionally, your protocols should specify how you will clean and analyze the data.

5. You need to create the *questionnaire*, pilot test it, and then make needed refinements based on the results.

These five steps complete the planning stage; then it is time to seek and obtain approval from your Internal Review Board (see Chapter Three). We cover each of these five domains in great detail, as they constitute the essence of survey research.

Determining the Sampling Frame, Sampling Technique, and Modality

As with all good research, the foremost guide to successful planning is always the same: carefully follow the intent of your research question. It is important to understand that if your research question involves an entire country (for example, "to determine the prevalence of soda consumption among children under the age of 15 who reside in the United States"), you are obligated to find a sampling frame that serves the purpose of your study. Recall that the sampling frame is a list of all possible sampling elements (people) who can be accessed by the researcher. This task is daunting even when the population is only one state, for instance, rather than the entire United States. Normally this daunting task is handled through a multi-stage cluster sampling technique as described in Chapter Six. However, other techniques such as simple random probability sampling or one-stage sampling are available and can be used. The sampling technique used to reach your targeted population will depend upon the nature of the sampling frame— the larger the sampling frame, the more limited your options. Moreover, if a sampling frame does not exist—meaning that there is not an actual list of some sort containing information related to all of the people constituting the population (such as all men who have sex with men and who reside in the Deep South)—then you are certainly limited in your sampling options.

IN A NUTSHELL

The sampling technique used to reach your targeted population will depend upon the nature of the sampling frame—the larger the sampling frame, the more limited your options.

A plausible alternative to random sampling methods that is especially useful when no true sampling frame is available involves approaching people in streets, city parks, and other public areas and asking them if they are members of your population. One drawback is that this method is not random and therefore survey results will not be generalizable to the larger population. To interject more rigor into this method, the Centers for Disease Control and Prevention has widely applied a technique known as **venue-day-time (VDT) sampling**. VDT sampling works by researchers' randomly selecting and visiting venues on specific days (the primary sampling units), and systematically intercepting and collecting information from consenting members of the target population. This allows researchers to construct a sample with known properties and make statistical inference to the larger population of venue visitors. Venues for consideration are defined as public, semi-private, or private locations and

venue-day-time (VDT) sampling used when there is not a known sampling frame, this technique generates a sample using randomly selected days, times, and venues to create a unique combination of recruitment opportunities

may include city parks, malls, movie theaters, cafes and restaurants, health clubs, social and religious organizations, bookstores, high-traffic street locations, community recreation centers, or housing projects. As standard protocol for VDT sampling, after the initial list of venues is developed, venue proprietors are approached and asked for permission before any recruitment events are scheduled. As an example, VDT has been used in the National HIV Behavioral Surveillance (NHBS) to survey MSM across 22 metropolitan areas in the United States (MacKeller, Gallagher, Finlayson, Sanchez, Lansky, and Sullivan, 2007). VDT sampling has also been used in many community-level evaluations and has considerable advantages over the use of more traditional sample survey methods that yield low numbers of eligible respondents (Doherty, Minnis, and Auerswald, 2007; MacKellar et al., 2007; Muhib et al., 2001; Remafedi, Jurek, and Oakes, 2008). In an ever-expanding number of studies, the use of VDT has resulted in recruitment of high numbers of study participants in relatively short time spans.

survey modalities
the chosen methods of
collecting the data for a
particular survey

Once the sampling technique is selected, the next task is to balance the choice of sampling techniques with the pros and cons of various possible **survey modalities**. A survey modality is the chosen method of collecting the data. Because the sampling technique constrains and defines the survey modality, the process of balancing the two selections is often time-consuming, yet it is extremely critical. To aid in this process, Box 13.1 provides a summary of the potential sampling techniques that could be used for each of the three modalities (again, these are computer-administered, interviewer-administered, or self-administered). As you study this information, note that that the modality you select will in turn inform your options for sampling.

BOX 13.1. ALIGNMENT OF MODALITY WITH SAMPLING TECHNIQUES

Modality One: Computer-Administered

Sampling Options

1. Random sampling via the Internet

2. Random sampling via phone

Modality Two: Self-Administered

Sampling Options

1. Surveys mailed to randomly selected households

2. Questionnaires completed by students in randomly selected schools

Modality Three: Interviewer-Administered

Sampling Options

1. Random sampling via phone

2. VDT sampling

We suggest that you use Box 13.1 to align the sampling technique that will be best for reaching your population with your choice of modality. Once this decision is made, you can identify the specific method of data collection. Box 13.2 displays the pros and cons regarding data collection for each of the three modalities. This information should be kept in a prominent location until you and the research team make the ultimate choice of modality.

BOX 13.2. PROS AND CONS OF THREE MODALITIES

Modality 1: Computer-Administered

Pros

Interactive voice recognition can be used.

Data are automatically uploaded to a spreadsheet.

Skip patterns are automatically navigated.

Logic checks can be programmed into the survey to detect false answers.

Cons

Definitions may not be detailed enough for all respondents.

Connectivity issues may cause premature discontinuation.

Some people may not trust confidentiality of responses submitted via the Internet.

Respondent identity cannot be definitively known.

Modality 2: Interviewer-Administered

Pros

The interviewer can probe and assist people to accurately recall behavior.

Constant use of responses such as "don't know" may be less likely.

Skip patterns are automatically navigated.

Definitions of terms or clarification of entire questions can be offered.

Cons

Respondents may not fully self-disclose sensitive or personal behaviors.

Interviewer bias may be a factor.

Surveys of large samples may not be possible.

Modality 3: Self-Administered

Pros

Disclosure of sensitive or personal behaviors may be optimal.

Technology is not required.

This modality can be used for large samples.

This modality is good for populations with low computer literacy.

Cons

Respondents may easily skip large numbers of questions.

Writing may be unclear or even entirely illegible.

Skip patterns will be problematic for many respondents to navigate.

Definitions may not be adequate, and entire questions may be unclear.

IN A NUTSHELL

The choice of your data collection method depends upon the population you are surveying; the available resources for the survey, such as staff; and the context in which the research will be conducted.

Your choice of data collection method depends upon the population you are surveying; the available resources for the survey, such as staff; and the context in which the research will be conducted. For example, you may want to consider using an interviewer-administered modality if respondents in your population have low literacy or low writing or typing skills or issues with their sight, tire easily, or have low motivation to complete the survey, or if the research context makes it difficult for them to complete the survey. A self-administered survey, on the other hand, would be conducive to surveying populations with high literacy, high writing or typing skills, and a high level of motivation.

One data collection method used often in survey research that falls under the category of being interviewer-administered is **random digit dialing** (RDD). A unique advantage of RDD is that it also serves as a sampling technique. Random digit dialing was first developed in 1972 and has stood the test of time for over five decades as a way to generate a random probability sample as well as a method to collect the data from respondents. RDD involves generating random telephone numbers using a legitimate local exchange (also area codes and country codes if targeting specific geographical areas) and then dialing the telephone numbers to survey potential respondents. One clear advantage of RDD is that everyone with a telephone number has an equal chance of being selected, thus meeting the defining criterion of a random probability sample, as households whose telephone numbers are unlisted could also be selected. **List-assisted random digit dialing**, which applies when sampling frames are a subset of the larger sample frame, may also be used to increase the efficiency of regular RDD methods. Although the exact procedural details and parameters used to implement list-assisted RDD vary, the data sources used to determine the portions of the frame to be retained are fairly standard and are derived from household databases compiled from local telephone directories. The term "list-assisted" is derived from the method's reliance on lists or databases of directory-listed telephone households to define the sampling frame. It is important to note, however, that the term list-assisted does not imply that the resultant sample contains only listed telephone households. Rather, "list-assisted" is descriptive of the data source used to define, truncate, and restrict the sample frame itself. List-assisted RDD is an improvement on RDD in that it increases the efficiency of RDD, and it is still used today.

Due to the widespread abandonment of landlines, RDD techniques now include cell phone numbers to avert noncoverage bias. Over the years, **response rates** (the ratio of the number of people who agree to participate to the total number contacted) to RDD surveys have declined markedly for several reasons, such as survey burnout, increased use of cell phones with caller identification, and do-not-call lists. Using RDD as your sampling technique is relatively straightforward (essentially generating random numbers), but you have to accept the shortcomings of the data collection method, such as low response rate, frequent cut-offs, and **coverage bias.** Coverage bias is indicated when the sampling frame is incomplete, as would be the case in telephone surveys when the sampling frame excludes those who have cellular phones but not those with landlines.

As stated previously, computer technology can be applied to both self-administered and interviewer-administered modalities. In the case

random digit dialing
selection of people for survey research by randomly generating telephone numbers

list-assisted random digit dialing
a technique that increases the efficiency of RDD by using a database or "list" against which the RDD-generated numbers are compared to determine whether they are working or nonworking telephone numbers

response rates
the number of people who participate in the survey divided by the number asked to participate

coverage bias
bias resulting from deficits in the sampling frame

of the interview-administered modality, computer-assisted telephone interviewing (CATI) software can be used to increase efficiency and accuracy. CATI software generates random numbers, calls the numbers, and then allows the interviewer to administer the survey questions to the respondent and automatically record the answers.

A popular and fairly new data collection method used for self-administered modalities is the online survey. Online survey platforms (for example, Qualtrics.com, PsychData, SurveyGizmo) have proliferated in recent years; they provide an efficient and convenient method for respondents to complete surveys. The researcher programs the survey items using a variety of available preprogrammed templates that include a high degree of functionality such as complex skip patterns. Once the survey is programmed, a URL is generated and then respondents can access the survey at a time and location convenient for them by using the link.

IN A NUTSHELL

Mail-based surveys still have a place in survey research because postal addresses are a matter of public record, thereby making a sampling frame available to the researcher.

Although use of mail-based surveys is far less popular since the advent of the Internet, they still have a place in survey research because postal addresses are a matter of public record, thereby making a sampling frame available to the researcher. For instance, an entire county of residential households could be the sampling frame, given that a comprehensive listing of all mailing addresses is already assembled. Once the sample is selected, the survey instrument is sent to selected households. The package must also include a letter inviting study participation, a preaddressed and postage-paid envelope for return of the completed questionnaire, and perhaps an incentive to complete the questionnaire. For example, Takahashi et al. (2011) conducted a needs assessment using questionnaires mailed to a convenience sample of Micronesian and Polynesian residents in Los Angeles, Orange, and San Diego Counties in southern California. The questionnaire focused on HIV knowledge, HIV testing behavior, and experience with intimate partner violence.

Although mail-based surveys may appear simple, it is critical to note that achieving respectable response rates with mail-based surveys requires sending follow-up requests (and new packages) to persons nonresponsive to the initial mailing. The need for repeated mailings and follow-up often becomes cumbersome and costly.

A great deal of time and attention should be dedicated to learning as much as possible about the methods you are thinking about using. Keep in mind that professional journals are replete with past examples, and reading about the successes (and failures) of others is an important first step as you begin your study.

Estimating the Required Sample Size

The classic children's story "Goldilocks and the Three Bears" contains the ideal metaphor for estimating sample size. As Goldilocks tastes porridge from various bowls belonging to the absentee bears, she finds that one is too hot, one is too cold, and one is just right. The same is true for sample size. You can have too many respondents in your survey ("too hot") or too few ("too cold")—either instance can be problematic. To understand why this is true in survey research, it is important to return to the opening of this chapter and recall a primary distinction of survey research: that it provides a population-level estimate of a single variable. Consider, for example, the importance to public health policy of knowing what percent of Americans on Medicare report finding a doctor who accepts their insurance. The answer to the question will stem from a survey administered to 500 Americans on Medicare, and it will be reported as a simple percentage, ranging from 0 to 100. Let's assume the answer is 29.3 percent. Next comes the real question: How confident are we that the 29.3 percent is a true estimate rather than an artifact of chance within the process of sampling the respondents? To determine the degree of confidence in our estimate requires us to understand the amount of sampling error and that sampling error is a function of sample size. The degree of confidence in our estimate equates with the widely accepted and statistical standard used, the 95-percent **confidence interval** (CI)—that is, the range around a statistic or measurement that conveys how precise it is.

The CI is constructed to yield plus or minus a value that must always be reported in tandem with the estimate—in this case, 29.3 percent. In this example, the CI was ± 2; Thus the CI would equal 27.33–31.33, suggesting a small degree of sampling error. It may be important to note that the CI reported in survey research relates to a single point estimate of one variable ("percent of people on Medicare who report being able to find a doctor to accept their insurance"). As the confidence interval is a measure of precision, a wider confidence interval equates with less precision than more narrow intervals. Box 13.3 provides you with a bit more practice with the idea of using CIs in survey research.

confidence interval
interval that sets off a low range and a high range as possible limits of an estimate and represents the precision of the estimate

IN A NUTSHELL

As the confidence interval is a measure of precision, a wider confidence interval equates with less precision than more narrow intervals.

BOX 13.3.   TEEN BIRTH RATES, PER 1,000, ACROSS FIVE SURVEYS REPEATED EVERY
TWO YEARS

2005	63.1 ← 67.1 → 71.2
2007	60.0 ← 62.5 → 65.0
2009	56.3 ← 59.5 → 62.7
2011	55.0 ← 57.4 → 59.8
2013	51.1 ← 53.1 → 55.1

In Box 13.3, the point estimates (shown in the middle of the 95-percent CIs) suggest a steady decline in teen pregnancy rates between 2005 and 2013. However, the data in the box also show that the decline is never significant between survey rounds. This is because the CIs all overlap as the larger decline occurs. For example, the lower limit of the 2011 point estimate (55.0) falls within the upper limit of the 2013 interval (55.1), thereby violating the dictum that significance is achieved only when the intervals being compared do not overlap at all. This same rule, however, would tell us that the decline from 2005 to 2009 was significant (because 63.1, the lower limit of 2005, falls above 62.7, the upper limit of 2009). This is similarly true for comparisons of 2007 to 2011 and 2009 to 2013.

Two methods of calculating CIs are used in survey research. One is used after collecting the data (standard error method) and the other is used before collecting the data (the margin of error). The standard error method could also be used before the data are collected, but doing so would entail guessing the possible **point estimate**. The point estimate is the value of a given variable in a population (for example, 23.2 percent of Americans smoke cigarettes). Guessing the point estimate can be achieved through reading published studies of similar populations and health issues.

Once you identify a likely point estimate, calculating a 95-percent CI around the point estimate is a fairly straightforward procedure. The **standard error** is a statistical term that measures the accuracy with which a sample represents the population. The smaller the standard error, the more representative the sample will be of the overall population. The standard error is also inversely proportional to the sample size; the larger the sample size, the smaller the standard error, because the statistic will approach the actual value. The standard error is the value that will be used to calculate the 95-percent CI. Two standard errors above the point estimate represent the upper limit of the CI. Similarly, two standard errors below the point estimate represent the lower limit of the CI. The formula

point estimate
the value given to a variable in a population

standard error
measurement of the accuracy with which a sample represents its corresponding population

for the standard error is defined as

$$\text{Standard error} = \sqrt{(p(1-p))/n}$$

where p is the percent of a population that you predict will have the quality, disease, opinion, or the like that is the object of your study, and n is the number of people surveyed. The math required to calculate the standard error is nothing more than a multiplication procedure ($p \times (1-p)$), one division (the product of $p \times (1-p)$ divided by n), and then determining the square root of the quotient. As you may have guessed, 1-p is simply the remainder of 100 percent after p is accounted for in your calculation. So let's assume, after a review of the literature, that 38.5 percent of Americans eat too much refined sugar. In this example, p would equal 38.5 percent and $1-p = (100 \text{ percent} - 38.5 \text{ percent} = 61.5 \text{ percent})$. Because you are determining the CI based on the sample size for your study, the formula uses n as the denominator. Let's try the value of $n = 100$.

$$\text{Standard error} = \sqrt{(38.5(61.7))/100}$$

As you can see from this example, the sample of 100 survey respondents yields a standard error of 4.866. This would mean that the resulting 95-percent CI would be ($4.866 \times 2 = 9.73$): 28.77 percent through 48.23 percent. This may be considered a wide interval, suggesting that the precision may not be high in the point prevalence estimate of 38.5 percent. This lack of precision could be improved with perhaps 500 people in the sample. Thus the next equation uses the value of 500 in the denominator.

$$\text{Standard error} = \sqrt{(38.5(61.5))/500}$$

Now the new estimated standard error is 2.17, which is smaller (and therefore more precise) than the estimate based on a sample of only 100 respondents. With 500 survey respondents, the 95-percent CI is 34.16 through 42.84. This is much smaller indeed! But is it small enough? In many cases, the point prevalence estimate does not need to be extremely precise. However, in trend studies there is a great need for precision in order to determine whether the point prevalence estimate changes significantly from one year to the next.

IN A NUTSHELL

In trend studies there is a great need for precision in order to determine whether the point prevalence estimate changes significantly from one year to the next.

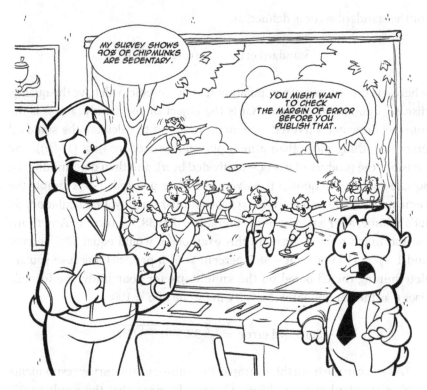

The Case of Too Few Respondents

Copyright 2014 by Justin Wagner; reprinted with permission.

For example, going back to our example of Americans on Medicare whose doctors accept their insurance, imagine that one year after doing the first survey (that included 500 respondents) you repeat the survey and find that instead of the 29.3 percent you found in the first survey, 27.5 percent of your respondents report that their doctors accept Medicare insurance. Do you then declare that fewer people on Medicare can find doctors willing to take this form of payment? No, because the value of 27.5 percent was within the estimate you obtained in the previous year (recall that the 95-percent CI in that first survey was 27.3 through 31.33). Thus, with only 500 people in your first survey, a decline of nearly 2 full percentage points in your second survey would have to be declared nonsignificant. Practically speaking, however, a decline of nearly 2 percent applied to the U.S. population on Medicare represents almost 1 million people. Thus it would be prudent to think about whether having more than 500 survey respondents would be a worthwhile investment. So let's try the calculation again, this time with 1,200 respondents.

$$\text{Standard error} = \sqrt{((29.3)(70.7))/1200}$$

After doing the math on this one, you will find that the standard error equals 1.31. This equates with a 95-percent CI of 27.99–30.61. This is a much more precise estimate; it would allow a drop (or increase) in the point prevalence estimate of 1.31 or greater, during a subsequent survey, to be classified as a significant trend.

As noted previously, the standard error method is best when applied *after* the data are collected. The margin of error (a much simpler procedure) is the method applied *before* the survey begins. At this juncture, it is important to note that the standard error of the point prevalence estimate is not the same as the **margin of error**. In fact, the terms are often misused and incorrectly taken to be synonymous. Margin of error expresses the maximum *expected* difference between the true population parameter and a sample estimate of that parameter.

margin of error
expresses the maximum expected difference between the true population parameter and a sample estimate of that parameter

The margin of error is calculated based only on sample size; it does not account for the differences in proportions. The formula involves using the value of 1.96 (which is a standard z-score value used to calculate 95-percent CIs). The value of 1.96 is the numerator in this calculation. The denominator is 2 × the square root of n, where n is the number of people surveyed. Thus the expression looks like this:

$$\text{Margin of error} = \frac{1.96}{2\sqrt{n}}$$

If, for example, your sample size was 100, the margin of error would be plus or minus .098 or 9.8 percent (note, the denominator is 20—simply 2 × the square root of *100*). For example, if a study estimates that 51 percent of Americans have ever been screened for cancer, and that study samples 1,200 people, then the new report might read something like this: "Between 48% and 54% of Americans have ever been screened for cancer." In this case, if you are more than happy with the approximate 3-percent margin of error, you may want to consider saving resources and reducing your sample size even further. In essence, confidence comes at a price, so you need to decide how much you can afford. Figure 13.1 provides you with a precalculated set of sample sizes that may serve as an important reference to you for your future survey research; they are based on an acceptable margin of error (1 percent to 5 percent) and the researcher's chosen CI (95 percent or 99 percent).

Constructing the Manual of Operations

The manual of operating procedures (MOP) will be needed throughout your study. The MOP describes all protocols that apply to the modality

Required Sample Size								
	Confidence = 95%				Confidence = 99%			
Population Size	Margin of Error				Margin of Error			
	5.0%	3.5%	2.5%	1.0%	5.0%	3.5%	2.5%	1.0%
10	10	10	10	10	10	10	10	10
20	19	20	20	20	19	20	20	20
30	28	29	29	30	29	29	30	30
50	44	47	48	50	47	48	49	50
75	63	69	72	74	67	71	73	75
100	80	89	94	99	87	93	96	99
150	108	126	137	148	122	135	142	149
200	132	160	177	196	154	174	186	198
250	152	190	215	244	182	211	229	246
300	169	217	251	291	207	246	270	295
400	146	265	318	384	250	309	348	391
500	217	306	377	475	285	365	421	485
600	234	340	432	565	315	416	490	579
700	248	370	481	653	341	462	554	672
800	260	396	526	739	363	503	615	763
1,000	278	440	606	906	399	575	727	943
1,200	291	474	674	1,067	427	636	827	1,119
1,500	306	515	759	1,297	460	712	959	1,376
2,000	322	563	869	1,655	498	808	1,141	1,785
2,500	333	597	952	1,984	524	879	1,288	2,173
3,500	346	641	1,068	2,565	558	977	1,150	2,890
5,000	357	678	1,176	3,288	586	1,066	1,734	3,842
7,500	365	710	1,275	4,211	610	1,147	1,960	5,165
10,000	370	727	1,332	4,899	622	1,193	2,098	6,239
25,000	378	760	1,448	6,939	646	1,285	2,399	9,972
50,000	381	772	1,491	8,056	655	1,318	2,520	12,455
75,000	382	776	1,506	8,514	658	1,330	2,563	13,583
100,000	383	778	1,513	8,762	659	1,336	2,585	14,227
250,000	384	782	1,527	9,248	662	1,347	2,626	15,555
500,000	384	783	1,532	9,423	663	1,350	2,640	16,055
1,000,000	384	783	1,534	9,512	663	1,352	2,647	16,317
2,500,000	384	783	1,536	9,567	663	1,353	2,651	16,478
10,000,000	384	784	1,536	9,594	663	1,354	2,653	16,560
100,000,000	384	784	1,537	9,603	663	1,354	2,654	16,584
300,000,000	384	784	1,537	9,603	663	1,354	2,654	16,586

Figure 13.1 Sample Size by Margin of Error for Survey Research

of data collection that you select. At least five categories may be relevant to the MOP: eligibility screening, procedures for "cutoffs," procedures for determining response rate, hiring and training interviewers, and handling missing data (nonresponse).

Eligibility Screening

Regardless of the modality you select, your MOP must specify exactly who is eligible to be a survey respondent and, more important, how that determination will be made. For example, if your research question is about colorectal cancer screening, your population may be limited to people age 50 or older. Further, because screening is a preventive measure, your population would exclude persons already diagnosed with colorectal cancer. You may also want to restrict your population to people who speak and read a given language, as you may not have the resources to make the survey available in multiple languages. With these three criteria in mind, the tough question then becomes "How do I screen potential study participants?"

One method that can be used to screen for eligibility is to create a brief set of survey questions that capture the key criteria you have established for the study. This screening tool can be self-administered or interviewer-administered, using a number of techniques. First, after briefly describing the study, you can require potential participants to agree to be screened. Participants' responses are important, because each "yes" answer will represent one more person screened for eligibility, thereby adding to an ongoing count kept as a permanent study record. Once a person is screened, then careful records must be kept detailing the number who were eligible and the number who were ineligible based on each of the stated criteria.

> **IN A NUTSHELL**
>
> Participants' responses are important, because each "yes" answer will represent one more person screened for eligibility, thereby adding to an ongoing count kept as a permanent study record.

Procedures for Determining Nonresponsiveness

Respondents hanging up the phone (disconnecting) or failing to complete an internet-based survey may be considered nonresponsive, depending on the rules you establish. Before the survey is administered you should determine what constitutes a completed survey. For example, if a person answers 60 percent of the questions asked, would you consider that a completed interview? Ideally, the solution is that only the people answering all of the questions are considered completers. However, with internet-based research rapidly replacing phone surveys, this question becomes more nuanced, because with online surveys many people may begin taking the survey and then prematurely end their participation due to respondent fatigue or perhaps feeling that the survey involves a higher level of commitment than thought initially. Because discontinuation of the survey leaves the researcher with only partial data, the MOP must specify how partially completed surveys will be used in the final analysis (if at all) and what degree of completion constitutes enough data to count the respondent as one more person toward the targeted enrollment goal. Bear in mind that you do have a target sample size to fill (recall that this is based on the margin of error) and that it relies on having a 100-percent completion rate, which may be unlikely.

Procedures for Determining the Response Rate

All survey research, like all research, is judged for rigor. A key indicator of rigor is the response rate; the inverse of the response rate is called the nonresponse rate. The response rate matters because a low rate suggests that sample bias may be high. If, for example, only 30 percent of all those screened actually go on to participate and complete the survey, would you be confident in generalizing the study findings to an entire population? At a 30-percent response rate, as you progress toward reaching your recruitment goal of, for example, 1,200 completed surveys, you would need to find 9,600 people who are study-eligible. The nagging question then becomes quite clear: Are the 8,400 people who declined to begin or complete the survey somehow different from the 1,200?

Because the response rate is vital, the researcher must prespecify how that rate will be mathematically determined. Several well-established methods for this calculation exist. For example, the Behavioral Risk Factor Surveillance System (BRFSS), the largest example of survey research in the world, uses a standard formula to calculate the response rate. Here is an excerpt from their MOP:

> The Cooperation Rate (aka, response rate) is the proportion of all respondents interviewed of all eligible units in which a respondent was selected and actually contacted. Non-contacts are excluded from the denominator. This rate is based on contacts with households containing an eligible respondent. The denominator of the rate includes completed interviews plus the number of non-interviews that involve the identification of and contact with a selected respondent. A Cooperation Rate below 65 percent may indicate some problem with interviewing techniques. [Available at ftp://ftp.cdc.gov/pub/data/brfss/2010_summary_data_quality_report.pdf]

The BRFSS, which uses a telephone methodology, is one example of how to calculate a response rate. Other ways include, for example, keeping records of the number of impressions made when people view a banner ad asking them to complete survey research on the Internet. For street-based surveys using methods such as VDT (described previously in this chapter), researchers must decide what denominator will be used for the response rate. Regardless of the number of challenges to generating a response rate, the MOP must precisely define and describe exactly how these challenges will be met.

Hiring and training interviewers. A common source of bias in interviewer-administered survey research is known as **interviewer bias**, which stems from effects of the person doing the interview (judgmental tones, leading, probing, and so on). The interviewer's opinion or prejudice shown during the interview can affect respondents' responses, which in turn can affect the outcome. Interviewer bias is to be avoided whenever possible. A question that is often germane to hiring an interviewer is, Does the gender, age, or race/ethnicity of an interviewer have a significant influence on how people respond to survey questions? Unfortunately, there is very little empirical data to address this empirical question. However, the scant evidence that does exist suggests that these demographics become largely unimportant factors in contrast to personality traits of the interviewer, such as warmth, expression, openness, and the appearance of being nonjudgmental (see Figure 13.2). Hiring an effective interviewer involves role-playing during the job interview to give you (as the hiring agent) a better picture of the presence or absence of key personality traits that will lead to more effective responses from survey participants. Because it is

interviewer bias
any bias expressed by the person conducting the interview that may influence the respondent's answers to questions

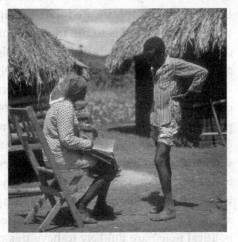

Figure 13.2 Respondent Being Interviewed
Source: "Nederlands: Dia" by Tropenmuseum of the Royal Tropical Institute (KIT). Licensed under Creative Commons Attribution-Share Alike 3.0 Unported License.
http://creativecommons.org/licenses/by-sa/3.0/deed.en.

IN A NUTSHELL

Hiring an effective interviewer involves role-playing during the job interview to give you (as the hiring agent) a better picture of the presence or absence of key personality traits that will lead to more effective responses from survey participants.

illegal to hire based on gender, age, or race/ethnicity, the MOP should specify the most important characteristics of the ideal interviewer.

Once the interviewer is hired, your MOP will be used as a guide for her training. The MOP should specify what skills should be taught to the interviewer(s), the methods that will be used to teach the skills, and the objectives that will be used to assess whether the skills have been acquired.

Handling Missing Data

imputation
the process wherein
missing values are
replaced with substituted
values

Missing data is the plague of all research, including survey research. One effective method to compensate for this problem is **imputation**, a process wherein missing values are replaced with substituted values. Although there are many sophisticated statistical imputation techniques, a common imputation method is to use the mean of the sample for any one question or item as the surrogate value for missing responses. Although this may appear to be a simple solution, the MOP should nonetheless specify how much imputation is allowed for any given variable. For example, if a survey question asks, "How many different people have you had sex with in the past 12 months?" it may well be that imputation for 20 percent or more of the sample is necessary. Thus the question becomes whether you are willing to impute one of every five cases. A final point is highly relevant here: short surveys are far more likely to yield 100-percent compliance than longer surveys. Therefore extremely lengthy surveys, such as the BRFSS, are prone to missing data, whereas those that are extremely short (such as political polls) are unlikely to have this problem. The lesson is that when you construct your questionnaire (more properly known as the survey instrument) you need to balance survey length against the increased risk of missing data.

Creating the Survey Instrument

The survey instrument should be constructed based on attention to question sequence, overall appearance (if written), wording of individual items, wording of response options, and a concept known as "survey burden." Instrument development is an art and a science. It is an art because repeated experience will, over time, make you better at the process; it is a science because the development process must always include pilot testing followed by data-guided alterations to the original instrument. It is important to note that survey research, unlike studies that test specific hypotheses, rarely uses scales or indexes as described in Chapter Seven, because the purpose of survey research is typically to estimate values of single variables, such as the number of people in a population who eat red meat at least 3 times per week or the percentage of women over age 40 who have never had a mammogram.

One caveat to the development of your survey instrument is vital to consider before you begin drafting the questionnaire items. This caveat is best presented as a question: How will your collected data be transferred to a computer spreadsheet for data analysis? This is a critical decision because even a low rate of keystroke errors from manual data entry can be problematic. Moreover, manual data entry is time-consuming and therefore expensive. Computer-based methods typically circumvent these issues; however, some software programs can be challenging to use and manage. There is no simple solution to the problem. As a rule, however, we suggest that you design your survey instrument with ease of data transfer in mind.

Item Wording

Unlike research designed to test hypotheses, survey research is designed to make estimates of single variables as they exist in an entire population. A good example of survey research is determining the number of women 21 and older who have had a Pap test in the past three years. Suppose you are in charge of women's health for an entire state. Using the BRFSS, you could access this estimate to determine trends in your state and then increase the promotion of Pap testing accordingly. Your allocation of personnel time and resources will ultimately hinge on a single question that was asked of hundreds (or even thousands) of women. As you can imagine, the wording of that single item must be exact! Imprecise wording will always result in poor decision making for the professionals who apply the results of survey research. Thus a question worded as, "In the past 3 years, have you had a Pap test?" may not be as effective as its face value may suggest. First, the word "Pap" may not always be known to women (especially if they have never had one). When taken in the context of completing a long survey (as most are), many women who are not entirely familiar with this term may quickly think of almost any gynecological procedure as a Pap test, so the data will overestimate prevalence. Second, the phrase "past 3 years" creates an expectation for the survey respondent; it seems to suggest that this is a rule or guideline for care and thus prompts the compliant answer of "yes." Upon reflection, then, a much better question would read:

IN A NUTSHELL

The choice of using a self-administered method of data collection versus an interviewer-administered method automatically creates differences in the wording of your questionnaire items.

"A Pap test involves a nurse/doctor collecting cells from your vagina. When was the last time you had a Pap test?"

☐ I have never had a Pap test

☐ More than 5 years ago

☐ Between 3 and 5 years ago

☐ Between 2 and 3 years ago

☐ Between 1 and 2 years ago

☐ Less than 1 year ago

Item wording plagues most health promotion research. Consider the following example of questionable item wording. A survey question is designed to assess the prevalence of smoking in a population. The item reads, "Are you a smoker?" Although the item is easy to comprehend and simple to read, you should pause for a moment and ponder what an answer of "no" could potentially imply. "No" may imply any of the following:

- A person smokes only on rare occasions, such as when stress levels are high; he does not classify the behavior as "being a smoker."

- A person uses tobacco as a party drug—smoking only during times of drinking with others during planned events; she does not classify the behavior as "being a smoker."

- A person smokes daily, but does so far less than most other people known to him; he does not classify the behavior as "being a smoker."

Given just these three possibilities, it would appear that the wording of this item is problematic because it would underestimate the true prevalence of "smoking" in the population. An initial step in formulating the question is of course identifying the health concern. In this case, given the overwhelming evidence of even short-term ill effects of smoking on health, the issue may be any use at all. The question would therefore be reframed as: "Have you smoked cigarettes, cigars, or other forms of tobacco?" Now the question makes more sense, but the problem is that it does not have a time-bound element. Because the effects of tobacco use on health are indeed reversible over time, a better indicator of health status would be to ask the question this way: "In the past 12 months, have you smoked cigarettes, cigars, or other forms of tobacco?" Although you may be tempted to declare that the question is now survey-ready, you still need to consider the purpose of the item from a health viewpoint. Are you concerned about the effects of tobacco on respiratory illness or are the effects on heart disease also important to you? If indeed heart disease is important, then your question is flawed because it does not account for smokeless tobacco use. A revised version is once again in order: "In the past 12 months, have you used cigarettes, cigars, smokeless tobacco, or other forms of tobacco?" While this question now seems to be "perfect," note that we have expanded from the original item of 4 easy words to an item that now has 17 words (many of which are multisyllabic). The teaching point here is the inherent tradeoff between simplicity (fewer words and syllables) and precision (more details and words) (see Figure 13.3).

IN A NUTSHELL

The teaching point here is that an inherent tradeoff exists between simplicity (fewer words and syllables) and precision (more details and words).

A final word of caution about item wording is in order. Always ask yourself whether the question collects data that are worthwhile to your study. A question taken from the Behavioral Risk Factor Surveillance System (BRFSS) is quite illustrative of this principle.

Would you say that in general your health is

1. Excellent
2. Very good
3. Good
4. Fair
5. Poor

In the context of survey research, this questionnaire item is unlikely to provide any meaningful data. The loss of meaning occurs because the question measures a personal perception rather than an objective standard. An overweight, diabetic person, with hypertension, for example, who resides in a community where these three health issues are normative may rate her

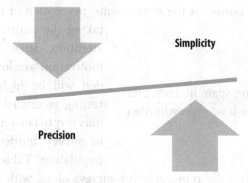

Figure 13.3 Trade-off between Simplicity and Precision

health as "Good" or even "Excellent." Conversely, an objectively healthy person could easily respond with "Fair" or even "Poor" if the respondent feels that his health is not as good as that of other peers or family members. Moreover, some people answering this question may think about only physical health when responding, whereas others may think about mental and social health. Ultimately the aggregate variable will not represent a unitary construct.

Pilot Testing

pilot testing
a very small-scale version of the survey research, used to ensure that the research protocols are effective

The process of resolving the tension depicted in Figure 13.3 involves **pilot testing**. Pilot testing is nothing more than a small-scale test of the item with likely survey respondents. Focus groups or an in-depth, one-to-one interview both work quite well for this purpose, and for this reason a working knowledge of qualitative research (see Chapter Eight) is very helpful. The small sample must include the full range of likely respondents. This is especially true for the dimension of literacy. Even if the interview is being read to respondents, literacy in the language used for the interview is vital. For example, the term "smokeless tobacco" may well be familiar to you, but youth responding to your survey may have never been exposed to this "high-class" term. They may know smokeless tobacco only as "dip." Your entire 17-word question, however, may test well in your qualitative investigation! You may feel fully confident in your newly created item, but unfortunately, confidence is all too often an illusion when creating a survey instrument.

It should be noted that the term "survey instrument" is distinct from "survey" because the former accurately describes the tool used to collect data, while the latter is a much larger process. The survey instrument is the entire collection of single items; while your pilot tests evaluate the wording of each item, they must also evaluate the concept of **survey burden**. Survey burden is the respondents' perception of the difficulty of taking the entire survey. When attention span, literacy, and motivation are low, survey burden will be high. Again, pilot testing is crucial as this is the only way to fairly judge the degree of survey burden for a given population. Table 13.1 provides examples of nationally representative surveys along with the number of questions included in the entire survey.

survey burden
a perception that the survey is too long or complex to reasonably complete with full attention

IN A NUTSHELL

When attention span, literacy, and motivation are low, survey burden will be high.

Table 13.1   Examples of National Surveys Conducted in the United States

National Survey	Length of Survey
Behavioral Risk Factor Surveillance Survey (BRFSS). BRFSS collects state data about U.S. residents regarding their health-related risk behaviors and events, chronic health conditions, and use of preventive services. BRFSS also collects data on important emerging health issues such as vaccine shortage and influenza-like illness. For example, since September 2009, federal, state, and local health agencies have used BRFSS to monitor the prevalence rates of influenza-like illness to help with pandemic planning. Interviewers administer the annual BRFSS surveys continuously through the year.	Core survey: 86 items with 34 optional modules.
National Longitudinal Study of Adolescent Health (Add Health). Add Health is a longitudinal study of a nationally representative sample of adolescents in grades 7–12 in the United States during the 1994–95 school year. The Add Health cohort has been followed into young adulthood with four in-home interviews, the most recent in 2008, when the sample was aged 24–32. Add Health combines longitudinal survey data on respondents' social, economic, psychological, and physical well-being with contextual data on the family, neighborhood, community, school, friendships, peer groups, and romantic relationships, providing unique opportunities to study how social environments and behaviors in adolescence are linked to health and achievement outcomes in young adulthood.	The current wave of data collection involves more than 200 pages of questions—the number of questions that people answer is a product of multiple skip patterns.
Youth Risk Behavior Surveillance System (YRBSS). YRBSS monitors six types of health risk behaviors that contribute to the leading causes of death and disability among youth and adults, including • Behaviors that contribute to unintentional injuries and violence • Sexual behaviors that contribute to unintended pregnancy and sexually transmitted diseases, including HIV infection • Alcohol and other drug use • Tobacco use • Unhealthy dietary behaviors • Inadequate physical activity YRBSS also measures the prevalence of obesity and asthma among youth and young adults. YRBSS includes a national school-based survey conducted by CDC and state, territorial, tribal, and local surveys conducted by state, territorial, tribal, and local education and health agencies and tribal governments.	131 items for state surveys and 136–142 items for national surveys.
National Health and Nutrition Examination Survey (NHANES). NHANES is a program of studies designed to assess the health and nutritional status of adults and children in the United States. The NHANES interview includes demographic, socioeconomic, dietary, and health-related questions. The examination component consists of medical, dental, and physiological measurements, as well as laboratory tests administered by highly trained medical personnel.	Survey items cover over 30 topic areas (for example, smoking, alcohol, physical activity, nutrition) and include over 150 items administered via ACASI or CAPI.

Motivating Complete Responding

A final aspect of questionnaire development involves attention to factors that will encourage people to complete the entire survey, regardless of the amount of survey burden. Bear in mind that people completing your survey are volunteers; they do not need to do anything beyond their level of motivation. Consequently, one critical task is to build motivation into your design. Dillman (1991) has created what is termed the "total design approach." This approach suggests that attention to the ease of survey completion, the aesthetics of the survey instrument, and even the clarity of instructions may all contribute to whether any given respondent will trudge through to the end of the questionnaire.

Grouping questions according to topic increases ease of completion. This prevents respondents from having to constantly switch back and forth from one set of thoughts to another. For example, questions related to diet should all be placed in the same section of the survey; this allows people to think about their past dietary behaviors only once during the course of completing the survey. In any given topical section, the items should be asked such that the response formats are also presented in groups. For instance, items asking respondents to use a five-point scale (such as "strongly agree" = 1 and "strongly disagree" = 5) should all be placed together within the set of questions pertaining to one topic. As the response formats change, the survey instrument should provide clear yet concise instructions to help people understand exactly what they are being asked to do. Overly complex or (at the opposite extreme) cryptic instructions are likely to cause a loss of motivation to complete one section, or possibly the remainder of the survey. So as people respond to each successive set of survey questions, it is important to provide some indication of their progress towards completion, such as "You are doing great—only 40 questions remain!" Cartoons, white space, and distinct boxes that separate one question set from another are all examples of aesthetic details that may also increase motivation to complete the entire questionnaire.

Data Weighting and Analysis

Because survey research is intended to generate estimates that pertain to an entire population, it is imperative that the sample of respondents creates a demographic profile that mirrors the actual population. For example, about 12 percent of all U.S. residents are Black/African American. Therefore, if after your data set is cleaned and ready for analysis you find that only 6 percent of the respondents have identified as Black/African American, then you may want to count each of these records

IN A NUTSHELL

Because survey research is intended to generate estimates that pertain to an entire population, it is imperative that the sample of respondents creates a demographic profile that mirrors the actual population.

as "double," meaning that your weighted data now accurately reflect the true portion of Black/African Americans in the population. This is why most nationally representative surveys have data sets that contain some type of **weighting**. Weights are used to make adjustments to the data so that the data better represent the population from which the sample was drawn. Various types of weighting techniques (for example, sampling or probability weights, frequency weights, or analytic weights) can be implemented depending on the sample and situation; however, in survey research, most often post-stratification weights are used. By applying these weights, you may greatly multiply the number of people in your sample, but bear in mind that this yields an artificial inflation of your sample size (n) and that making interpretations in absolute numbers (rather than percentages) is fallacious. A detailed description of how to generate and apply weights and then analyze weighted data can be found in a textbook entitled *Applied Survey Research Analysis* (Heeringa, West, and Berglund, 2010).

weighting
technique of making artificial but systematic adjustments to the data

Summary

Survey research is unique and vital to public health. The basic function of this type of research is to provide population estimates that inform the allocation of health promotion efforts and guide policies relevant to prevention. The process of survey research does rely on some of the skills you have acquired (or will acquire) by reading this textbook; however, the skills you learned in this chapter are specific to conducting this "one variable" type of investigation. The key to achieving rigor in survey research is always to optimize the odds that your sample represents your population and to take great care in how you recruit respondents, measure behaviors or other health indicators, and interpret and represent the data.

KEY TERMS

Confidence interval	Random digit dialing
Coverage bias	Response rates
Imputation	Sampling frame
Interviewer bias	Standard error
List-assisted random digit dialing	Survey burden
Margin of error	Survey modalities
Pilot testing	Survey research
Point estimate	Venue-day-time (VDT) sampling
Probability sampling	Weighting

For Practice and Discussion

1. This chapter informed you that all survey research is based on probability sampling. Think about this statement and then describe (in one paragraph) why this is so. Some hints may be helpful: (a) think about the purpose of survey research as opposed to observational or experimental research, and (b) think about the one thing that you can do with probability sampling that is not possible with nonprobability sampling.

2. Locate and read a journal article that reports original findings from a study you would classify as behavioral survey research. Then answer the following four questions.

   a. Were the data weighted to account for differences between the sample and the population?

   b. Were point estimates and 95-percent CIs included? If so, were the CIs narrow enough to inspire your confidence in the estimates?

   c. What flaws (all studies have at least one) did you observe in the study methodology?

   d. How much overall confidence do you have that the primary estimates of behavior can be used to make judgments about the entire population? Elaborate on this answer.

3. Locate and read a journal article that reports the use of venue-day-time sampling applied to a survey research study. Find a colleague who is also learning research methods from this textbook. Pass along the article you found to that person. Make annotations on this article concerning what the researchers did and did not do correctly relative to this method. Then ask your selected colleague to do the same thing (without seeing your annotations beforehand). Finally, compare and contrast your annotations with those of your colleague and come to consensus to resolve differences in opinion.

4. Participation rates in the Behavioral Risk Factor Surveillance System (BRFSS), conducted by the Centers for Disease Control and Prevention (CDC), are notoriously low. This phone-based survey may not be the ideal method of capturing the health-protective behaviors of the people residing in the United States. Thoughtfully suggest an alternative to this phone-based methodology that CDC should consider for subsequent administration of the BRFSS. Compose a one-page defense of your answer.

References

Dillman, D. A. (1991). The design and administration of mail surveys. *Annual Review of Sociology, 17*, 229–245.

Doherty, I. A., Minnis, A., Auerswald, C. L., et al. (2007). Concurrent partnerships among adolescents in a Latino community: The Mission District of San Francisco, California. *Sexually Transmitted Diseases, 34*(7), 437–443. PMID:17195772.

Food and Agriculture Organization of the United Nations. (2013). The U.N. State of Food and Agriculture Report. Retrieved from http://www.scribd .com/doc/153178439/The-U-N-State-Of-Food-and-Agriculture-Report.

Heeringa, S. C., West, B. T., and Berglund, P. A. (2010). *Applied survey data analysis*. Boca Raton, FL: CRC Press.

MacKellar, D. A., Gallagher, K. M., Finlayson, T., Sanchez, T., Lansky, A., and Sullivan, P. S. (2007). Surveillance of HIV risk and prevention behaviors of men who have sex with men—a national application of venue-based, time-space sampling. *Public Health Report, 122*(Suppl 1), 39–47. PMID:17354526.

Muhib, F. B., Lin, L. S., Stueve, A., Miller, R. L., Ford, W. L., Johnson, W. D., . . . Community Intervention Trial for Youth Study Team. (2001). A venue-based method for sampling hard-to-reach populations. *Public Health Reports, 116* (Suppl 1), 216–222. PMID:11889287.

Remafedi, G., Jurek, A. M., and Oakes, J.M. (2008). Sexual identity and tobacco use in a venue-based sample of adolescents and young adults. *American Journal of Preventive Medicine, 35*(6 Suppl), S463–470. PMID:19012840.

Takahashi, L. M., Kim, A. J., Sablan-Santos, L., Quitugua, L. F., Lepule, J., Maguadog, T., . . . Young, L. (2011). HIV testing behaviour among Pacific Islanders in Southern California: Exploring the importance of race/ethnicity, knowledge, and domestic violence. *AIDS Education and Prevention, 23*(1), 54–64.

PART FOUR

DATA ANALYSIS

CHAPTER 14

STATISTICAL TECHNIQUES FOR ANALYZING OBSERVATIONAL RESEARCH IN HEALTH PROMOTION

Richard A. Crosby
Laura F. Salazar
Ralph J. DiClemente

Ultimately, all of the hard work and financial resources devoted to the research process are either justified or lost based on the quality of the data analyses. Decision making during the analytic phase is vital to the overall rigor of the study. Although at times there may be some discretion when choosing the type of statistical analysis to conduct, when answering certain research questions that involve specific types of data, the analysis is typically prescribed. This chapter is designed to help you make sound analytic decisions when you reach this all-important phase of your research study.

Students often experience a great deal of anxiety over the topic of data analysis. Although a modest level of anxiety may be helpful, this chapter is designed to alleviate the anxiety associated with statistics. Indeed, statistical methods applied to health promotion research do not need to be highly sophisticated (or complicated) to be effective. Although the research process is often labor-intensive and time consuming, data analysis can be a fairly short process that is straightforward by comparison. The caveat, however, is that the selection of analytic tools must be exact and the analyses must be precise. Without these two conditions—selection and precision—the entire research process is jeopardized.

LEARNING OBJECTIVES

Learning Objectives
- Understand how and when to use three basic bivariate tests.

- Understand how and when to use logistic regression versus linear regression.

- Explain the principles of the normal curve.

- Explain and calculate measures of dispersion.

- Explain and calculate effect size.

- Understand the determinants of statistical power and articulate the relationship between statistical power and effect size.

IN A NUTSHELL

Data that tell a story worth hearing need not be "tortured" to achieve a valuable analysis.

As noted in Chapter One, parsimony is a critical concern with respect to data analysis. Data that tell a story worth hearing need not be "tortured" to achieve a valuable analysis. On the contrary, data analyses require the application of three basic procedures. First, the data should be described. This initial procedure is nothing more than a representation of the data in the form of frequency counts and, if applicable, means with their standard deviations. Some research questions do not require data analysis beyond this point.

Second, bivariate associations between variables should be calculated and statistical significance determined. The term **bivariate** refers to a relationship between two variables. Typically, in health promotion research, the bivariate association would be between one Y variable (the outcome variable) and one X variable (the predictor variable); however, you may be interested in calculating bivariate associations between two predictor variables. When testing whether these bivariate associations are statistically significant, the **P-value** (the probability that a finding occurred by chance given the null hypothesis is true) must be calculated. Calculating P-values is a long-standing tradition in the behavioral and social sciences.

Again, some research questions do not require further analysis. The problem, though, is that bivariate relationships seldom capture the complexity of health behaviors. Most health behavior is rarely, if ever, predicted by only one predictor variable. In fact, health behaviors often have complex determinants that can only be understood when a large number of X variables are taken into consideration. Studies of behaviors such as overeating require multiple X variables. For example, a study of youth by Goossens and colleagues (2011) found that depression during early adolescence was significantly associated with continued overeating after being treated for weight problems. Four other X variables were simultaneously tested and found to be not significantly associated with overeating, namely a construct termed dietary restraint, and concerns about overeating, shape, and weight. In this case, because of the use of multiple X variables, it can truly be said that depression was independently associated with overeating after accounting for other predictors. This is an example of a multivariate analysis (referred to by some scholars as "multivariable"). Thus the third and final basic procedure is to conduct a multivariate analysis of the data. In this chapter, the term "multivariate" will be used to represent a statistical analysis involving multiple predictors or X variables and a single outcome or Y variable.

bivariate
refers to a relationship between only two variables

P-value
the probability that a finding occurred by chance given the null hypothesis is true

After presenting these basic procedures (description, bivariate analyses, and multivariate analyses), the chapter will also provide an overview of other related statistical issues such as power, sample size, and effect size, as these affect testing the research question. This presentation will be modest in scope. Readers who are interested in a more comprehensive treatment of these topics are encouraged to consult a text authored by Cohen (1988). The overall approach of this chapter is to provide a conceptual basis for applying analytic procedures that are commonly used in health promotion research. This chapter will serve as a springboard into statistics for observational research. Fortunately, a large number of very well-written statistics textbooks are readily available (for example, Pagano and Gauvreau, 2000; Siegel and Castellan, 1988; Tabachnick and Fidell, 1996).

Descriptive Analysis

Observational data analysis seeks to describe and explain characteristics of defined groups. Ideally, these are representative samples of priority populations (see step one in Chapter One). An initial goal of descriptive analysis is to characterize the group through the use of appropriate statistics. In this section, we will use an example of an observational study of adolescents residing in detention facilities, which was conducted by the editors of this textbook, to highlight the different descriptive statistics. In this particular example, one of the research questions involved assessing the prevalence of 34 different health risk behaviors. After collecting the data, we produced the graphic shown in Figure 14.1. The figure shows the distribution of scores and thus provides a useful overview of the data.

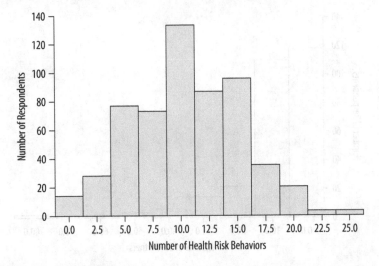

Figure 14.1 Distribution of Health Risk Behaviors for 569 Detained Adolescents

The Normal Curve

normal curve

when scores on a variable produce a symmetrical curve shaped like a bell

parametric tests

tests relying on data being represented by continuous distributions

nonparametric tests

tests relying on data being represented by categorical distributions

skewness

refers to the length of tails in a given distribution

kurtosis

refers to the shape of a distribution at the top

A **normal curve** represents scores that are distributed normally and produce a distribution that, when graphed, create a specific, symmetrical curve shaped like a bell that follows a particular mathematical function. Often the normal curve is referred to as a bell-shaped curve, although, strictly speaking, not all bell-shaped curves are normal. However, any distribution that is not symmetrical cannot be a normal curve. It is important to determine whether or not your data are approximately normally distributed, as this characteristic is an assumption that must be met for many statistical analyses to be performed correctly and accurately. Statistical analyses that require data to be normally distributed (for instance, linear regression) fall into the category of **parametric tests**. Other tests that do not require the data to be normally distributed (for example, a chi-square test) are deemed **nonparametric tests**.

A curve's deviation from normality can be judged based on two properties: **skewness** and **kurtosis**. Skewness is a measure of the lack of symmetry in the curve. Specifically, it assesses the degree to which scores in the distribution fall disproportionately on one side, creating a curve with a "long tail." Although by graphing and visually inspecting a distribution we have a gross indicator of a distribution's skewness, it should be evaluated statistically. Most statistical software programs will determine whether or not skewness exceeds that of a normal distribution. The distribution shown in Figure 14.2 illustrates a positively skewed distribution in that most of the scores fall to the left side (in other words, most of the study participants reported having sex with 10 or fewer partners), creating a long

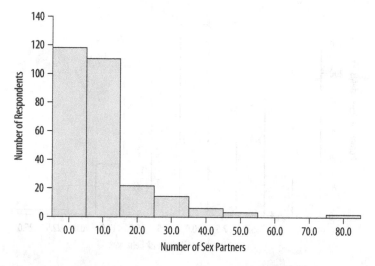

Figure 14.2   Number of Sex Partners (Lifetime) Reported by Detained Adolescents

tail extending to the right. Whether or not a distribution is positively or negatively skewed depends on the direction of this tail. Many variables assessed in health promotion research will have a positive skew. Some examples include number of pregnancies, number of times diagnosed with a sexually transmitted disease, use of illicit substances, and frequency of driving while intoxicated.

An example of a distribution that is negatively skewed is shown in Figure 14.3. As indicated, the majority of scores are clumped together on the far right, leaving a long tail that extends to the left (the negative direction of the number line). The graph shows that most women in the sample reported having approximately 12 or more Pap tests in their lifetime.

Kurtosis measures whether the data are peaked or flat relative to a normal distribution. In other words, it refers to the shape of the distribution from top to bottom rather than side-to-side. A distribution with a preponderance of cases clustered in the middle—making a very tall peaked shape—is called **leptokurtic**. Conversely, a distribution with a relatively flat shape (an absence of scores grouped around the mean) is called **platykurtic**. Again, by graphing and visually inspecting a distribution we can have a gross indicator of a distribution's kurtosis; however, it should be evaluated statistically. Most statistical software programs will also determine whether or not kurtosis exceeds that of a normal distribution.

leptokurtic
term for a tall spike in the middle of a distribution

platykurtic
term for a flat top of a distribution

The Mean

A mean can be calculated for any distribution assessed using **ratio-level** or **interval-level** data. *Ratio-level* data are assessed such that the distance

ratio-level
describes data that are one step better than interval-level data because they also have a true zero point, a feature not described by interval data

interval-level
describes data that are continuous; they are not based on categories, and the separation between points on the continuum is always equal

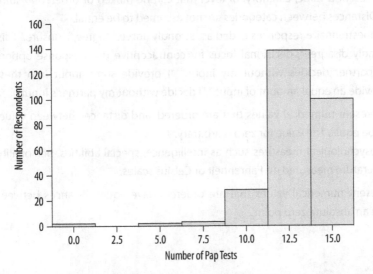

Figure 14.3   Number of Pap Tests (Lifetime) Reported by 273 Women

between possible values is always equal and an absolute (rather than arbitrary) zero point exists. Age is a good example of a ratio-level measure. *Interval-level data* assume an equal distance between values, but an absolute zero point is not present (see Box 14.1 for more information about levels of measurement). The obtained distribution portrays the health risk behavior profile of the entire sample of 569 adolescents (Figure 14.2). Of 34 possible risk behaviors, some adolescents engaged in no risk behavior, whereas others engaged in as many as 25. The arithmetic average, or the *mean*, was 10.6. It is important to note that the mean does not pertain to any one person; instead, it represents the average score of the group. Because it is an average score of the group, the mean is vulnerable to any extreme scores or outliers. For example, in a study of 141 high-risk men, frequency of crack cocaine use was assessed for the past 6 months. The mean number of uses was 29.1. Of interest though, one man indicated using crack 1,000 times. Upon converting this score to "system missing" (as it is quite difficult to place full confidence in this extremely high value) the mean was reduced to 22.1 (a much truer representation of the group).

BOX 14.1. FOUR LEVELS OF DATA

1. *Nominal data* represent discrete categories that are not ordered in any particular way.

    Examples: sex, religion, reasons for not having a mammogram, types of illicit substances used in the past 30 days, and outcome of health promotion program (for example, improved or did not improve).

2. *Ordinal data* represent a value, category, or level that can be ranked or ordered in some particular way. Distances between categories are not assumed to be equal.

    Examples: questionnaire responses coded as "strongly agree," "agree," "unsure," "disagree," or "strongly disagree"; decisional focus for contraceptive use (response options might be "my partner decides without my input," "I provide some input into these decisions," "I provide an equal amount of input," "I decide without my partner's input").

3. *Interval data* represent numerical values that are ordered, and distances between values are assumed to be equal. The value for zero is arbitrary.

    Examples: psychological measures such as intelligence, special abilities, personality, and so on; temperature measured on Fahrenheit or Celsius scales.

4. *Ratio data* represent numerical values that are ordered, have equal distances between values, and have an absolute zero point.

Examples: age, inches, weight, dollars, number of times a person used alcohol in the past month, number of times a person has had their blood serum cholesterol checked, number of vaccinations given by voluntary health organizations, percentage of body fat.

Note: Sometimes data can be converted from one type to another. For example, age (a ratio measure) can be converted to an ordinal measure by assigning scores that fall below 45 to a category named "young" and scores that equal or fall above 45 to a category named "old."

Spread

One important aspect of the group scores is characterized by their distribution or spread. It is important to understand two elemental indicators of spread: the **range** of the scores (in other words, the lowest score subtracted from the highest score) and the **dispersion** (that is, how much each score differs from the mean). Both the range and the dispersion are sensitive to extreme scores. For example, the initial range in the study of men who use crack was 1,000 (1,000−0). After excluding the extreme score of 1,000, the range decreased to 250 (250−0), indicating a much narrower degree of spread.

range
the distance between the lowest and highest scores in a given distribution

dispersion
the difference between scores and the mean of a distribution

The Standard Deviation

Because the goal is to characterize the group, it is useful to calculate an average measure of dispersion. This is called the **standard deviation**; it indicates how much, on average, the scores in this sample deviate from the mean. The standard deviation can be derived by first subtracting each score (all 569) from the mean, squaring them, and then summing each of the squared deviations from the mean. Because a negative deviation score will cancel out positive deviation scores, the sum of all these deviations would produce a value of zero, so the deviations are squared. Then, to obtain an average of the deviations, the sum of the squared deviations is divided by the total number of study participants minus 1 (569 − 1 = 568). To return to the original metric, the square root is then calculated. The obtained value is known as the standard deviation and is always a positive value.

standard deviation
the average dispersion from the mean

Like the mean, the standard deviation provides a great deal of clarity to the description of a group. It too is sensitive to the influence of extreme scores. In the example of men who use crack, before excluding the score of 1,000, the standard deviation was 88.4 (this is a very large standard

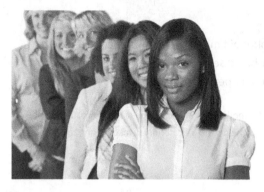 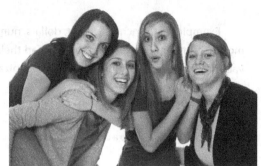

Figure 14.4   Demographic Heterogeneity or Homogeneity

deviation). After excluding the extreme score, the standard deviation becomes much more reasonable (32.2). It is important to note that size does matter. When the standard deviation is small, this statistic indicates that the group is very similar relative to the variable being studied. For example, a group of young women of the same race or ethnicity and same age, and perhaps similar in socioeconomic status, as pictured in Figure 14.4 on the right, would most likely have very similar political attitudes, that, if measured, would result in a small standard deviation. A degree of similarity in characteristics for a sample is called **homogeneity**. Conversely, when the standard deviation is large, this statistic indicates that the group is very diverse relative to the variable being studied. We can refer to this level of diversity as **heterogeneity**; the women pictured on the left would be more heterogeneous compared to the women on the right, due to their differences in race/ethnicity.

homogeneity
classifies a sample of people who share a great deal of similarity for a specified variable

heterogeneity
classifies a sample of people who are quite diverse in terms of a specified variable

The standard deviation can be used as a tool to characterize distributions that are relatively symmetrical. Returning to the previous example, recall that the mean is 10.6 and the standard deviation is 4.8. Moving in both positive and negative directions from the mean by one standard deviation (plus or minus 1 SD) will account for approximately two-thirds of the scores (about 68 percent). Stated differently, slightly more than two-thirds of the sample will have scores between a low value of 5.8 (10.6 minus 4.8) and a high value of 15.4 (10.6 plus 4.8). Furthermore, moving in both directions from the mean by two standard deviations accounts for 95 percent of scores. Therefore 95 percent of the scores would fall between scores of 1.0 (10.6 minus [4.8 times 2]) and 20.2 (10.6 plus [4.8 times 2]).

median
the score occurring at the midpoint of a ranked distribution of scores

The Median

The **median** is the score occurring at the midpoint of a ranked distribution of scores; it should be used when data are skewed or when the data are measured using an *ordinal scale* (again, ordinal measurement means that the scores can be ranked from low to high, but the distance between scores is not known to be equal; see Box 14.1 for more information about levels of measurement). For example, in the United States a distribution of income would have a strong positive skew, meaning that most people have low income levels whereas a small minority has extremely high income levels. Thus the mean is not an accurate indicator of the "middle" income level for all people residing in the United States. In this instance, the median would be a better statistic to use to describe income distribution levels, as it separates the ranked order distribution at the middle. In health promotion research, many health-related variables are not always amenable to interval- or ratio-level measurement. Instead, ordinal-level measures are quite common. For example, to characterize a group with regard to satisfaction levels of physician-patient relationships when the difference between satisfaction levels are unknown and should not be assumed to be equal is conducive to the use of the median to describe the distribution of scores.

Frequency Distributions

When nominal-level data are collected, statistics are not available to characterize a distribution. Nominal-level measurement means that discrete categories are being assessed (such as male and female; Black and White; former smoker, current smoker, and never smoked); therefore ranking from low to high or ordering in a particular way is not possible nor is it logical (again, see Box 14.1 for more information about levels of measurement). Because nominal data are not ranked, a median would be an inappropriate statistic for describing these distributions (a mean, standard deviation, or other statistic is also not applicable). Instead, simply enumerating the number of occurrences for each attribute of the nominal measure is appropriate; this is called a "**frequency distribution**." An example of a computer-generated frequency distribution is shown in Table 14.1. Notice that four columns appear in this table. The first provides the actual number of study participants categorized into each of the listed attributes. For example, 219 adolescents self-identified as Black and non-Hispanic. Notice in this column that data are missing for 13 adolescents. This observation is important because it suggests that converting the frequency counts into percentages could be achieved by using one of two possible denominators. The second column shows percentages based on the entire sample as the denominator (in this case 569). The third column also shows the percentages, but these are based only on the number of valid cases (meaning that the thirteen missing cases are not included in the denominator). Thus when data are missing (which is generally unavoidable) the values in the third column will always be greater than the values in the second column. The

frequency distribution
an ordered list of scores for one variable

Table 14.1   Frequency Distribution of Race or Ethnicity for a Sample of 569 Detained Adolescents

Valid			Cumulative	
Race or Ethnicity	Frequency	Percentage	Percentage	Percentage
White-not Hispanic	223	39.2	40.1	40.1
Black-not Hispanic	219	38.5	39.4	79.5
White-Hispanic	32	5.6	5.8	85.3
Black-Hispanic	42	7.4	7.6	92.8
Asian American	4	.7	.7	93.5
Native American	6	1.1	1.1	94.6
Other	30	5.3	5.4	100.0
Total	556	97.7	100.0	
Missing	13	2.3		
Total	569	100.0		

fourth column is merely a running subtotal of the third column. This can be useful for descriptive purposes. For example, inspection of this column reveals that 92.8 percent of the sample self-identified as either White or Black.

Bivariate Analysis

Before we describe a few selected types of bivariate analyses, it is important to clarify in general why statistical tests are performed. The tests yield two critical pieces of information that must be considered to answer the research question. First, the test informs us if a finding may have occurred by chance. In this context, chance is determined by a probability value that when conducting statistical tests is judged against the **alpha level**. The alpha level can be conceptualized as a cut-off point to determine the statistical significance of a test; by convention it is set at .05 or less. Depending on any given journal's adopted convention, uppercase P and lowercase p may be used to denote the probability level associated with a particular statistical test. The second piece of critical information that statistical tests provide is a quantitative indicator of strength in relationships. The exact value of P is generated by statistical software programs used often in health promotion, such as SAS, SPSS, and STATA.

When embarking on a bivariate analysis, a key step is to select an appropriate statistical test. Three of the most basic options in health promotion research are (1) an independent groups t-test, (2) a Pearson's chi-squared test, and (3) the Pearson Product Moment Correlation Coefficient. The t-test is a statistical test that determines the differences between two means in relation to the variation in the data and then the likelihood

alpha level
the probability that, given that the null hypothesis is true, the results observed occurred by chance

of the differences occurring due to chance. The *t*-test is used when the research question has a grouping variable that identifies only two groups (for example, male/female, treatment/control group) and an outcome variable measured at an interval- or ratio-level. Pearson's chi-square test assesses the likelihood of any observed differences being due to chance. A chi-square test also can be used with a grouping variable, but the variable can have two or more levels (for example, White/Black/Asian, single/married/divorced), but is appropriate for when the outcome variable is nominal (such as HIV+/HIV−). Finally, the Pearson Product Moment Correlation coefficient is a measure of the degree to which two variables are related—that is, how much the scores for one variable covary with the other variable. The Pearson Product Moment Correlation is used when both variables are represented with interval- or ratio-level measures.

T-Test Example

A common goal of observational research in health promotion is to compare subgroups of a sample (defined by a "grouping" variable) with respect to a second variable. Imagine, for example, that your research question involves comparing males and females on an index of health risk behavior. The grouping variable would be sex, and the second variable would be the score on an index. Consider the distribution shown in Figure 14.2. Because this was assessed with a ratio-level measure, a *t*-test would be an appropriate method of addressing a research question involving sex differences. The test answers a basic question that is essential to all statistical tests: Are observed differences between the two groups "real" or due to chance? By convention, real differences can be attributable to chance no more than 5 times out of 100 tests. This corresponds to an alpha of .05. In some research studies, a more restrictive *P*-value may be used, such as .01 (real differences can be attributable to chance no more than once out of 100 tests). Of interest, the *P*-value of .05 corresponds to values of the test statistic that are greater than two standard deviations above or less than two standard deviations below the mean. This relationship is explained in Box 14.2.

BOX 14.2. CONFIDENCE INTERVALS

Intervals—defined by lower and upper boundaries—can be used to define a given level of confidence that a mean (or a similar estimate) is accurate. For example, a statement might read, "The mean was 19.2 (95 percent CI = 9.2–29.2)." The statement provides a range of confidence for the mean—implying 95-percent confidence that it is, in reality, a value that falls between 9.2

and 29.2. Values beyond this range (in either direction) would be attributable to chance—note, then, that chance is set at 5 percent (corresponding to a P-value of .05). If a 99-percent confidence had been reported, then chance would be set at 1 percent (corresponding to a P-value of .01).

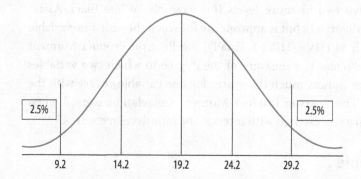

The confidence interval (CI) is defined by standard deviations. Adding and subtracting two standard deviations from the mean defines the 95-percent confidence interval (three standard deviations defines the 99-percent CI). Given a standard deviation of 5.0, the 95-percent CI would be defined according to the picture shown here. The 2.5 percent of the cases that fall at either extreme would be "outside" of the defined interval. Wide intervals imply less precision (or confidence) in the estimate, so a narrow CI is a desirable standard. For example, what if the standard deviation had been 2.0 percent rather than 5.0 percent?

Confidence intervals can also be applied to test statistics. An odds ratio, for example, is always shown with a corresponding 95-percent CI. Again, narrow intervals are desirable. The interval can be used to compare the relative strength of two odds ratios. If the lower limit of the interval with the higher odds ratio overlaps the higher limit of the lower odds ratio, then the two odds ratios are not significantly different from each other. However, if they do not have overlapping values between their CIs, they are indeed different, and the value of the larger odds ratio is significantly greater than that of the lower odds ratio.

The t-test will compare a mean risk score for females to the mean risk score for males. Dispersion of each distribution (one pertaining to females, the other to males) plays an important role in the calculation of the t-statistic; small standard deviations will produce a larger t-value. The number of study participants in each group also plays an important role in the calculation of the t-test; larger numbers of participants will produce a larger t value because sample size is used to calculate the standard deviation, and a larger "N" would equate with a smaller denominator and hence a larger t-value. The formula for the t-test follows; it represents the difference between the two means in the numerator, divided by the square root of the sum of each sample's standard deviation squared (S^2), which is also the variance, divided by each sample size.

$$t = \frac{\overline{X}_1 - \overline{X}_2}{\sqrt{\frac{S_1^2}{n_1} + \frac{S_2^2}{n_2}}}$$

$\overline{X}_1$ = Mean of first set of values

$\overline{X}_2$ = Mean of second set of values

S_1 = Standard deviation of first set of values

S_2 = Standard deviation of second set of values

n_1 = Total number of values in first set

n_2 = Total number of values in second set

In this example, 276 males had a mean of 11.3 (SD = 4.5) and 283 females had a mean risk score of 9.9 (SD = 5.0). Therefore the t-test = (11.3 – 9.9)/ SQ RT of (5^2/283) + (4.5^2/276) and equals 3.48. Output from a statistical program will generate a P-value for this t-value. In fact, in this case the output indicated a P-value of .001, suggesting that, given no sex differences, the findings would be attributable to chance only 1 out of 1,000 times! So what can be concluded from this bivariate analysis? Given that the test was significant, it can be said that the mean for males is significantly greater than the mean for females (in other words, the observed difference between 11.3 and 9.9 has a low probability of being a chance occurrence). The conclusion might read, "The average level of risk was significantly greater for males as compared to females."

Chi-Square Example

Suppose that a research study is examining whether family history of breast cancer (that is, the predictor) is related to practicing breast self-exams on a regular basis. The nature of the research question demands that women with a history be contrasted to all other women (these are two discrete categories). Those women practicing breast self-exam on a regular basis—perhaps defined as once a month—would then be compared to those engaging in the practice less frequently (again, these are two discrete categories). The public health outcome of interest here is clearly breast self-exam; thus the predictor variable is family history of breast cancer (none versus history). Table 14.2 is a contingency table presenting data that address this research question.

Table 14.2   Contingency Table of Data Pertaining to a Study of Breast Self-Examination Practices

	Monthly	Less Than Monthly	Total
Family history of breast cancer	79	14	93
No family history of breast cancer	66	19	85
Total	145	33	178

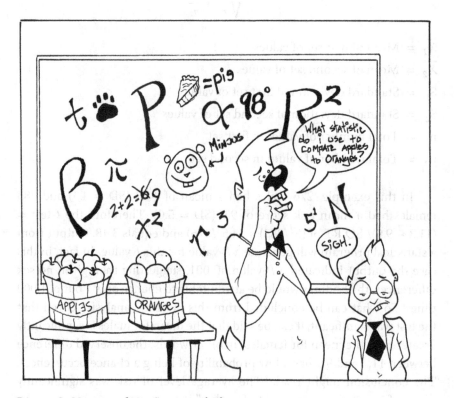

Dincus Is Unsure of His Statistical Plan

Copyright 2005 by Justin Wagner; reprinted with permission.

As shown, the contingency table has four cells. These tables have an endless array of uses in health promotion research and therefore deserve extensive study by the new investigator. The outcome is shown in columns and the predictor is shown in rows. Each column and row has a total. The row totals and the column totals must, by definition, sum to the same value (in this case the value is 178; this is a "grand total"). The most basic function of the table is purely descriptive. Notice, for example, that among the 93 women with a family history of breast cancer, 14 (15.1 percent) did not practice breast self-exam on a monthly basis. Among the 85 women without a family history of breast cancer, 19 (22.9 percent) did not practice breast self-exam on a regular basis.

Although the descriptive value of a contingency table is important, the question that arises is identical to that posed earlier in the t-test example: How likely is it that the difference between 15.1 percent and 22.9 percent is due to chance alone? This question can be addressed by the chi-square statistic (shown as χ^2). The formula for the chi-square statistic is as follows:

$$\chi^2 = \sum \frac{(O - E)^2}{E}$$

O = Observed value

E = Expected value

Using the row and column totals, a value expected by chance (the expected value) can be calculated for each of the four cells. For example, the upper left cell has a corresponding row total of 93 and a corresponding column total of 145. To obtain the value expected by chance for this cell, this formula is used: (row total × column total)/Grand Total. In this example, we multiply 93 by 145 and divide the product by the grand total of 178. The expected value for the upper left cell is 75.75, whereas the observed value is 79. Herein lies the key to the chi-square test: the difference between the obtained value of 79 and the value expected by chance is 3.25. Across the four cells in Table 14.3, we have computed the expected values; these differences (observed-expected) would then form the *conceptual* basis for the calculations needed to arrive at the χ^2 value.

If you do the math, then in this example the chi-square = 1.57. After obtaining the χ^2 value, the final step is to evaluate it for statistical significance. Again, a corresponding P-value of .05 or less would typically be counted as evidence that the difference between 15.1 percent and 22.9 percent is not readily attributable to chance. A χ^2 value of 1.57 and with 1 degree of freedom (df) has a corresponding P-value of .21. (Note: the chi-square distribution table will provide an estimate of P that corresponds to ranges of chi-square values, or you can use an online calculator for an exact value.) Thus 15.1 percent and 22.9 percent are not significantly different values. The conclusion for this study might then read: "The chi-square test

Table 14.3   Frequency of Breast Self-Examination with (Expected Values)

	Monthly	Less Than Monthly	Total
Family history of breast cancer	79 (75.75)	14 (17.25)	93
No family history of breast cancer	66 (69.24)	19 (15.76)	85
Total	145	33	178

revealed that the percentage of women who practiced breast self-exam and who had a family history of breast cancer was not significantly different from the percentage of women who do not have a family history of breast cancer."

Before leaving this discussion of the chi-square test, it is useful to discuss the concept of a **median split.** A median split is literally "splitting" a distribution at its median point into two groups and can be a useful procedure that results in the ability to apply a chi-square test. The median can be used to split a nonnormal distribution of interval- or ratio-level data into two distinct parts (for example, high versus low, healthy versus unhealthy, more frequent versus less frequent). This median split is a very useful tool for describing a group in relationship to a second variable. Consider the following research questions:

median split

when a continuous distribution is divided in half, using the median as the "breaking point"

- Does a measure of attitude toward preventive practices predict the intention to get a colonoscopy?

- Does a measure of attitude toward preventive practices predict the intention to be tested for HIV?

- How do people diagnosed with depression differ from those not having this diagnosis with respect to whether they use tobacco?

In each question, the predictor variable (that is, attitude toward prevention or, in the latter question, depression level) necessitates the use of a scale measure (see Chapter Seven). However, as noted previously in this chapter, the obtained distribution for such measures may be markedly skewed (as shown in the examples displayed in Figures 14.2 and 14.3). In such cases, the lack of a normal (or nearly normal) distribution violates typical assumptions of statistical tests that might be used for these ratio-level measures. Moreover, the people represented by the skew (the long tail) are a potentially important focal point. If a median split was performed on each of these predictor variables, then the analyses could all be addressed by chi-square tests. (Note: in each test a contingency table with four cells—like that displayed in Table 14.2—could be created.)

Correlation Examples

When interval- or ratio-level data are available, the Pearson Product Moment Correlation is an efficient method of representing the strength of a linear relationship (correlation) between variables. The correlation coefficient is represented by a lower case r. The values of r range from negative 1.0 to positive 1.0, with a perfect correlation being found at either extreme (in other words, both negative 1.0 and positive 1.0 are perfect correlations). A positive and significant value of r means that the two variables being compared each increase together; this is known as a **direct relationship**. Consider, for example, self-efficacy for engaging in aerobic exercise (X) and the average number of aerobic workouts per week (Y). As scores on the measure of X (presumably a paper-and-pencil assessment) increase, an increase (to some corresponding degree) in Y would be expected. Because the value of r provides an indicator of how strong the correspondence is between X and Y, an r of positive 1.0 would mean they rise in perfect synchrony. However, this is only a theoretical possibility; in reality the two variables may rise together at a level of .20 or .30 or higher. Note also that r does *not* address causality; that is, X may be influencing the corresponding rise in Y, or Y may be influencing the corresponding rise in X. Sometimes a researcher can rule out the possibility that Y could be "causing" X by knowing that X cannot be changed (age, gender, and race are good examples). However, if X and Y are related, this still does not establish that X must cause Y (as there could be unknown variables that actually cause Y).

A negative and significant value of r means that an increase in one variable corresponds to a decrease in the other variable; this is known as an **inverse relationship**. Consider, for example, a relationship between age (X), ranging from 14 to 45, and the average number of health risk behaviors (Y) assessed by an index. A study may have obtained an r-value of $-.35$ for this correlation. Given that this value was significant (it had an acceptably low probability of occurring by chance), the value provides an indicator of how strongly (strength) the two variables are connected inversely. The direction of this relationship (that is, negative or inverse) is not surprising, and the magnitude (that is, .35) is modest. This latter point regarding magnitude, however, warrants further consideration.

Figure 14.5 displays two scatterplots. A scatterplot is a collection of bivariate data points. A bivariate data point represents the intersection of locations on an X-axis (an abscissa) and a Y-axis (an ordinate). Through visual inspection of these data points, two observations can be made

IN A NUTSHELL

A positive and significant value of r means that the two variables being compared each increase together; this is known as a direct relationship.

direct relationship
occurs when one variable rises or falls in value in tandem with a second variable

IN A NUTSHELL

A negative and significant value of r means that an increase in one variable corresponds to a decrease in the other variable; this is known as an inverse relationship.

inverse relationship
occurs when the value of one variable increases while the value of the second variable declines

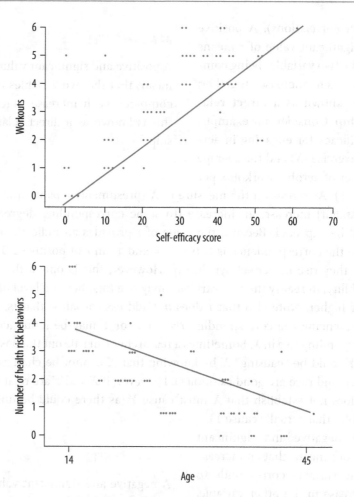

Figure 14.5 Scatterplots Illustrating Direct and Inverse Correlations

related to determining the magnitude of the linear relationship. First, a conceptual line should be "drawn" that indicates whether the two variables may be linearly related. Second, the conceptual line may be steep or flat, indicating a perfect linear relationship or no linear relationship, respectively.

In the first scatterplot displayed in Figure 14.5, it can be seen that a conceptual line superimposed on the data rises from left to right in a relatively steep slope. Because the purpose of the line is to depict a linear relationship and compare how close the corresponding data points are to the line, it appears that the correlation is quite high: the closer the data points are to the line, the greater the correlation, whereas data points that are quite distant from the conceptual line indicate a low correlation. In the second example in Figure 14.5, although the data points are close to the conceptual line, the line is not as steep as in the first example. Consequently, the correlation must be lower. Notice also that the line descends as it moves from left to right. This means that the correlation is inverse.

A caveat to each of the bivariate procedures must be disclosed. After the two variables have been identified, it is critically important to determine which one is the outcome measure and which one is the predictor variable. (Note: the term *"predictor variable"* technically only applies to prospective studies; in cross-sectional studies a preferred term is *"correlate."*) This determination is made based on the research question and the nature of the variables. In the preceding example, which compares males and females on an index of health risk behaviors, the determination is simplified because gender cannot possibly be a logical outcome variable (that is, we could not possibly expect scores on the health risk index to be a determinant of gender, but we could fairly expect that gender would be a determinant of health risk behavior). For that reason we urge that great caution and careful logic be applied when interpreting bivariate findings; causality is often elusive and difficult to determine!

A second caveat is in order. Imagine a graphic display of bivariate data points that takes the shape of an inverted "U." In this case, the correlation may be nonsignificant and very weak—approaching zero. This does not mean that X and Y are unrelated! This is true because not all relationships are linear. In this example, the relationship could be *quadratic*. A **quadratic relationship** between variables means that the two variables do not rise or decline in synchrony; rather, at some point along the X-axis the relationship changes. A classic example of a quadratic relationship is anxiety (X) and performance (Y): at low levels of X, performance is low; at medium levels of X, performance is high; at high levels of X, performance is low.

> **IN A NUTSHELL**
>
> After the two variables have been identified, it is critically important to determine which one is the outcome measure and which one is the predictor variable.

quadratic relationship occurs when two variables do not rise or decline in synchrony; rather, at some point along the X-axis the relationship changes

Multivariate Analysis

Although several forms of multivariate analyses are available, two of the most widely selected are linear and logistic regression. Linear regression (a parametric test) attempts to model the relationship between two variables by fitting a linear equation to observed data. Linear regression is appropriate for outcomes that are interval-level or ratio-level data. Similarly, logistic regression (a nonparametric test) attempts to predict the outcome of a dependent variable based on one or more predictor variables but is used when the outcome is a binary variable (that is, can take on one of two possible values).

Linear Regression

The Pearson Product Moment Correlation forms the basis for simple linear regression. In simple linear regression, you are calculating an equation that determines the Y-intercept and slope of the best-fitting line involving only one predictor. The best-fitting line refers to an actual line generated from the data that minimizes the distance from the data points to the line. The Y-intercept and slope are termed **parameter estimates** of this equation. In turn, multiple linear regression is an extension of this test; however, as opposed to only one predictor variable, multiple linear regression involves several predictors.

parameter estimates
numerical estimates of the characteristics of the population

Basically, regression serves several purposes: (1) test the nature of the linear relationship between X variable(s) and a given outcome Y, (2) test the strength of the relationship, and (3) formulate prediction equations based on sample data that can be applied to the population. All three purposes can be achieved by generating the equation for the regression line.

One key concept in regression is the parameter estimation of the slope that reveals what the association is between X variable(s) and Y. The **slope estimate**, which is referred to as b, gauges how much Y would increase given a one-unit increase in X. This involves a brief understanding of *rise-to-run*. The estimate for slope is an **unstandardized parameter estimate**, meaning that it is read in the original metric of the variable. Interpretation of slope estimates is as follows: "a one-unit change in X corresponds to a change in Y of b units." For example, a regression equation that was generated to examine the relationship between self-efficacy and number of days per week people exercise had a slope of 1.5. In practical terms, this means that for every 1 unit increase in self-efficacy (the X variable shown on the abscissa, the run), people exercised 1.5 more days (the rise). Alternatively, if the relationship is inverse, the question becomes, How much does Y *decrease* for a one-unit increase in X?

slope estimate
a measure of how much Y would increase given a one-unit increase in X

unstandardized parameter estimate
estimate expressed in the original metric of measurement

The concept of slope is actually one that you see everyday. When a contractor builds the roof on a home, the roof will have a slope. A common roof slope is known as a 5–12 pitch. This simply means that for every 12 inches that is measured from either end of the roof line the slope of the roof will rise by 5 inches. This is the identical concept (and mathematical values) as the self-efficacy and exercise example, described in the previous paragraph.

standardized regression coefficient or beta (β) weight
a measure of the strength of the association between X variable(s) and the outcome Y

Another function of regression is to provide standardized values of the slope estimate. Standardizing a variable places the measure on a common metric. The **standardized regression coefficient or beta (β) weight** is a measure of the strength of the association between X variable(s) and the outcome Y. Standardized regression coefficients are standardized so that their variance = 1. Imagine three X variables: self-efficacy, age, and depression. An important question might be which of these three variables has the strongest relationship with an outcome of "attitudes toward getting a colonoscopy." Imagine further that the obtained beta weights are .30, .21, and .15, respectively. Because they are standardized, these beta weights can be directly compared with each other. The strongest variable in this case would be self-efficacy, followed by age and then depression.

Another purpose of linear regression is to generate equations used for prediction. As mentioned earlier, multiple linear regression models will generate a value for a "constant" and the unstandardized parameter estimates (symbolized as *b*) that can be used to predict *Y*. The assumption here is that the sample data can be applied to make inferences about the population. The equation may look familiar: $Y = $ constant plus b_1 ($X1$) plus b_2 ($X2$) plus b_3 ($X3$), and so on. Using the constant and the unstandardized parameter estimates, the information from this model could then be applied to persons who were not included in the sample, in order to make predictions of *Y*.

Multiple linear regression is also used to determine how well a set of variables collectively is related to *Y*. Specifically, multiple linear regression can be used to judge the collective strength of the *X*-variables in explaining **variance** in *Y* relative to using the mean of *Y* scores. Variance is another measure of dispersion that is essentially the standard deviation squared. In multiple regression, the variance refers to the dispersion of data points around the horizontal line that represents the mean and also the dispersion of data points around the regression line. Accounting for variance is an important goal of multiple regression because it tells how well our *X* variables do in predicting scores in *Y* over and above how well the mean score does. The statistic used to represent this value is R^2.

R^2 ranges from 0 to 1.0. The value of R^2 typically does not exceed the sum of the r^2-values representing the bivariate relationships between the assessed *X*-variables and the given *Y*-variable, at least when the *X*-variables are **intercorrelated**. Intercorrelation means that significant values of *r* exist between

IN A NUTSHELL

Multiple linear regression can be used to judge the collective strength of the *X*-variables in explaining variance in *Y*.

variance
the squared standard deviation

IN A NUTSHELL

The value of R^2 typically does not exceed the sum of the r^2-values representing the bivariate relationships between the assessed *X*-variables and the given *Y*-variable, at least when the *X*-variables are intercorrelated.

intercorrelated
descriptor indicated by significant correlation between predictor variables

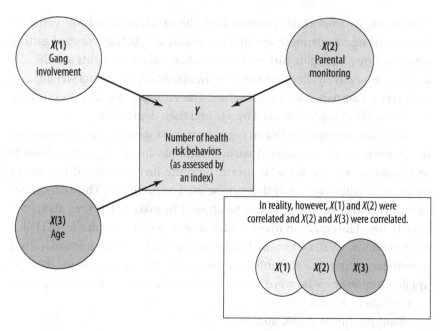

Figure 14.6 The Sum of Pearson r-Values Does Not Necessarily Equate with R^2

Note: Bivariate correlations: $X(1)r = .33, r^2 = .11; X(2)r = .30, r^2 = .09;$ and $X(3)r = .10, r^2 = .01$ (all are significant at $P < .05$).

two or more of the X variables. Figure 14.6 provides an illustration of this principle, using three X-variables: level of gang involvement, level of parental monitoring, and age (the outcome of interest [Y] is number of health risk behaviors). Although the Pearson correlations were all significant, two were modest in strength, while the magnitude of strength for age was very weak.

While a quick glance at the r-values might suggest that R^2 would be about .21, the box in the lower right-hand corner of Figure 14.6 shows the common, multivariate reality. In fact, the R^2 for this model was .09. The diminished value occurs because of intercorrelation among the X-variables. When the correlations among the X-variables are strong, this

multicollinearity
effect manifested when the correlations among the X-variables are strong

effect is referred to as **multicollinearity.** This effect can be undesirable because when there are strong correlations among the X-variables, then the standard error associated with each correlation coefficient becomes inflated, and what would have been a significant effect on Y becomes nonsignificant. As indicated in Figure 14.6, parental monitoring was significantly correlated (inverse) with the level of gang involvement. Parental monitoring was also significantly correlated with age (direct). Thus the three X-variables exert a collective effect on Y but overlap between variables represents a joint influence on Y. Of course, the overlap cannot be counted twice. Researchers must then determine which variable (X_1 versus X_2, for example) is "credited" for explaining variance in Y relative to the region of overlap. The answer is determined by the research team and takes the form of an analytic decision relative to the order of entering X variables into the regression model. Although entry methods are beyond the scope of this introductory chapter, the curious reader should consult an excellent textbook authored by Tabachnick and Fidell (1996).

Logistic Regression

In linear regression, the Y-variable must be an interval- or ratio-level measure. Analyses that rely on outcomes that are assessed with interval- or ratio-level measures are termed parametric. Conversely, nonparametric analyses use outcome measures that are assessed with a **categorical variable**. Categorical data have values that can be only one of a fixed number of nominal categories (for example, "White=1; Black=2; Native American=3; Asian=4") or the data have been converted into that form (such as a median split of a self-efficacy scale Low=1; High=2). A common form of nonparametric analysis in health promotion research is logistic regression, used when the outcome variable is **dichotomous** (meaning it has only two possible values, such as "yes or no" or "present or absent"). Of course, the number of research questions in health promotion that necessitate a dichotomous outcome measure is nearly infinite, so assessing the presence or absence of a disease, condition, or risk behavior is clearly part of a research question that lends itself to the use of logistic regression.

For the purposes of this introductory chapter, it can be said that the basic principles of multiple linear regression apply to multiple logistic regression. The principle behind the procedure is that an exponent (a constant value) is raised to a power of beta (β), yielding an adjusted odds ratio. The model will then classify a given percentage of the cases correctly, based on the collective X-variables that achieve multivariate significance. Keep in mind, however, that the odds of classifying the outcome correctly are 50 percent by chance alone. So, for example, classifying 60 percent of the cases correctly would result in classifying only 10 percent beyond that expected by chance alone.

Interpreting odds ratios is an important prerequisite to understanding research findings from logistic regression. An **odds ratio** (OR) is a measure of association between a measure of exposure (such as unprotected sex)

categorical variable
a variable that exists as a group or classification or a variable that represents ranked categories or classifications

dichotomous
having only two dimensions

IN A NUTSHELL

The principle behind multiple logistic regression is that an exponent (a constant value) is raised to a power of beta (β), yielding an adjusted odds ratio.

odds ratio
a measure of association between an exposure and an outcome

and an outcome (such as sexually transmitted disease). The OR represents the odds that an outcome will occur given a particular exposure, compared to the odds of the outcome occurring in the absence of that exposure. ORs are estimates of added risk for Y based on the knowledge of an X-variable. For example, text in a manuscript might read as follows: "Adolescents identifying as members of a minority group were more than three times as likely to test positive for a sexually transmitted disease (OR = 3.12; 95-percent CI = 1.31–7.43)." This OR can be judged for significance based on its 95-percent CI. Simply put, CIs that exclude the value of 1.0 are significant. An OR of 1 has to be nonsignificant because it means "one time as likely," which of course means the same as or equally likely (1 times anything is itself). Alternatively, the **relative risk ratio** is similar to the odds ratio but is defined as the ratio of the cumulative incidence rate among those exposed to the rate among those not exposed. Relative risk is appropriate for cohort or prospective studies in which incidence can be determined; then the relative risk ratio is equal to the OR. In either instance, a higher value represents a greater degree of risk for Y. An exception to this occurs when an X-variable is inversely associated with Y. Consider, for example, parental monitoring (from the previous example used in Figure 14.6). A high level of parental monitoring might be associated with a decreased risk of teen pregnancy. Therefore the obtained OR would be protective (meaning that high monitoring would equate with *lower* risk of a negative outcome). Protective ORs range from 0 to .99. A protective OR of .50, for example, would mean that teens with high monitoring were one-half as likely as those with low monitoring to become pregnant (if female) or cause a pregnancy (if male). As before, the significance of a protective OR is judged by whether its 95-percent confidence interval excludes 1.0.

relative risk ratio
the cumulative incidence rate among those exposed relative to the incidence rate among those not exposed

A Warning about *P*-Values

Even seasoned researchers sometimes become confused about the meaning of a significant *P*-value. Simply stated, a *P*-value less than the established alpha level means that the related finding is deemed statistically significant, indicating that the association had a low probability of occurring by chance alone, assuming that the null hypothesis is true (that is, there is no association). The *P*-value is *not* a measure of substantive effect (that is, the strength of association between X and Y); thus the *P*-value tells us nothing about whether the effect was large or trivial.

The confusion comes from a tendency to equate diminishing *P*-values (those such as .01, .001, and .0001) with progressively larger associations. This is not the case. Indeed, a large (and important) association may have a high probability of occurring by chance (yielding a nonsignificant *P*-value).

Conversely, a rather weak (and unimportant) association may have a very low probability of occurring by chance alone (thus the *P*-value would be significant). How is this possible? The difference is a function of sample size. The lesson here is quite simple: *P*-values speak only to the question of the probability or likelihood that an association can be attributed to chance alone. To understand this concept in greater detail, it is important to have a basic understanding of statistical power and effect size.

Statistical Power and Effect Size

When considering observational research, **power** is the ability of a statistical test to detect true associations (effects) between variables. Power is influenced by the following:

power
the ability of a statistical test to detect true associations between variables

- Sample size (this is a direct relationship)
- Effect size
- Dispersion or variance (this is an inverse relationship)
- The alpha level selected for the study (a lower, more stringent *P*-level gives less power)
- The use of a one-tailed rather than a two-tailed test of significance (more power with one tail)

Effect size can be conceptualized as the magnitude of association between two variables. For example, suppose that 22 percent of teens who reported low parental monitoring had ever been pregnant. In comparison, only 11 percent of those reporting high parental monitoring had ever been pregnant. Teens who had low parental monitoring were two times as likely to get pregnant than teens with high parental monitoring. The "two-times" is the OR and is a measure of effect size in this example.

effect size
the magnitude of association between two variables

As empirical values, effect sizes allow readers to judge whether statistically significant results are also meaningful at a practical level. Stated differently, effect size captures the true impact of an association, whereas significance testing merely provides a determination of whether or not the association is a chance occurrence. Unlike other determinants of power, effect size is not influenced by anything other than the observations that are collected from the

IN A NUTSHELL

Effect size captures the true impact of an association, whereas significance testing merely provides a determination of whether or not the association is a chance occurrence.

research participants. Power, on the other hand, can be affected by the researcher and can be increased (for example, by using a very large sample size or a high alpha level). By the same token, power may be low due to a small sample size.

Large effect sizes require less power than medium or small effect sizes. Conversely, small effects require a great deal of power to detect them. An important and perhaps never-ending question in health promotion research is, When are small effects that are deemed statistically significant, substantive? The flip side to this question is, When are large effects mistakenly declared nonsignificant due to low levels of power? These questions correspond to two classic forms of error in analysis. When an effect is deemed significant but is not real ("false positive"), the result is termed a *Type 1 error* and is in fact represented by alpha. Recall that alpha is the probability of results occurring by chance, given that there are no real effects. When large effects are mistakenly declared nonsignificant (based on problems with low power), the result is termed a *Type 2 error* ("false negative") and is represented by β. Power is equal to $1 - \beta$. Both types of error unfortunately are common. Studies with very large sample sizes (for example, more than 1,000 participants) may be prone to Type 1 errors and, of course, studies with very small sample sizes (for example, fewer than 200 participants) may be prone to Type 2 errors. These errors along with alpha and power are shown in Figure 14.7.

This somewhat abridged discussion of power and effect size is important for several reasons. First, a fair test of a research question implies that the power is not too high and not too low (by convention, 80-percent power is considered a "fair test" criterion). Of note, power can be adjusted before the study begins (by planning sample size) or after the study has

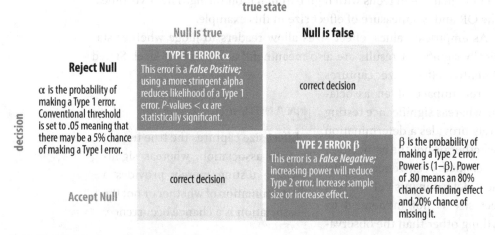

Figure 14.7 Hypothesis Testing and Associated Errors

concluded (by adjusting alpha upward). Second, power problems in small studies that have already been completed may not be resolved; thus effect size may be an especially important value to report. Third, as previously mentioned, in studies that have high power due to a large sample size, the effect size is an important indicator of whether the findings have substantive significance. Finally, studies should be planned to detect a reasonable effect size that is not unrealistically large but is substantive, and this planning should culminate in an empirical estimate of the sample size requirement. Several software packages are available for free on the Internet (for example, http://www.epibiostat.ucsf.edu/biostat/sampsize.html) that can calculate sample size requirements based on estimated effect sizes and the determinants of power shown in the previous bulleted list. Furthermore, after a study is done these programs can be used to calculate the available power (based on effect sizes obtained) and the determinants of power as previously described.

Applied Examples

To give you a bit of practice applying what you have learned so far in this chapter, two examples from published journal articles are provided. The first illustrates the use of linear regression; the second illustrates the use of logistic regression.

A study published in *Prevention Science* provides a good application of linear regression to observational research in health promotion. Cain and colleagues (2012) used linear regression to assess the effects of visiting an establishment that serves alcohol and using alcohol in predicting HIV risk behaviors in 1,473 people living in South Africa. The outcome variable was HIV risk behaviors; using anonymous community surveys to collect information regarding alcohol use and attendance of establishments serving alcohol, the researchers assessed the predictor variables. The researchers compared 1,210 participants who had patronized establishments serving alcohol in the past month with 263 participants who did not patronize establishments serving alcohol. Results demonstrated higher rates of the frequency of alcohol use, higher rates of the quantity of alcohol consumed, more sexual partners, and higher rates of vaginal intercourse without condoms for the participants who had patronized an establishment that served alcohol compared to those who did not. Multiple linear regression analysis found that attendance in an establishment that served alcohol in the preceding month predicted greater sexual risk for HIV regardless of demographic characteristics and alcohol use.

A study published in the *Journal of Acquired Immune Deficiency Syndromes* provides a good application of logistic regression to observational research in health promotion. Hua and colleagues (2013) selected a group of HIV-infected heroin users who were currently in drug rehabilitation treatment in Yunnan, China. The researchers investigated suicidality risk in 204 HIV-positive and 202 HIV-negative injection heroin users in treatment. Suicidality risk correlates were largely composed of scale measures (each assessed using interval- or ratio-level data). The outcome variable was the presence or absence of HIV. Multivariable logistic regressions examined predictors of suicidal ideation separately in HIV-positive and in HIV-negative treated heroin users. The critical alpha level was set at 0.05 for statistical significance, and all comparisons were two-tailed. Among the entire cohort (both HIV-positive and HIV-negative), factors significantly correlated with current suicidal thinking included being unmarried or unemployed and having a lifetime (past) history of major depression or a lifetime alcohol use disorder or heroin use disorder (all $P < 0.0001$). Among HIV-positive heroin users, experiencing HIV-relevant stress was significantly associated with current suicidality ($P = 0.0041$). The correlation between social support and HIV stress was small but significant ($P = 0.0009$). In the HIV-positive group, past major depression was associated with a six-fold increase in risk of current suicidal ideation [OR: 6.12; CI: 1.68–22.33]. In the HIV-negative group, both prior history of major depression ($P < 0.01$) and prior alcohol use disorder ($P < 0.001$) were uniquely significant.

Thoughtfully Writing about the Analytic Findings

Writing the research report ("the manuscript") is an obligation of conducting science. We provide detailed guidelines in Chapter Seventeen; for now, know that the manuscript is essentially a historic record of all that you did to collect the data and all that you did to analyze the data. When you write about the data analysis, it is important to show that you optimized "fairness" (meaning that falsification of the hypotheses was possible). Indeed, good research is brought to life by a fair analysis, including a sample size that offers adequate statistical power. A carefully crafted study is designed to identify effect sizes that can be detected without having to sample an unduly high number of participants. Certainly, assurances that Type 1 and Type 2 errors have been avoided are important when writing about your findings. It is important to note that many journal editors are now requiring authors to report associated effect sizes because, as we pointed out, P-values do not equate with effect size. You should also show that you used the correct tests and applied each in the prescribed manner. This is a type of analytic vigilance. Vigilance in analysis sometimes requires the assistance of qualified statisticians. The statistician may apply tests that you had not planned on using (or that you do not even know about). The use of unplanned tests in experimental research (see Chapter Fifteen) is generally discouraged. However, it should be noted that observational research is quite distinct from experimental research. In the latter, analyses are prescribed by the study design. In observational research, however, analyses can be conceived before and after the data have been collected. Furthermore, observational research can be used to answer two distinct varieties of research questions. First (and probably most common), the research can be designed to predict Y (meaning that correlates or predictors of one given outcome are identified). Most examples provided previously in this chapter have been patterned using this approach. Second, the research can begin with only a single X-variable and then determine the relationship of this variable to multiple outcomes that are pertinent to public health. Although less common, this approach can be an effective means of addressing a broad range of health promotion outcomes as opposed to a monolithic goal. As a maxim, it can be said that data derived from observational research should be used to its fullest potential. In fact, you should bear in mind that when study participants volunteered and provided consent, they were told that their assistance would "benefit science." Your task, then, is to ensure that this is indeed the case, and your manuscript—aided by appropriate analyses—is the method for keeping that promise.

Summary

Data analysis is a turning point in the research process. This chapter has presented a few of the most basic techniques that are applied to the descriptive, bivariate, and multivariate analyses of data collected in the field of health promotion. One key thread that deserves attention is that not all data are created equal. In fact, data typically follow a divide between parametric and nonparametric camps. The former involves interval- or ratio-level outcome measures and is generally based on means, standard deviations, and variance. A t-test is a common example of bivariate parametric analysis, and multiple linear regression is a common example of a multivariate parametric analysis. Alternatively, nonparametric analyses are used for data with nominal- or ordinal-level outcome measures. Frequency distributions and medians are quite useful for describing nominal and ordinal data, respectively. A common example of a bivariate nonparametric analysis is the chi-square test. Logistic regression is often used to handle nonparametric multivariate analyses pertaining to health promotion research. These tools should be used with great caution and with careful attention to precision and to issues relevant to power and effect size.

KEY TERMS

Alpha	Nonparametric
Beta (β) weights	Normal curve
Bivariate	Odds ratio
Categorical variable	P-value
Dichotomous	Parameter estimates
Direct relationship	Parametric tests
Dispersion	Platykurtic
Effect size	Power
Frequency distribution	Quadratic relationship
Heterogeneity	Range
Homogeneity	Ratio-level
Intercorrelated	Relative risk ratio
Interval-level	Skewness
Inverse relationship	Slope estimate
Kurtosis	Standard deviation
Leptokurtic	Standardized regression coefficient
Median	Unstandardized parameter
Median split	estimates
Multicollinearity	Variance

For Practice and Discussion

1. As a consequence of taking this course and reading this chapter you become known to others as somebody who can help with statistics. A person approaches you for help and asks what bivariate tests should be used in her study investigating the effects of aging and housing status (rent, own, or homeless) on a scale measure of life satisfaction. Remember, she is asking only for help identifying the appropriate bivariate tests. What would you recommend and (more important) why?

2. Locate and read a journal article that reports an original investigation of a health promotion topic using an observational research design. Be sure to find one that includes a bivariate and a multivariate analysis based on regression. Then respond to the following:

a. What was the outcome variable (or variables, if more than one was analyzed) and was the chosen bivariate test (or tests) appropriate to this measure?

b. List the correlates or predictors and identify the metric (nominal, ordinal, interval, or ratio) for each one.

c. Describe and critique all aspects of the regression model. What did this model do that you cannot yet understand after reading this chapter? Identify those issues that you were not able to understand and then reread the chapter to see if you can resolve these points.

3. Using the Internet, learn more about the pros and cons of using a median split in your data analysis plan. Make a list of each and then write a one-paragraph opinion that comes out either decidedly for or against this practice (be decisive).

4. Setting alpha at .05 is a long-standing tradition in the behavioral sciences as well as the medical sciences. Under what circumstance would you be compelled to make this *more* stringent, such as .01? Similarly, under what circumstance would you be compelled to make this *less* stringent, such as .10? In both cases, describe and justify your answer.

References

Cain, D., Pare, V., Kalichman, S., . . . Mwaba, K. (2012). HIV risks associated with patronizing alcohol serving establishments in South African townships, Cape Town. *Prevention Sciences, 13*(6), 627–634.

Cohen, J. (1988). *Statistical power analysis for the behavioral sciences* (2nd ed.). Hillsdale, NJ: Erlbaum.

Goossens, L., Braet, C., Verbeken, S., Decaluwe, V., and Bosman, G. (2011) Long-term outcome of pediatric eating pathology and predictors for the onset of loss of control over eating following weight loss treatment. *International Journal of Eating Disorders, 44*, 397–405.

Hua, J., Atkinson, J., Duarte, N., . . . Heaton, R. (2013). Risks and predictors of current suicidality in HIV-infected heroin users in treatment in Yunnan, China: A controlled study. *Journal of Acquired Immune Deficiency Syndromes, 62*(3), 311–316.

Pagano, M., and Gauvreau, K. (2000). *Principles of biostatistics* (2nd ed.). Pacific Grove, CA: Duxbury Thompson Learning.

Siegel, S., and Castellan, N. J. (1988). *Nonparametric statistics for the behavioral sciences* (2nd ed.). Boston: McGraw-Hill.

Tabachnick, B. G., and Fidell, L. S. (1996). *Using multivariate statistics* (3rd ed.). New York: HarperCollins.

CHAPTER 15

PRINCIPLES OF STATISTICAL ANALYSIS FOR RANDOMIZED CONTROLLED TRIALS IN HEALTH PROMOTION RESEARCH

Ralph J. DiClemente
Laura F. Salazar
Richard A. Crosby

Implementing a randomized controlled trial requires attention to detail and adherence to rigorous protocols to ensure integrity and internal validity. A critical part of the planning process before implementation of the randomized controlled trial is determining the data analytic plan. Without an appropriate sample size and strategy for analyzing the data, the results may not be valid or precise. The aim of this chapter is to provide an overview of the fundamental statistical principles and data analytic techniques useful in the analysis of randomized controlled trials in health promotion.

As mentioned previously in Chapters Five and Ten, a randomized controlled trial (RCT) is a specific type of scientific experiment, involving randomization and at least two groups, that is used to test the efficacy and/or effectiveness of various types of interventions. Often used in medicine to test the efficacy of new therapeutic agents as well as new medical devices, the RCT is equally appropriate as a research design to evaluate the effects of health promotion programs. RCTs are considered to be the gold standard of research designs. Results derived from an RCT are considered the most reliable form of scientific evidence in the hierarchy of evidence because RCTs reduce spurious causality and bias.

LEARNING OBJECTIVES

- Learn how to develop a data analytic plan for randomized controlled trials.

- Learn how to use appropriate statistical techniques for describing the data.

- Understand the importance of assessing comparability between groups and determining if randomization worked.

- Name and describe different statistical techniques used for dichotomous or categorical outcome variables.

- Name and describe the different statistical techniques used for continuous outcome variables.

- Understand the importance of limiting post-hoc subgroup analyses.

Even though RCTs are the most rigorous experimental designs, the results are meaningful only if the appropriate data analytic techniques are used. Think of your data analytic strategy as the last few pieces of a 5,000-piece jigsaw puzzle—without these, there will be a gap and the puzzle will be incomplete and of no value. Moreover, forcing a piece into a puzzle where it doesn't really fit may result in erroneous findings that detract from the quality of the research. It is critical to fit the analysis to the research question.

The old adage "An ounce of prevention is worth a pound of cure" is certainly applicable when discussing analysis of RCTs. Statistical analysis, although conducted after all data have been collected, should actually begin much earlier in the research enterprise. Indeed, it should be considered simultaneously with the research design. The data analysis is directly related to the design of the study and how well the study has been implemented.

IN A NUTSHELL

No matter how well designed, clever, or sophisticated a data analytic plan, it cannot compensate for a poorly implemented RCT.

No matter how well designed, clever, or sophisticated a data analytic plan, it cannot compensate for a poorly implemented RCT. Conversely, a poorly conceived data analytic plan may obscure detection of meaningful findings or obscure interpretation of the resultant findings, or both.

A data analytic plan entails (1) conducting a power analysis to determine the appropriate sample size needed to detect a prespecified statistical difference, (2) ensuring that measurements are administered in a timely and appropriate fashion, (3) specifying a procedure for handling participant attrition, and (4) selecting the statistical techniques most appropriate for the design and research question. Thus proper planning and execution of the study as well as the statistical analysis are critical to yielding reliable and valid results. Throughout this book, we have described various research designs, including the randomized controlled trial design (see Chapters Five and Ten); however, without appropriate attention to proper implementation on the front end of the RCT during planning and design, the data analysis on the back end can become overly complex or confusing, or defy interpretation. Forethought is forewarned—be careful that the data analysis is not planned ex post facto of the study implementation.

Although we covered RCT design and implementation in Chapter Ten, the primary purpose of this chapter is to help you put those last puzzle pieces into place. We describe the underlying statistical techniques used for RCTs, with an emphasis on selecting appropriate statistical techniques for enhancing understanding and interpretation of data derived from an RCT.

Specifically, we provide an overview of the data analytic process, which entails describing the data, assessing comparability between groups, and understanding different types of dependent variables.

Describing the Data

Once the data are obtained by following the data analytic plan, it is useful to examine the underlying characteristics of the scores for the variables collected before proceeding to more complex analyses. The first analytic activity is usually the generation of simple descriptive statistics (for example, mean, median, standard deviation, range, frequencies). These descriptive statistics are used to evaluate how scores on various variables are distributed. These variables include the dependent variables, the participants' sociodemographic characteristics, and other key predictors (in other words, theory-derived mediators of the dependent variables). A visual inspection of the data, especially histograms, may reveal underlying deviations from normality of which the investigator should be aware prior to progressing to the selection of statistical techniques for the data analysis. Generation of these statistics also serves as the last quality control and quality assurance activity in data management. A critical step for RCTs is to compute summary statistics for all measures separately for each arm of the trial.

Assessing the Comparability between the Study Groups. The major strengths of the RCT are randomization and having the pretest assessment, which permits comparison between groups before a treatment such as a health promotion program (HPP) is implemented. The concept of assessing comparability between the HPP group and the control group is sometimes difficult for novice investigators to understand. They often ask, Why assess comparability between groups that were created through randomization of participants in the first place? Doesn't the fact that participants were randomized, using appropriate allocation techniques, obviate the need to assess comparability? It is important to remember that randomization does not ensure that the study groups are equivalent; it only ensures that there is no systematic bias in the assignment of participants to the two study conditions. Indeed, for relatively small samples, it is likely that the groups may not be comparable

IN A NUTSHELL

Randomization does not ensure that the study groups are equivalent; it only ensures that there is no systematic bias in the assignment of participants to the two study conditions.

on all variables (dependent variables, sociodemographics, and mediators). Thus a critical step in the data analytic plan is to assess the comparability between the study groups with respect to sociodemographics, dependent variables, and other mediators of interest. An example from the authors' research may be illustrative.

We conducted an RCT to test the efficacy of a behavioral intervention to increase condom use among African-American female adolescents, 14 to 18 years of age. As participants completed their baseline assessment, they were randomized to one of two study conditions using a computer-generated randomization algorithm, complying with established conceal-ment of allocation techniques. Comparisons between the study conditions were made for variables, including sociodemographic characteristics, other potential predictors of sexual behavior, psychosocial mediators of sexual behavior, and sexual behaviors. We compared the conditions using *t*-tests for continuous dependent variables (such as age and scale scores) and chi-square tests for categorical variables (for instance, whether participants' families were recipients of public assistance). Results of these analyses are presented in Table 15.1.

Examination of Table 15.1 reveals that randomization was effective. The HPP condition and the general health education control condition were similar with respect to sociodemographic characteristics, psychosocial mediators that serve as secondary dependent variables, and sexual behaviors that serve as the primary dependent variable. In general, it is valuable to include a range of variables when assessing comparability between study conditions. If there are imbalances between the groups (for example, in this case, if there was a statistically significant mean difference for the variable "age" between conditions), then it is important to control for this age difference in the analysis. Differences between the study groups for other variables that may be potential confounders (that is, variables theoretically or empirically associated with the dependent variables) could also be controlled for in subsequent data analyses.

Understanding Different Types of Dependent Variables

In all studies there are different types of dependent variables. Two types often collected as part of an RCT are categorical and continuous variables.

categorical dependent variables

sometimes called nominal variables; there are two or more categories in no intrinsic order

Categorical Dependent Variables

Categorical dependent variables refer to the classification of participants into one of several categories according to some predefined evaluation criteria. In its most elemental form, categorical data can assume a binary format, meaning there are two independent categories. These categories might be labeled as "has a disease or is disease-free," "changed behavior

Table 15.1 Comparability of the HIV Risk-Reduction and General Health Promotion Conditions

Characteristic	HIV Prevention Condition			General Health Promotion Condition			P
	Mean (sd)	Percentage	(N)	Mean (sd)	Percentage	(N)	
Sociodemographics							
Age	15.99 (1.25)		(251)	15.97 (1.21)		(271)	.87
Education (did not complete tenth grade)		45.80%	(115)		48.70%	(132)	.51
Recipients of public assistance		17.90%	(45)		18.50%	(50)	.86
Living in single-family home		74.10%	(146)		72.30%	(162)	.68
Living with someone other than a parent		21.50%	(54)		17.30%	(47)	.23
Employed		16.10%	(40)		19.70%	(53)	.28
Psychosocial Mediators							
HIV knowledge	8.88 (3.25)		(248)	9.13 (3.03)		(267)	.38
Condom attitudes	36.02 (4.22)		(250)	35.62 (4.42)		(271)	.29
Condom barriers	42.23 (14.16)		(243)	43.13 (14.30)		(267)	.48
Communication frequency	8.61 (4.10)		(251)	8.37 (4.50)		(271)	.54
Condom use self-efficacy	30.74 (9.30)		(249)	30.52 (9.73)		(264)	.79
Condom use skills	2.91 (1.30)		(248)	3.03 (1.18)		(268)	.25
Put condom on partner	1.49 (1.01)		(232)	1.46 (0.98)		(246)	.77
Sexual Behaviors							
% Condom use, past 30 days	0.79 (0.38)		(232)	0.77 (0.38)		(246)	.68
% Condom use, past 6 months	0.72 (0.37)		(232)	0.70 (0.38)		(245)	.53
Unprotected vaginal sex, past 30 days	1.12 (2.84)		(226)	0.84 (2.01)		(241)	.22
Unprotected vaginal sex, past 6 months	4.81 (16.01)		(232)	4.23 (10.25)		(245)	.64
Consistent condom use, past 30 days		40.27%	(60)		43.35%	(75)	.58
Consistent condom use, past 6 months		43.53%	(101)		48.57%	(119)	.27
Condom use, last time had sex		31.90%	(74)		32.11%	(79)	.96

or did not change behavior," or "consistent or inconsistent condom use." They are based on participants' responses, test scores, and/or medical examinations. For example, in a study of vegetable consumption, a primary dependent variable could be the incidence of a heart attack over the follow-up period. The research question is whether or not more heart attacks were observed among participants in the control group relative to the HPP group. Thus for any participant in the study, the range of potential values for the dependent variable "heart attack" is 1 "Yes (experienced a heart attack over the course of the follow-up)" or 0 "No (did not experience a heart attack over the course of the follow-up)." In a study designed to test the effects of an HPP on reducing alcohol use among adolescent drivers and, as a consequence, reducing the risk of an automobile accident, we could have a categorical dependent variable of alcohol-related vehicular accidents. In this case, for any participant in the study, the range of potential values that could be obtained for the dependent variable "alcohol-related auto accident" is 1 "Yes (experienced an alcohol-related automobile accident over the course of the follow-up)" or 0 "No (did not experience an alcohol-related automobile accident over the course of the follow-up)."

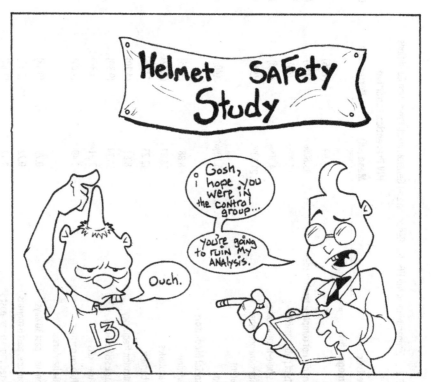

Mincus Uses "No Head Lump = 0" and "Head Lump = 1" for the Dependent Variable

There are circumstances when it may be desirable to have multiple levels of the categorical dependent variables. This is a logical extension of the **binary categorical dependent variable** described earlier. Dependent variables with more than two levels are deemed **polychotomous dependent variables**. For example, we could examine different sites within the body for buildup of extracoronary plaque and use this information to create a polychotomous outcome variable as a proxy for heart attack. This variable could have four levels (none, 0, 1, 2), with each value corresponding to the number of sites with the presence of plaque. Also, it is possible to have an **ordered categorical dependent variable**—usually called an "ordinal variable." This ordered categorical dependent variable would assume the form of a hierarchy or gradient. For example, in a study designed to test the effects of a stress-reduction class (the HPP) on reducing the severity of headaches among college students during final exams, we could have an ordinal dependent variable of "headache severity." In this case, for any participant in the study, the potential values for the dependent variable "headache severity" could be 1 "mild," 2 "moderate," and 3 "severe." Often we would be tempted to treat these data as continuous when in fact the data are ordinal and should be treated as such.

Continuous Dependent Variables

A second type of dependent variable is a **continuous dependent variable**. Continuous variables are distinct from categorical or ordinal variables in that the data represent a continuous scale of measurement assessed using interval or ratio scale metrics (such as temperature, height, blood pressure, weight). In health promotion research, our interest is often in enhancing mental health. Let's return to our study of how stress reduction may reduce the severity of headaches among college students during final exam week. RCTs, in general, have primary dependent variables, in this case, "severity of headaches." They may also have secondary dependent variables, which could include other variables that the HPP is hypothesized to affect. In this study, for example, we may hypothesize that participation in a stress-reduction class not only would reduce severity of headaches (the primary dependent variable) over the course of final exam week (the follow-up period) but also may have the collateral benefit of reducing depressive symptoms (a secondary dependent variable). In this example, we could collect participants' self-reports of depressive symptoms with a depression inventory at baseline, randomize them to the stress-reduction-class condition (the HPP) or no stress-reduction-class condition (control), then administer the same depression inventory at the scheduled follow-up assessment at the end of the final exam week. The depression inventory provides a continuous dependent variable, with the hypothesis that

binary categorical dependent variable
variable with only two levels

polychotomous dependent variables
variable with more than two levels

ordered categorical dependent variable
a categorical variable for which the possible values are ordered

continuous dependent variable
a variable that can assume any value between its minimum value and its maximum value

participants in the HPP will have fewer depressive symptoms during the final exam week than participants in the control condition.

IN A NUTSHELL

One reason for transforming a continuous dependent variable is that the underlying distribution of the continuous variable violates assumptions of normality necessary for performing parametric statistical analyses.

Continuous dependent variables can also be transformed into categorical variables. One reason for transforming a continuous dependent variable is that the underlying distribution of the continuous variable violates assumptions of normality necessary for performing parametric statistical analyses. For example, if we were also interested in hypothesizing that participation in a stress-reduction class (the HPP) would not only reduce the severity of headaches and depressive symptoms but also result in less weight gain over the course of final examinations week, we could measure a participant's weight at baseline and at follow-up and examine changes in his or her weight as a function of his or her group assignment. While we have a continuous dependent variable—weight in pounds—this variable can be transformed into a categorical dependent variable with the following categories: "gained weight," "lost weight," or "no change in weight." What was a continuous dependent variable is now a categorical dependent variable.

There are some issues to consider in categorizing a continuous dependent variable. In general, use of a categorical dependent variable derived from continuous data may entail some loss of detail in describing each participant when a range of scores is reduced to only two or three categories. The issue is potential loss of statistical power. A continuous variable implies certain statistical tests that rely on variability and normality within the data for performing those tests. When a continuous variable is transformed into a categorical dependent variable, the variability in the dependent variable is markedly reduced and it can no longer be normally distributed. Thus when a reliable continuous dependent variable exists and it meets statistical assumptions necessary for parametric statistical analyses, it is usually best not to transform the data.

Selection of Statistical Techniques

While there are numerous statistical techniques for testing whether an HPP is effective relative to a control group, we will focus on those that are most readily applicable in health promotion research. More complex research designs, by their very nature, require the use of more complex statistical techniques. We propose a decision strategy based on the type of dependent variable (categorical or continuous) as an overarching framework to facilitate understanding, identifying, and selecting the most appropriate statistical technique.

Data analysis is a process. At each juncture in the data analytic process, the investigator (that is, you) will be faced with making decisions regarding what statistical technique is most appropriate for analyzing the type of dependent variable collected. The decision-mapping approach is based on an understanding of the types of data to be analyzed and the qualities and characteristics of those data. The type of statistical approach used is directly dependent on the type of data represented by the dependent variable.

Analysis with Categorical Dependent Variables

Categorical dependent variables in RCTs can have multiple categories but are often dichotomous, meaning the data assume only two levels or categories. An example would be a long-term study (say, with a 10-year follow-up) of the health-promoting effects of stress-reduction classes for men, ages 50 to 59, at high risk for a heart attack because they have a low density lipoprotein (LDL) over 250, they are overweight by 20 pounds, and they report no regular physical exercise. The primary dependent variable for this study is a dichotomous variable representing "heart attack." Thus for any participant the range of potential values for the variable "heart attack" is 1 (experienced a heart attack over the course of the follow-up) or 0 (did not experience a heart attack over the course of the follow-up).

The hypothesis associated with the primary aim is that participation in the HPP would reduce the risk of heart attacks relative to the control group. The basic approach to testing this hypothesis is to compare the proportion of participants in each condition who experience a heart attack over the follow-up period. This can be done using a **nonparametric statistic** such as a simple chi-square test of proportions. Nonparametric statistics do not make distributional assumptions about the underlying normality of the distribution of dependent variables. If we compare the proportion of participants in each condition experiencing a heart attack and find statistically significant differences, with the HPP group having a lower proportion of participants experiencing a heart attack, we can conclude that the HPP was effective in reducing the risk of a heart attack (see Figure 15.1).

nonparametric statistic

a statistical test wherein the data are not required to fit a normal distribution

As Figure 15.1 indicates, 5 men in the HPP group reported having a heart attack compared with 20 men in the control group. This corresponds to 2.5 percent of the HPP participants compared with 10 percent of the control participants. The question is whether this proportional difference

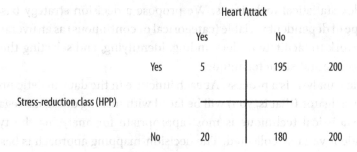

Figure 15.1 Number of Participants Experiencing a Heart Attack in a Stress-Reduction Program and a Control Condition

is statistically significant. In analyzing the study, the investigator is required to make a determination as to what statistical technique is most applicable to these data. To assist you, we have developed a simple decision map to guide the selection of a statistical test. This map is depicted in Figure 15.2.

Let's use our decision map as we would use a roadmap and see where it takes us. We have a categorical dependent variable (heart attack, "yes" or "no"), and there is no need for adjustment for other sociodemographic

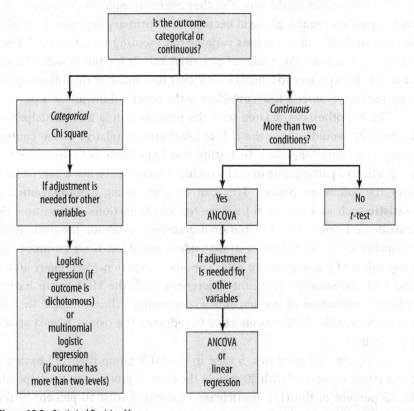

Figure 15.2 Statistical Decision Map

or predictor variables based on our examination of the baseline data (essentially, the groups are comparable). Following our guide, a simple chi-square test would be the test statistic. The chi-square can determine whether the difference observed in the proportion of participants having a heart attack between conditions is statistically significant (that is, there is a high probability that any difference observed cannot be attributed to chance alone). Statistical significance is expressed as a probability (P), relative to chance. The customary criterion for determining statistical significance is $P < .05$.

In our example, the results are statistically significant ($P < .05$). The findings support the hypothesis that stress-reduction classes can reduce the risk of a heart attack among high-risk men ages 50 to 59. Note the specificity of reporting the result. We may not be able to generalize the findings to populations with different sociodemographic characteristics, such as women, younger men, men of a particular ethnic or racial group, or men without risk indicators. **External validity** or **generalizability** refers to the capability to generalize the findings and is related to how we select our sample and the setting in which the RCT is conducted; it is not related to the type of test statistic used or the validity of the findings.

external validity
the extent to which the results of a study can be generalized to other situations and to other people

IN A NUTSHELL

External validity or **generalizability** refers to the ability to generalize the findings and is an issue related to how we select our sample and the setting in which the RCT is conducted; it is not related to the type of test statistic used or the validity of the findings.

While the P-value is useful, it does not provide a full assessment of the effects of the HPP. Indeed, it describes the findings relative to chance. However, our hypothesis is that the HPP will reduce risk of heart attack. To capture more fully the effect of the HPP on the risk of heart attack, it is useful to consider calculating a measure of **effect size** (ES). Effect size measures the strength of association between two variables or the magnitude of the difference in outcomes between two groups. In an RCT designed to test the efficacy of a heart attack HPP, the two groups are treatment (the HPP) and control, and the dependent variable is whether or not the participant had a heart attack. In this case there are two measures that could be calculated. One is the percentage (or the proportion) difference that results from subtracting the percentage of participants who had a heart attack in the HPP (2.5 percent) from the percentage who had a heart attack in the control condition (10 percent), resulting in a percentage difference of 7.5. A second measure of ES is called the **relative risk** (RR), defined as those

effect size
a quantitative measure of the magnitude or strength of an association

relative risk
the ratio of the probability of an event's occurring (for example, developing a disease) in an exposed group to the probability of the event occurring in a comparison, unexposed group

who experienced a heart attack in one group relative to the other group. In this example, RR = 4 and is calculated as (20/200 = .10) divided by (5/200 = .025), which indicates that participants in the control group had four times the risk of having a heart attack relative to the HPP. Alternatively, if we invert the groups in the calculation, the RR could be expressed as .25, which is (5/200) divided by (20/200), indicating that participants in the HPP condition had only one-quarter the risk of having a heart attack compared with participants in the control condition. Either calculation of RR is correct, depending on how you prefer to present your findings.

The RR as a measure of intervention (or treatment) effect has a number of advantages. First and foremost, it is readily interpretable. In public health and health promotion research we commonly refer to "risk" for a specified dependent variable. For example, dependent variables might include the risk of a heart attack, the risk of having an automobile accident while driving under the influence of alcohol, or the risk of developing ovarian cancer with estrogen use. Second, the RR is a "true" measure of the strength of the effect of the HPP, not a measure of chance. Third, the RR is invariant with respect to sample size. This latter advantage may require some further discussion. Simply put, if the sample size was increased in each group, but the same proportions of participants in each study condition were identified with a heart attack, the *P*-value would get smaller, attributable to the increased sample size, while the RR would be exactly the same! This latter advantage is important not only when considering whether an HPP is efficacious, but also in identifying the magnitude of efficacy.

confidence interval

a measure of the reliability of an estimate

In addition to measuring the magnitude of the HPP effect (using the RR), it is also recommended that the **confidence interval** (CI) around the RR be calculated. The confidence interval provides a measure of the precision of the effect. To illustrate what this means, let's suppose we did the exact same study one hundred times; the 95-percent CI (the customary statistic) would inform us that in 95 of those 100 times, the RR would be between the lower and upper confidence limits. When the confidence intervals are relatively narrow, we have more confidence that our RR calculation is precise. Conversely, relatively wide intervals detract from our confidence that our RR calculation is precise. For example, an RR of 2.1 with a confidence interval of (1.9, 2.3) suggests that the estimate is very close to its limits. An RR of 2.1 with a confidence interval of (1.2, 3.5) would not have the same degree of precision.

An example of a study that calculated an RR was conducted by Lee, Landry, Jones, Buhrmann, and Morley-Forster (2013) in a university hospital in Ontario, Canada. Lee and colleagues conducted an RCT in which the HPP was a smoking cessation intervention. The primary outcome of the smoking cessation intervention was to reduce smoking rates;

the secondary outcomes were in-surgery complications and immediate after-surgery complications. Patients were randomly assigned to either the control group (N=84) or the smoking cessation intervention group (N = 84) at least 3 weeks prior to a scheduled surgical operation. The control group received no information on smoking cessation. The intervention group received brief counseling by a nurse, brochures on smoking cessation, referral to a smoker's helpline, and a free six-week supply of a nicotine replacement drug. Results showed that smoking cessation occurred in 12 patients in the intervention group (12/84 = .142) compared to 3 patients in the control group (3/84 = .035). In this study, the authors also calculated an RR ratio: (.142/.035) = 4.0. Thus stated another way, patients participating in a smoking cessation program were four times as likely to quit smoking as patients not in a smoking cessation program.

In analyzing and interpreting data from an RCT to test the efficacy of an HPP, two statistical indicators should be calculated: (1) the intervention ES using the RR and (2) the precision of the effect using the confidence interval around the RR. In keeping with our advice, note in Table 15.2 that we have calculated the statistical indicators necessary to describe the HPP effects for an HIV risk-reduction program designed to enhance consistent condom use and reduce the number of sex partners. These statistical indicators may be presented when describing the results.

Interpreting the Results

Now that we have calculated the appropriate statistics to describe the effects of the HPP, the next step is to interpret them. As shown in Table 15.2, the findings would be interpreted as follows: relative to participants in the control condition, participants in the HIV risk-reduction intervention were 1.76 times (95-percent CI = 1.07–3.19, P = .04) more likely to report

Table 15.2 Effects of an HIV Risk-Reduction Intervention on Adolescents' Sexual Behaviors

	6-Month Follow-Up Assessment		
	RR	(95-percent CI)	P
Consistent condom use (past 30 days)	1.76	(1.07–3.19)	.04
Consistent condom use (past 6 months)	2.46	(1.44–4.21)	.001
Condom use, last time had sex	3.94	(2.06–6.42)	.0001
Sex with new partner (past 30 days)	0.30	(0.11–0.78)	.01

using condoms consistently in the 30 days prior to assessment, 2.46 times (95-percent CI = 1.44–4.21, P = .001) more likely to report using condoms in the prior 6 months, 3.94 times (95-percent CI = 2.06–6.42, P = .0001) more likely to report condom use at last sexual intercourse, and .70 times (95-percent CI = 0.11–0.78; P = 0.1) less likely to have a new sex partner in the prior 30 days. The use of these statistics provides a rich description of effects of the HIV intervention (the HPP), one that includes a measure of the strength of the HPP effect that is invariant with respect to sample size (the relative risk), one that provides a measure of precision of the ES (the confidence limits around the relative risk), and, of course, one that includes the traditional measure of statistical significance relative to chance, the P-value.

Multivariable Models with a Categorical Dependent Variable

covariates

variables that may be predictive of the outcome under study; they may be of direct interest or may be a confounding or interacting variable

As we noted earlier, a key step in preparing for the analysis of any RCT is to examine whether the groups are comparable at baseline on sociodemographics and other predictor variables. In the event that differential selection is a threat (that is, there are differences between groups on sociodemographic variables or other study variables), we may want to control for these differences statistically, otherwise our findings may not be valid. Controlling for variables statistically means including these variables as **covariates** in the model so that we can examine the effect of the IV (treatment) on the dependent variable (DV) over and above these differences. Covariates are factors that vary in conjunction with the dependent variable, are not manipulated in the RCT but were observed, and can affect the relationship between the IV and the DV. Including multiple variables in a statistical model that predicts a single dependent variable is considered to be a multivariable analysis. In intervention analyses, this implies the independent variable plus any identified covariates. An analytic strategy that controls for the effects of these covariates while testing for intervention effects on a dichotomous DV could be logistic regression. Logistic regression is used for categorical dependent variables that are dichotomous (Hosmer and Lemeshow, 1989); other analyses (for example, multinomial regression) would have to be employed for categorical dependent variables with more than two categories or levels (see Figure 15.2).

logistic regression

a type of probabilistic statistical classification model typically used to predict a binary response from a categorical predictor, based on one or more predictor variables

Logistic Regression. **Logistic regression** is a statistical technique that allows for the testing of an independent variable (in other words, the HPP) in the presence of identified covariates. This process "controls" for the effects of covariates on the categorical dependent variable. To control in this context essentially means that the influence of the intervention on the dependent variable is determined while accounting for any effect the covariates may have on the dependent variable, so that differences between groups on the covariates are addressed.

Like linear regression, logistic regression yields several parameter estimates. However, the primary estimate of interest is the odds ratio. If a logistic regression equation that had condom use as the dependent variable, and a variable representing the HPP condition, along with several covariates, yielded an odds ratio of 3.9, it would be interpreted as "the odds that participants in the HPP group would report condom use at last sexual intercourse were 3.9 times greater than participants in the control group." In addition to the odds ratio for the HPP, we would also like to calculate the 95-percent CI and the corresponding *P*-value for the HPP.

A note of caution is impor-tant here. The odds ratio (OR) may overestimate HPP effects when the outcomes are com-mon. To correct for this potential inflation of effect, we recommend converting ORs to RR whenever feasible, using procedures described by Zhang and Yu (1998).

IN A NUTSHELL

The odds ratio (OR) may overes-timate HPP effects when the out-comes are common.

A three-arm RCT conducted by Walton and colleagues (2010) exam-ined the effects of an intervention that addressed alcohol use and violence among adolescents who visited an urban emergency department (ED) in Michigan. The independent variable was intervention group and the depen-dent variable was alcohol use and violence. A total of 729 ED patients were randomized to either a control group (receipt of a brochure with com-munity resources) or a therapist-led or computer-based alcohol/violence intervention, each consisting of 35 minutes of motivational interviewing and skills training. Patients were assessed at baseline and completed a 3-month and a 6-month follow-up that included self-reported measures of behaviors and consequences such as peer aggression and violence, con-sequences of violence, alcohol use, binge drinking, and consequences of alcohol use. Results at the 3-month follow-up showed that compared to controls, participants in the therapist-led intervention showed self-reported reductions in the occurrence of peer aggression (RR = .74; 95-percent CI = 0.61–0.90), peer violence (RR = .70; 95-percent CI = 0.52–0.95), and consequences of violence (RR = .76; 95-percent CI = 0.64–0.90). Results at the 6-month follow-up showed that compared to controls, partici-pants in the therapist-led intervention showed self-reported reductions in the occurrence of consequences of alcohol use (OR = .56; 95-percent CI = .34–.91). In addition, participants in the computer intervention also showed reductions in alcohol consequences compared to the control group, (OR = 0.57; 95-percent CI, 0.34–0.95).

Multiple Follow-Up Assessments

Although the pretest-posttest RCT is the basic research design to assess change as a function of exposure to an HPP, there are, as you might expect, more complex designs and, of course, comparably more complex statistical approaches to analyze data derived from these complex designs. It is beyond the scope of this chapter to address the range and complexity inherent in these advanced RCTs, but we consider it important for students of health promotion to be aware of them.

One way to extend the basic pretest-posttest design is to incorporate multiple follow-up assessments. Investigators are often curious about the sustainability or maintenance of HPP effects. Although we may expect that people would change their behavior, attitudes, and beliefs as a function of participating in an HPP, these changes may begin to show decay over time (DiClemente, Brown, Sales, and Rose, 2013). We may therefore want to assess people on several occasions over a protracted time period. This design could be depicted as shown in Figure 15.3.

generalized estimating equation
a technique that estimates the parameters of a generalized linear model with a possible unknown correlation between outcomes

Analysis of this design with a categorical dependent variable can be accomplished through a variety of statistical techniques. One statistical approach that is gaining popularity is the use of **generalized estimating equation** (GEE). The GEE logistic regression model is an extension of the simple logistic regression model discussed in the previous section and can be used when the categorical dependent variable is dichotomized. With the GEE logistic model, all variables are measured on multiple occasions. Because repeated observations (measurements) collected for the same participant (for instance, measuring a participant's weight at two or more time points) are not independent of each other, a correction must be made for these within-participant correlations. This approach permits an adjustment for repeated within-participant measurement and the correlation between the participant's measurements over time (Hardin and Hilbe, 2003).

time-invariant variable
a variable that does not change over time, such as a person's race

The overall model design includes a **time-invariant variable**, which represents a variable that is not expected to change during the experimental period. In an RCT, a time-invariant variable is the variable representing

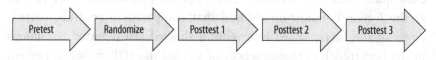

Figure 15.3 Standard Pretest-Posttest Design

the program, such as the HPP. Also, the model will include **time-variant variables** (these are other predictors in addition to the dependent variable that are expected to change). Additionally, a variable representing the number of time periods involved is also included in the model to differentiate the temporal order of the repeated measures. The resultant statistics are adjusted ORs and 95-percent confidence intervals. Although we have simplified, for heuristic purposes, the rationale and format of a GEE logistic model, it is important to note that not all popular computer statistical packages offer this statistical routine as part of their package.

For example, a school-based RCT at a single elementary school was analyzed using GEE by Sandora, Shih, and Goldmann (2008). In this study, the researchers assessed the effectiveness of a multifactorial intervention, which included alcohol-based hand sanitizer and surface disinfection, in reducing absenteeism caused by gastrointestinal and respiratory illnesses. Classrooms that were randomized to the intervention received alcohol-based hand sanitizer and disinfecting wipes to use at school daily for 8 weeks; control classrooms followed usual hand-washing and cleaning practices. Parents of students completed a pre-intervention demographic survey. Absences were recorded along with the reason for absence. Swabs of environmental surfaces were evaluated by bacterial culture and polymerase chain reaction for norovirus, respiratory syncytial virus, influenza, and parainfluenza 3. The primary outcomes were rates of absenteeism caused by gastrointestinal or respiratory illness. GEE was used to compare absenteeism rates between intervention and control groups, accounting for potential correlations among students and controlling for covariates: family size, race, health status, and home sanitizer use. In total, 285 students participated in the study. Controlled GEE analyses showed that the absenteeism rate for gastrointestinal illness remained significantly lower in the intervention group compared with the control group; the rate ratio was 0.91 (95-percent CI = 0.87–0.94). The adjusted absenteeism rate for respiratory illness was not different between groups; the risk ratio was 1.10 (95-percent CI = 0.97–1.24).

time-variant variables
variables that change over time, such as a person's income

Analysis with a Continuous Dependent Variable

Analysis with a continuous dependent variable is often more familiar to investigators in health promotion and health education research than is analysis with other variable types. In this case, the dependent variable assumes a range of scores rather than a binary response. Examples of commonly used dependent variables in health promotion research include blood pressure (either diastolic or systolic), weight, a score on an aptitude test, a score on a scale measuring depressive symptoms, number of servings of fruits and vegetables consumed, and so on. As you can see, the range of continuous dependent variables is almost limitless.

Student's *t*-test

a statistical hypothesis test in which the test statistic follows the Student's *t* distribution if the null hypothesis is supported; used to determine whether two sets of data are significantly different from each other

The **Student's *t*-test** is one statistic that may be familiar, often learned in introductory statistics courses and used to assess group differences on continuous DVs. In the case of an RCT, the student's *t*-test provides a statistic that compares the means of two samples. Let's use an example to illustrate a simple analysis. In the HIV risk-reduction intervention described previously, a secondary dependent variable was to increase positive attitudes toward condom use (a continuous secondary dependent variable) among the participants in the intervention group. Attitude was assessed using a well-established scale, with higher scale scores reflecting more positive attitudes toward using condoms during sexual intercourse. Participants were then randomized to either the risk-reduction group or a control group. Subsequent to participating in the intervention or control group, we asked all participants to return after 6 months and complete a follow-up (posttest) assessment. The goal, of course, was to determine if condom attitude scores were different in the HIV risk-reduction group relative to the control group. The question is, How do we test for this important difference?

null hypothesis

refers to a general statement or default position that there is no relationship between two measured phenomena, or that a potential treatment has no effect

Let's assume that at follow-up (posttest), the participants in the HIV risk-reduction group had a mean condom attitude score of 32.65 (the scale ranged from a low of 10 to a high of 40). The control group had a mean condom attitude score of 22.40. The *t*-test assesses whether these observed means for the two study groups are statistically different from each other. It is important to note that in the case of this RCT we are using an independent groups *t*-test. In our example, the results were statistically significant ($P < .05$). The findings support the hypothesis that HIV risk-reduction intervention increases participants' positive attitudes toward condom use.

motivator or alternative hypothesis

refers to a general statement that there is a relationship between two measured phenomena or that a potential treatment has an effect

In general, a hypothesis may be proposed as being either a **null hypothesis** (that is, there are no differences between groups) or a **motivator or alternative hypothesis** (that is, there are differences between groups, and the direction of the difference is specified). However, as we noted in previous sections describing analysis of RCTs with a categorical dependent variable, although the *P*-value is useful, it does not provide an indication of the ES related to the HPP. Indeed, it describes the findings relative to chance. To capture more fully the effect of the HIV risk-reduction intervention on condom attitude scores (continuous secondary dependent variable), it is useful to calculate an ES.

As noted earlier, and certainly worth reiterating, an ES provides an index of the strength of the association between the HPP and the dependent variable. In this case, a measure that could be calculated is the mean difference (D) between the groups' condom attitude scores. Let's refer back to our example by examining Table 15.3.

Table 15.3 Differences in Condom Attitude Scores by Study Group

Group Assignment	Mean (at follow-up)	Mean Difference
HIV risk reduction	32.65	+10.25
Control	22.40	

We have calculated an absolute measure of effect on mean condom attitude scores attributable to the HIV risk-reduction intervention. On average, condom attitude scores in the HIV risk-reduction group are 10.25 units greater compared with the control group. As noted earlier, in addition to measuring the magnitude of the HPP effect (the mean difference) and the corresponding *P*-value to assess its statistical significance, it is also recommended that the confidence interval around the mean difference be calculated. The confidence interval provides a measure of the true effect of the HPP in the population. In other words, if the study was repeated 100 times, the 95-percent CI would indicate that in 95 of those 100 times the mean difference would be between the lower and upper limit. In Table 15.4, we have calculated all the statistics necessary to describe the HPP effects for an HIV risk-reduction intervention designed to enhance condom attitude scores.

Although Table 15.4 conveys a great deal of information about the effects of the HIV risk-reduction intervention on participants' condom attitude scores, it is important to understand that the statistic D is not a standardized measure of ES. If we wanted to compare a number of continuous dependent variables with different scale ranges, it would be problematic (like comparing apples to oranges). For example, the condom attitude scale had a range of possible scores from 10 to 40. Perhaps we want to examine another two scales as continuous secondary dependent variables—not an unreasonable thing to do. One scale measures HIV prevention knowledge and has a range of scores from 1 to 10 (higher scores indicate greater knowledge) and another scale measures self-esteem and has a range of scores from 1 to 5 (higher scores indicate greater self-esteem). Table 15.5 presents information regarding these new scales.

Table 15.4 Effects of an HIV Risk-Reduction Intervention on Condom Attitude Scores

Group Assignment	Mean (at follow-up)	D	95-% CI	P
HIV risk-reduction	32.65	10.25	(7.38–13.86)	.03
Control	22.40			

Notes: D = mean difference (HPP − Co).
95-% CI = 95-% confidence interval around D.

Table 15.5   Effects of an HIV Risk-Reduction Intervention on HIV Knowledge and Self-Esteem

Dependent Variable	Mean Posttest Scores				
	Intervention	Control	D	95-% CI	P
HIV knowledge	8.0	6.0	2.0	1.5–2.5	.04
Self-esteem	4.0	2.0	2.0	1.5–2.5	.04
Condom attitude	32.65	22.40	10.25	7.38–13.86	.03

Notes: D = mean difference (HPP − Co).
95-% CI = 95-% confidence interval around D.

Examining the differences between the HIV knowledge score and the self-esteem score, we note that the mean difference (D) is 2 in both instances. Hence, should we conclude that the effect of the HIV risk-reduction intervention is identical? Well, the answer is yes, if we are focusing only on the absolute difference. However, it is important to note that the HIV knowledge scale has a much larger range of potential scores (1 to 10) compared with the self-esteem scale (1 to 5). Thus the same difference (D = 2) observed for each of the scales may have a markedly different magnitude of effect if we consider the relative difference. One measure that permits a relative assessment of change is called the percent of **relative difference** (RD). The RD statistic provides a common metric for measuring the magnitude of change across different scale measures. The RD is calculated by dividing the value for D by the mean posttest score for the control group.

IN A NUTSHELL

One measure that permits a relative assessment of change is called percent *relative difference (RD)*. The RD statistic provides a common metric for measuring the magnitude of change across different scale measures.

relative difference

comparison of two quantities, taking into account the "sizes" of the things being compared; expressed as a ratio, it is a unitless number, and by multiplying these ratios by 100 they can be expressed as percentages

We can demonstrate the calculation and utility of this statistic. For example, the RD for HIV knowledge would be equal to 2/6 = .33. Likewise, for self-esteem, the RD would be 2/2 = 1.00. It may be easier if the RD is then converted to the percent RD by multiplying the value by 100. As the example demonstrates, the percent RD for knowledge was 33 percent and for self-esteem was 100 percent. Therefore the HPP had a relatively greater effect on improving mean self-esteem scores compared with HIV knowledge scores. Now that we are using the same metric, we can compare the efficacy of the HPP for both variables, whereas examining only the absolute differences in mean scores would obscure this important finding. As with the other measures of HPP effects, the 95-percent CI can also be calculated around the percent RD.

An RCT was conducted by McDermott et al. (2013) and calculated the mean difference (D). The RCT employed a home-based walking intervention that incorporated group support and self-regulated skills. A total of 194 patients with peripheral artery disease were randomized to either the home-based walking intervention or a control group. The primary outcome was the distance a participant was able to walk in 6 minutes. Secondary outcomes included amount of physical activity and scores on a self-health rated questionnaire. Prior to the intervention, the mean distance for the intervention group was 357.4 meters; following the intervention it was 399.8. Pretest mean distance for the control group was 353.3 meters; posttest, it was 342.2. The mean difference between groups was 53.5 meters, with a 95-percent CI of 33.2 to 73.8. These results showed that participants in the intervention group significantly increased the distance they were able to walk in 6 minutes compared to participants in the control group.

Interpreting the Results. Now that we have calculated the appropriate statistics to describe the effects of the HPP on continuous outcomes, we can interpret them. In the study of HIV risk-reduction intervention described earlier, the findings would be interpreted as follows: relative to participants in the control group, those in the HIV risk-reduction intervention had significantly higher mean scores on condom attitudes, HIV knowledge, and self-esteem. We concluded this based on the significant t-test. Moreover, the effect sizes indicated that the greater proportional difference was found for self-esteem, as assessed by the percent RD. The use of these statistics therefore provides a rich description of significant effects of the HIV intervention.

Multivariable Models with Continuous Dependent Variables

As we noted earlier for dichotomous dependent variables (DVs), if there are any differences between groups on study variables, we want to control for these differences statistically. This procedure is not any different if the DVs are continuous. The statistical analysis used to control for both the effects of covariates and, if necessary, the baseline value of the dependent variable is either **multiple linear regression** or its algebraic equivalent, **analysis of covariance** (ANCOVA).

Linear Regression and ANCOVA. Linear regression and ANCOVA are statistical techniques that allow for two or more variables to be included in a model with a continuous dependent variable. The HPP variable is included as the independent variable as well as covariates and the baseline measure of the continuous dependent variable. While the computation of the linear model is beyond the scope of this chapter, the interested reader is referred to Kleinbaum, Kupper, Muller, and Nizam (1998) for an eminently

multiple linear regression
an approach for modeling the relationship between a scalar dependent variable y and one or more explanatory variables denoted X

analysis of covariance
a measure of how much two variables change together and the strength of the relationship between them

IN A NUTSHELL

Multiple linear regression and ANCOVA can adjust for the effects of group differences that would otherwise obscure intervention effects as well as adjusting for the baseline value of the continuous dependent variable.

readable discussion of this approach. Multiple linear regression and ANCOVA can adjust for the effects of group differences that would otherwise obscure intervention effects as well as adjusting for the baseline value of the continuous dependent variable. Multiple linear regression and ANCOVA permit computation of adjusted means and mean differences (D) for continuous dependent variables similar to that discussed earlier in this section as well as constructing the 95-percent CI around these effect sizes (D).

An RCT was implemented and analyzed for continuous outcomes with ANCOVA by Buchan, Ollis, Cooper, Shield, and Baker (2013) to assess the effects of an exercise intervention on cardiovascular disease in adolescents who are healthy. The intervention employed a type of exercise known as "high-intensity training" (HIT), which involves sprints followed by periods of inactivity for recovery time. The intervention group performed exercise sessions 3 times a week over a 7-week period. The control group resumed their normal physical activity levels. A total of 89 adolescents were randomized to either the intervention or the control group. Pretest and posttest of all participants included blood pressure tests, four physical performance tests, and biochemical marker tests for cardiovascular disease. Buchan and colleagues used ANCOVA to determine the between-groups and within-group statistical differences. Results showed that participants in the intervention significantly improved their vertical jump (D = +1.0; 95-percent CI = 0.3–1.6) vs. (D = −2.1; 95-percent CI = −3.0–1.1) and their sprint times (D = −0.09; 95-percent CI = −0.12 to −0.05) vs. (D = −0.03; 95-percent CI = −0.01–0.06) after partitioning out baseline measures of sex, maturation, physical activity, and kcal/d.

Data Analytic Topics for Special Consideration

Prospecting for Results: "Data Mining." Statistical tests have become increasingly more sophisticated; this is partly attributable to the increasing power of computers to run more complex software. However, in an era with high-powered computers and sophisticated statistical software, some basic and enduring principles of analysis remain valid. Hypothesis-driven analyses—which are theory-driven, derived from an understanding of the relevant empirical literature, and specified in the protocol—should be afforded priority status for analysis. As a basic principle, the statistical analysis should focus foursquare on the hypothesis-driven analyses. Although there are myriad statistical procedures, complex statistics, and fast, powerful computers that can run these programs quickly, be wary of **data mining**. Data mining entails conducting many post-hoc analyses that are not related to the primary hypotheses. Data mining can appear attractive, but it can also lead to spurious findings that capitalize on chance. As a rule, results from analyses that have a firm basis in the original research question are more valid.

data mining
the computational process of discovering patterns in large data sets

Subgroup Analysis: "Less Is More." RCTs estimate a treatment effect averaged over the study participants; however, health promotion researchers are often interested in examining the effects of HPP for various subgroups of participants. For example, you may be interested in gender differences, racial/ethnic differences, age differences, or even differences based on a characteristic of the sample, say, depression scores. The rationale for conducting these subgroup analyses, referred to as moderation analyses, is to ascertain whether the effects of the HPP for participants with specific characteristics are different from the average HPP effects seen in the overall sample. In other words, moderation analyses determine whether certain variables of interest (such as race or gender) moderate or change the effects of the HPP.

Although subgroup analysis is scientifically intriguing and interesting, there is one serious problem: if many analyses are performed, it becomes likely that the results could be spurious; that is, statistically significant by chance alone. Allow us to illustrate. Suppose participants in an RCT with two conditions (HPP and the control) are partitioned into G mutually exclusive subgroups and a statistical significance test at $P = 0.05$ is conducted within each subgroup. In this instance, even if there is no true effect, the probability of at least one significant result is equal to $1 - (1-P)G$. For $P = 0.05$ and $G = 5$, this probability is 23 percent; for $P = 0.05$ and $G = 10$, the probability is 40 percent! The probability of observing a statistically significant effect, even in the absence of a true effect, increases markedly with the increasing number of subgroup analyses performed.

The reliability of subgroup analysis is often poor, partly because subgroups are generally smaller compared with the whole sample. A guiding principle is to keep the number of subgroup analyses to a minimum and prespecify them in the protocol. This allows readers to know how many subgroup analyses were performed. Furthermore, prespecification of subgroup analyses increases the credibility of findings, as hypothesis-driven analyses reflect a priori knowledge of biologic or other factors instead of a posteriori justification. Before you implement your RCT, you may want to consider how the HPP may differentially affect subgroups within your sample. Finally, when reporting subgroup analyses they should be interpreted as exploratory, hypothesis-generating analyses rather than definitive.

Summary

This chapter has provided an overview of the principles, logic, and statistical procedures involved in data analyses pertaining to testing whether an HPP is effective in a randomized controlled trial design. Planning and implementation of an RCT is critical to the integrity of the design. However, the data analysis should be viewed not as ancillary to the research process but as the final pieces of the puzzle. Without it, a study will never quite provide the complete picture. To assist you in the data analytic process, we provided a decision map, which can be used to determine the specific type of analytic technique appropriate for the type of dependent variable and to decide when other adjustments are necessary. It is critical that the decision map be followed, given the necessity of providing an accurate and valid test of the HPP, thereby avoiding biased (invalid) results. In addition to choosing the appropriate statistical technique for testing intervention effects, we also emphasized the importance of moving beyond the reporting of basic significance associated with the statistical test to include measures of effect size and confidence intervals to enhance the precision of estimated effects. Including these additional statistics provides breadth to the analysis that enhances description of the results while allowing for their comparability across other studies.

KEY TERMS

Analysis of covariance (ANCOVA)

Binary categorical dependent variable

Categorical dependent variables

Confidence interval

Continuous dependent variable

Covariates

Data mining

Effect size

External validity

Generalizability

Generalized estimating equations

Logistic regression

Motivator or alternative hypothesis

Multiple linear regression

Nonparametric statistic

Null hypothesis

Ordered categorical dependent variable

Polychotomous dependent variables

Relative difference

Relative risk

Student's t-test

Time-invariant variables

Time-variant variables

For Practice and Discussion

1. Locate three examples of RCTs by doing an electronic search. Be sure that your examples relate to health promotion rather than medical advances. You will notice that most RCTs are designed around questions in medical care such as drug effects or the effects of a new treatment procedure. Using the decision map shown in this chapter, determine if the authors of each study used an analytic strategy that is consistent with the map.

2. Again, using the decision map select an analytic approach for each scenario listed below.
   • The dependent variable is blood serum cholesterol level.
   • The dependent variable is having a Pap test in the past 2 years (women answered "yes" versus "no").
   • The dependent variable is an ordinal measure of cigarette use (participants responded with one of three options: "None," "Less than one pack per day," "At least one pack per day.")
   • The dependent variable is a continuous scale measure of depression.
   • The dependent variable is a scale measure of depression, and several covariates are critical to the analysis.
   • The dependent variable is contraceptive use (dichotomized as "yes" versus "no"), and several covariates are critical to the analysis.

3. As in Question 1, consider three RCTs of health promotion intervention that are of interest to you. Examine their data analysis section. What measures do the investigators report to justify their claim as to whether the intervention was efficacious or not? Pay particularly close attention to measures of effect were reported. Which measures of effect were reported? Are these appropriate, given the study design?

4. Select an HPP from the published literature that uses an RCT design, and critique the data analytic plan. What was the method of randomization? Did the authors present differences of groups at baseline? Did the data analysis match up to the design and the types of variables?

References

Buchan, D. S., Ollis, S., Cooper, S. M., Shield, J. P., and Baker, J. S. (2013). High intensity interval running enhances measures of physical fitness but not metabolic measures of cardiovascular disease risk in healthy adolescents. *BMC Public Health*. doi:10.1186/1471-2458-13-498

DiClemente, R. J., Brown, J. L., Sales, J. M., and Rose, E. S. (2013, June). Rate of decay in proportion of condom-protected sex acts among adolescents after participation in an HIV risk-reduction intervention. *Journal of Acquired Immune Deficiency Syndromes, 63*(Suppl 1), S85–9. doi:10.1097/QAI.0b013e3182920173. PMID: 23673893; PMCID: PMC3662369.

Hardin, J. W., and Hilbe, J. M. (2003). *Generalized estimating equations.* New York: Chapman and Hall/CRC.

Hosmer, D. W., and Lemeshow, S. L. (1989). *Applied logistic regression.* New York: Wiley.

Kleinbaum, D. G., Kupper, L. L., Muller, K. E., and Nizam, A. (1998). *Applied regression analysis and other multivariable methods.* New York: Duxbury Press.

Lee, S. M., Landry, J., Jones, P. M., Buhrmann, O., and Morley-Forster, P. (2013). The effectiveness of a perioperative smoking cessation program: A randomized clinical trial. *Anesthesia & Analgesia.*

McDermott, M. M., Liu, K., Criqui, M. H., . . . Rejeski, W. J. (2013). Home-based walking exercise intervention in peripheral artery disease: A randomized clinical trial. *Journal of American Medicine, 310*(1):57–65.

Sandora, T. J., Shih, M.-C., and Goldmann, D. A. (2008). Reducing absenteeism from gastrointestinal and respiratory illness in elementary school students: A randomized, controlled trial of an infection-control intervention. *Pediatrics, 121*(6), e1555-e1562.

Walton, M. A., Chermack, S. T., Shope, J. T., Bingham, C. R., Zimmerman, M. A., Blow, F. C., and Cunningham, R. M. (2010). Effects of a brief intervention for reducing violence and alcohol misuse among adolescents: A randomized controlled trial. *Journal of American Medicine, 304*(5), 527–535.

Zhang, J., and Yu, K. F. (1998). What's the relative risk? A method of correcting the odds ratio in cohort studies of common outcomes. *JAMA: The Journal of the American Medical Association, 280*(19), 1690–1691.

CHAPTER 16

METHODS AND PROCEDURES FOR ANALYZING QUALITATIVE DATA IN HEALTH PROMOTION

Laura F. Salazar
Alejandra Mijares
Richard A. Crosby
Ralph J. DiClemente

Whether it is quantitative or qualitative, positivist or interpretivist, good research entails a lengthy and involved process. Once a quantitative study has been successfully implemented and data are collected, the next step is the statistical analysis. Quantitative analyses involve statistical assumptions not to be violated and statistical techniques prescribed based on the type of data and nature of the research question. In contrast, data analyses in qualitative studies typically do not wait until all the data have been collected, but rather are ongoing and can begin in the field during data collection. Qualitative analyses are dynamic, fluid, and process-oriented. There are basic techniques and procedures for qualitative analyses that, once mastered, can be applied to numerous types of qualitative research questions, intentions, strategies, and data. This chapter is designed to provide the knowledge and skills necessary to understand the basics and allow for the analysis of qualitative data.

Irrespective of type of inquiry (quantitative or qualitative), the culmination of any health promotion research project is typically the point where the participants have all been recruited, enrolled, interviewed, observed, assessed, or tested. If the project was an evaluation of a health promotion program, then ideally the program was implemented successfully without issue. All that is left are the

LEARNING OBJECTIVES

- Explain the importance, function, and elements of a data collection plan for qualitative research.

- Define concepts, patterns, codes, and themes.

- Describe the process of codebook development and of coding of data.

- Distinguish between grounded theory and theory-driven analyses.

- List the pros and cons of qualitative data analysis software.

- Identify the different approaches taken for triangulation of data.

- Describe the process used for interpretation of data.

data, patiently waiting to be analyzed so that knowledge can be generated. You may recall from Chapter Eight that qualitative modes differ from quantitative modes in the assumptions made about (1) the generation of facts, (2) their purposes, (3) their approaches, (4) the types of data, and (5) the role of the researcher. Thus you should have a good understanding that data analysis for qualitative research will be vastly different from data analysis for quantitative research. However, for many health promotion students and even seasoned researchers, there is one commonality: the emotional response of anxiety when faced with data analysis. Anxiety is the anticipation of a threat and is accompanied by a fear component. Quantitative analysis can create extreme anxiety due to anticipating the threat of having difficulty in understanding sophisticated, theoretical, or abstract mathematical concepts and in turn, the specific statistical principles and procedures involved. This "statistical" threat can also be coupled with fear of implementing the appropriate statistical techniques properly and interpreting the results correctly. Indeed, if you feel this way, you are not alone. Fear of statistics is a common anxiety: a research study found that it is experienced by as many as 80 percent of graduate students in the social and behavioral sciences (Onwuegbuzie and Wilson, 2003).

As is the case in conducting quantitative data analyses, anxiety is also a common response when faced with qualitative data analysis. The fear component is different in that the perceived threat stems from difficulty in managing voluminous amounts of data—pages of transcribed interviews, notes from participant observation sessions, sketches or pictures, news stories, and other sources—as well as a lack of prescribed statistical "tests" to use when analyzing. But the fear component is similar in that it derives from the need for interpretation—that is, the need to correctly interpret what the data mean.

It may allay these fears somewhat to realize that, whether quantitative or qualitative, results are always open to varying interpretations and may not always represent one absolute truth. Quantitative results can vary in interpretation because there are different statistical techniques that can be used to approach the same research question, which may lead to varying results. Qualitative results can also vary in interpretation because, as you may recall from Chapter Eight, qualitative research takes an interpretivist perspective, meaning the researcher is trying to socially construct the reality of the research participants; researchers coming from diverse backgrounds could come to different conclusions with the same set of data. In other words, the perspective of the researcher may have an effect on the conclusions drawn. Results will always be open to varying interpretations, but you should be prepared to back up the rationale used to support your choices in terms of procedures and techniques. So you can set aside your fears about arriving at a single correct interpretation in your data analysis. Of course, you will still need to address other anticipated challenges.

It is beyond the scope of this chapter to provide an in-depth discussion of qualitative data analysis; many textbooks have been written on the subject and should be consulted (for example, Lofland and Lofland, 1995; Miles and Huberman, 1984, 1994). In this chapter we provide the basic tools and procedures needed for you to cope with anticipated challenges associated with qualitative data analysis. We will describe ways for you to manage and organize your data and develop a reliable and valid code book that will help you answer your research questions, and explain how to code your data, identify emergent themes, and provide an interpretation. We also provide guidance on the write-up of results. We emphasize that this chapter is specific to qualitative research conducted within the context of health promotion; it is not meant to be on par with chapters written for textbooks specific to qualitative research methods or disciplines such as anthropology, whose predominant paradigm is interpretivist. In this chapter we provide an overview of the qualitative data analytic process with the suggestion that the best way to learn how to do qualitative data analysis is to actually do it. We realize that the first time it may seem like a formidable task. In fact, regarding qualitative data analysis, Miller and Crabtree (1999) pointed out: "Interpretation is a complex and dynamic craft, with as much creative artistry as technical exactitude, and it requires an abundance of patient plodding, fortitude, and discipline" (p. 128).

Reflexivity

There is an erroneous assumption among some researchers that quantitative research is not biased, because it is "objective," whereas qualitative research *is* biased, because it is subjective. We take the position that all research is biased to some degree and that the researcher's perspective affects all forms of research, whether it is bench science being conducted in a laboratory, quantitative research, or qualitative research. In fact, "a researcher's background and position will affect what they choose to investigate, the angle of investigation, the methods judged most adequate for this purpose, the findings considered most appropriate, and the framing and communication of conclusions" (Malterud, 2001, pp. 483–484). There is some form of bias in all research. In quantitative research, bias can take the form of formulating one's hypotheses, choosing a particular study design over another, using a certain type of measurement instrument, or deciding on a specific laboratory assay over another. These are all forms of bias and can affect the outcomes of the study. Although it is virtually impossible to eliminate all bias inherent in research, researchers should always strive to minimize bias and to acknowledge any sources of bias. In qualitative research, researchers should acknowledge that their preconceptions and perspective may introduce bias and affect the results. This is where the concept of **reflexivity** comes into play. Reflexivity is the process of examining both oneself as researcher and the research relationship. The reflexivity process involves (1) a self-examination of one's assumptions and preconceptions and how these affect research decisions—particularly the selection and wording of questions—and (2) examining one's relationship to the respondent and how the relationship dynamics affect responses to questions (Hsiung, 2010). In this chapter, in certain sections we will highlight steps for researchers to take to foster reflexivity, as it is essential in qualitative research.

reflexivity
the process of examining both oneself as a researcher and the research relationship

Data Organization and Analysis Preparation

Although Albert Einstein argued the logic of the adage that a cluttered desk is the sign of a cluttered mind (of what, then, is an empty desk a sign?), we cannot emphasize enough the importance of having an uncluttered and systematic data management system in place to handle the organization of the data being collected. During the data collection process, a detailed and well-articulated plan should have been devised to handle, catalog, and store voluminous amounts of data in a secure and reliable location. We suggest that it is possible "out of clutter to find simplicity," but you must be purposeful in doing so. Your data collection plan should entail a process for not only documenting the various types of data collected, but also for **annotating the data**. Annotating the data can mean to provide other notes or additional comments, such as interviewer ID, date, participant ID or initials if used, location or site where collected, and so on. Any identifying or relevant information associated with the data should be noted and attached to that datum. Whether the data are maps, handwritten field notes, interview notes, focus group audio, or archival records, each piece must be documented accordingly along with annotations and then stored.

annotating the data
a process used to provide other notes or additional comments to the datum

If you are unsure of what type of additional information should be documented, a useful tool is a 32-item checklist developed by qualitative researchers to promote consistency and quality in reporting of interviews and focus groups. Shown in Table 16.1, the checklist was designed to provide qualitative researchers with formal reporting guidelines; it highlights pertinent information across the following three domains (which should be included in written research reports and journal articles): (1) the research team and reflexivity, (2) the study design, and (3) the analysis and findings. As we see in the domain 1 section, the collection of this information is

Table 16.1   Consolidated Criteria for Reporting Qualitative Studies (COREQ): 32-Item Checklist

No	Item	Guide Questions/Description
Domain 1: Research team and reflexivity		
Personal Characteristics		
1.	Interviewer/facilitator	Which author/s conducted the interview or focus group?
2.	Credentials	What were the researcher's credentials? *e.g., PhD, MD*
3.	Occupation	What was their occupation at the time of the study?
4.	Gender	Was the researcher male or female?
5.	Experience and training	What experience or training did the researcher have?
Relationship with participants		
6.	Relationship established	Was a relationship established prior to study commencement?
7.	Participant knowledge of the interviewer	What did the participants know about the researcher? *e.g., personal goals, reasons for doing the research*
8.	Interviewer characteristics	What characteristics were reported about the interviewer/facilitator? *e.g,. bias, assumptions, reasons and interests in the research topic*
Domain 2: Study design		
Theoretical framework		
9.	Methodological orientation and Theory	What methodological orientation was stated to underpin the study? *e.g., grounded theory, discourse analysis, ethnography, phenomenology content analysis*
Participant selection		
10.	Sampling	How were participants selected? *e.g., purposive, convenience, consecutive, snowball*
11.	Method of approach	How were participants approached? *e.g., face-to-face, telephone, mail, email*
12.	Sample size	How many participants were in the study?
13.	Non-participation	How many people refused to participate or dropped out? Reasons?
Setting		
14.	Setting of data collection	Where were the data collected? *e.g., home, clinic, workplace*
15.	Presence of non-participants	Was anyone else present besides the participants and researchers?
16.	Description of sample	What are the important characteristics of the sample? *e.g., demographic data, date*
Data collection		
17.	Interview guide	Were questions, prompts, guides provided by the authors? Was it pilot tested?
18.	Repeat interviews	Were repeat interviews carried out? If yes, how many?
19.	Audio/visual recording	Did the research use audio or visual recording to collect the data?
20.	Field notes	Were field notes made during and/or after the interview or focus group?
21.	Duration	What was the duration of the interviews or focus group?

(continued)

Table 16.1 Consolidated Criteria for Reporting Qualitative Studies (COREQ): 32-Item Checklist

No	Item	Guide Questions/Description
22.	Data saturation	Was data saturation discussed?
23.	Transcripts returned	Were transcripts returned to participants for comment and/or correction?
Domain 3: Analysis and findings		
Data analysis		
24.	Number of data coders	How many data coders coded the data?
25.	Description of the coding tree	Did authors provide a description of the coding tree?
26.	Derivation of themes	Were themes identified in advance or derived from the data?
27.	Software	What software, if applicable, was used to manage the data?
28.	Participant checking	Did participants provide feedback on the findings?
Reporting		
29.	Quotations presented	Were participant quotations presented to illustrate the themes / findings? Was each quotation identified? *e.g., participant number*
30.	Data and findings consistent	Was there consistency between the data presented and the findings?
31.	Clarity of major themes	Were major themes clearly presented in the findings?
32.	Clarity of minor themes	Is there a description of diverse cases or discussion of minor themes?

Source: Tong, Sainsbury, and Craig (2007). Consolidated criteria for reporting qualitative research (COREQ): A 32-item checklist for interviews and focus groups. *International Journal for Quality in Health Care, 19*(6), 349–357. With permission.

related to reflexivity. So, for example, noting whether the interviewer had any relationship with the participant prior to the study and, most important, documenting the interviewer characteristics (such as assumptions, bias, reasons and interests in the research topic) will help ensure that the process of reflexivity has been implemented.

In addition to documenting additional information associated with the data and the research, any interviews or focus groups that were captured via a digital audio or video recorder should be transcribed. It is recommended that you transcribe soon after an interview so that you can start analyzing your data immediately, and any new concepts or ideas can be captured and subsequently explored in later interviews. This is one of the major advantages of qualitative research. The electronic word document containing the transcription of the interview or discussion becomes the data that will be stored; the electronic file should be documented along with the original audio or video files. Most institutional review boards dictate that researchers store audio or video files for a specified time frame (for example, "after transcription," "one year," "five years"), after which they must destroy them. Audio or video files are destroyed to protect the confidentiality of the research participants. Therefore it is extremely important to ensure that all transcriptions are safely and securely stored and properly documented. We provide some guidance for doing transcriptions in the next section.

When conducting transcript-based analysis, it is very important that the transcripts being coded are **verbatim** transcripts (that is, word for word). They should include any pauses, additional comments, half sentences, and the like. In addition, any social expressions (such as laughter) or incidents (such as interruptions) should be included in brackets. The transcript must capture any colloquial language that the speaker used, because it mirrors true speech. A verbatim transcript helps provide context about how participants think and feel about the issues being researched. In contrast to a verbatim transcription, a summarized or edited transcript may miss important information that could be key to the question you are trying to answer. If possible, data collectors (for example, the interviewer, moderator, the note-taker) should listen to the audio and transcribe the session together while it is still fresh and use any notes to capture nonverbal cues associated with the data collection method. If you are conducting focus groups, you could begin the focus group by asking participants to give themselves a pseudonym (such as Mr. Red). This will help the transcriber to more easily distinguish participants throughout the transcription process and help you identify whether a particular issue is being repeated by more than one participant (that is, whether that particular issue emerges as a theme). After the first draft of the transcript is completed, it is very important that you review the transcript alongside the recording, to ensure that it is accurate and captures everything participants said. Finally, if you conducted your study in another language, you should: (1) conduct transcription in the language in which data were collected and (2) translate the transcript into the language being analyzed. In the translation of a transcript, the most important instruction you can give your translator is that the translation "conveys meaning of the issues discussed rather than a *literal* translation of the words used. A literal translation may make little sense" (Hennink, 2007, p. 216) and important meaning could get "lost in the translation."

We highly recommend that you use a database to assist with organizing and managing all of the data, annotations, transcriptions, and other information. Ideally, this entire process of cataloging, documenting, and storing data and other relevant information has been ongoing during the data collection period. Once the data have been fully processed and annotated, the first step in analysis is to try to sort the data and impose some type

verbatim
transcription process in which the narrative is captured word for word

IN A NUTSHELL

A verbatim transcript helps provide context about how participants think and feel about the issues being researched.

of organization. This organization process should also be ongoing. You should not wait until all data have been collected to begin the process of organization; rather, this should occur parallel to data collection and be relevant to the goals of the study. Some researchers organize their data first by type (for example, interviews, field notes, archival records) and then within each type by research question, date, people, or places; however, generally for health promotion qualitative research, it is most useful to sort the data by research question and identify the relevant data sources that will be used to answer the research questions.

Multiple Analysts. The use of multiple analysts is another step used to enhance reflexivity. Having multiple analysts can promote dialogue that will lead to "the development of complementary as well as divergent under-standings of a study situation and provide a context in which researchers' (often hidden) beliefs, values, perspectives and assumptions can be revealed and contested" (Cohen and Crabtree, 2008).

Depending on the situation, in some instances the analysis team may have also participated in the data collection; in others, the interviewers and analysts are part of separate teams. Before you initiate your analysis, it is very important that training is provided to members of the anal-ysis team. The training should cover the study basics (that is, purpose and background of the research study), codebook review (that is, definitions and decision rules), coding guidelines (such as what to do when a new code emerges or needs modification), how to use the study qualitative data analysis (QDA) software to code and manage data, and practice sessions. Training of analysts will ensure that your data are coded consistently, accurately, and systematically. We recommend developing a QDA protocol that can be reviewed during training. This protocol should be a living document that can be modified as needed and includes guidelines on the following:

- Preparing transcripts for coding (that is, quality control and quality assurance steps)
- Codebook development
- Adding or modifying codes
- Coding process
- Performing intercoder reliability checks (such as two transcripts every two weeks)
- Adding memos and diagrams (such as adding initials, dating)

When the analysis protocol is modified, all team members should be in agreement. Make sure you date your revised protocol so that you can keep track of revisions.

Codebook Development

Codes are the building blocks for theory or model building and the foundation on which the analyst's arguments rest.

—*MacQueen, McLellan-Lemal, Bartholow, and Milstein (2008), p. 119*

In qualitative data analysis, the **codebook** should be considered the "Rosetta Stone" that assists with the process of "translating" and unlocking the meaning of the data. The codebook (1) organizes the data at a basic level, (2) allows the investigator to divide the data into fundamental categorical units, and (3) provides a record of how those categorical units are defined and interpreted. Developing the codebook can be viewed as a complex and ongoing iterative process that is integral to and part of data analysis, so we will attempt to break this process down into manageable steps. Generally, a **code** can be a descriptive word or short phrase used as a label and attached to units of data (such as a word, a sentence, or a paragraph) and that represents a **concept** observed by the analyst. In this context, concept refers to an idea or notion that is suggestive of the data. For example, women talking about their relationships with their friends and family—how their friends and family help them out in certain situations, provide emotional support when they are in trouble, lend them money, or babysit their children—could be suggestive of the concept of "social support" and could become a code "Social Support." Developing the codebook is essentially the beginning of data analysis. The codes associated with a qualitative dataset essentially constitute the codebook. In order for your analysis to be transparent, valid, and reliable, it is essential that you and your team develop a codebook that is operationally defined, structured, and clear. Once the codebook is developed, coding is the transitional process used to systematically classify the units of data in order to facilitate interpretation. Coding is the step the researcher takes to begin identifying relevant concepts and attaching codes to index them. Coding enables you to organize and then subsequently group similarly coded data into categories based on shared characteristics.

The first step in codebook development is to determine the intent of the research. How the codebook is developed and how the data are coded will depend on this intent. If the research is exploratory—for example, aiming to build a theory that helps explain real-world phenomena (such

codebook
a document that assists with the process of translating and unlocking the meaning of the data as part of the qualitative data analysis process

code
a descriptive word or short phrase that is used as a label and attached to units of data

concept
an idea or notion that is suggestive of the data

as a theory that helps explain the intersection of HIV and gender-based violence)—then the research approach should be driven by **grounded theory**. As stated previously in Chapter Eight, grounded theory is a general methodology for deriving a theory or theories from data systematically gathered and analyzed. It entails a process by which the analysts immerse themselves in the data so that the meanings and relationships within the data can emerge (Strauss and Corbin, 1990). When using grounded theory as the approach for a qualitative analysis, you can readily understand that the codebook would also have to emerge from the data and is an integral part of the data analysis process. Creating the codebook involves reading the data intimately and thoroughly, making notes of any concepts, patterns, or topics of interest related to the research, as well as potential explanations. These concepts or patterns of interest that develop can be captured by either a word, some type of label, or a short phrase; these essentially become codes. Although we like the building blocks analogy of MacQueen, McLellan-Lemal, Bartholow, and Milstein (2008), you may recall from Chapter One the "taking a road trip" analogy that we used to illustrate the research process. In keeping with this analogy, you can also think of codes as street signs that will help you navigate through unfamiliar neighborhoods (the vast amounts of text) and direct you to your final destination (theory development).

grounded theory
a general methodology for deriving a theory or theories from data systematically gathered and analyzed; it involves the analysts immersing themselves in the data so the meanings and relationships in the data can emerge

In contrast, if the research aims to answer a specific hypothesis, then the research approach should be **theory-driven**. In this instance, the theoretical constructs that guided the research methods and research questions can be mapped onto your codebook. Following the example we used in Chapter Eight, imagine that you are evaluating a family planning program in India and chose to use the Bruce-Jain framework to analyze transcripts from interviews with family planning nurses. This framework has been widely used to evaluate the quality of care in family planning programs around the world; it comprises six constructs (Bruce, 1990). You would use the constructs of this framework to map onto your research questions, as shown in Table 16.2.

theory-driven
an approach in which the research aims to answer a specific hypothesis

While you are determining the intent of your research, an important consideration is that, although QDA can be performed by one person, to ensure reliability and validity it is recommended that the codebook and the coding process occur in a team-based setting. In this chapter, we will guide you through a team-based approach to qualitative analysis of text-based data.

After the analysis approach is determined (theory-driven or grounded theory), the next step in developing a codebook is for two analysts to randomly select and read through thoroughly a subset of transcripts (approximately 10 to 20 percent). Through this independent review, each

Table 16.2 Example of Mapped Research Questions to Theoretical Main Codes

Research Question	Theoretical Main Codes
1. How are family planning services being provided in rural clinics?	Choice methods
2. What type of family planning information are patients receiving?	Information given to clients
3. How has the capacity to provide IUD services changed among nurse practitioners between 2005 and 2008?	Technical competence
4. What are the barriers experienced by nurse practitioners when providing family planning services?	Interpersonal relations
5. What are the strategies employed by nurse practitioners to encourage continuity of care?	Mechanisms to encourage continuity of care
6. What other types of services are being provided at rural clinics?	Appropriate constellation of services

analyst comes up with an initial list of codes and definitions. This independent review of codes is important, because it provides a mechanism for validating each code and a way to add detail on a definition that might have been missed by one analyst. When the two analysts meet to compare codes, they can effectively discuss and clarify definitions, remove redundant codes, and reach agreement on the master codebook (Hruschka, Schwartz, Cobb St. John, Picone-Decaro, Jenkins, and Carey, 2004; MacQueen, McLellan-Lemal, Bartholow, and Milstein, 2008; Patton, 2002). If applicable, this subset of transcripts should include different types of respondents. For instance, if your study includes physicians, patients, and hospital administrators, then your codebook should be developed from a mix of transcripts from these different types of respondents.

MacQueen, McLellan, Metzger, Kegeles, Strauss, and Scotti (2001) suggest following a codebook structure that includes the following components: the code, a brief definition, a full definition, guidelines for when to use the code, guidelines for when not to use the code, and examples. Each of these components helps the analysts determine whether the code is appropriate for a specific segment. Box 16.1 provides an example of a codebook entry that included these components, which was developed by MacQueen and colleagues as part of an analysis of *emic* (approaching the analysis from the perspective of a member of the community being studied; that is, an "insider") representations of "community" (MacQueen et al., 2001). In our studies, as many others have done, we have used a spreadsheet to develop our codebook. This helps with version control. As you may have been able to glean, codebook development is an iterative process, and you will undoubtedly have many versions until you agree upon the final codebook. Using a spreadsheet also allows the data manager to make and document changes, and it provides a template that can easily be shared with the rest of the team.

BOX 16.1. EXAMPLE OF CODEBOOK ENTRY

Code: MARGIN

  Brief. Definition: marginalized community members

  Full Definition: community groups that are negatively perceived as socially and/or physically outside the larger community structure. In marginalized groups, boundaries are imposed by others to keep "unfavorable" groups from participating in or interacting with the mainstream community groups.

  When to use: Apply this code to all references to groups of individuals that the larger community group has marginalized. These individuals or groups may be referred to as outcasts, extremists, and radicals or explicitly described as peripherals, strangers, outsiders, ostracized, bizarre, and the like.

  When not to use: Do not use this code for reference to community groups institutionalized for health or criminal reasons (see INSTIT) or for groups that have voluntarily placed themselves on the outer boundaries of community life (see SELFMAR).

  Example: "Then you got the outcast Blacks—drug dealers, junkies, prostitutes."

When you are using grounded theory, your codebook is developed as already stated, with both main codes and subcodes emerging from patterns in the data. For example, the first two authors in their study of African-American women who had experienced recent intimate partner violence and lived in high-risk areas for HIV infection found that women talked about how they responded to the abuse they incurred. This was an overarching concept that became a code "response to abuse"; however, several subcategories emerged and became subcodes (for example, "fights back," "leaves vicinity," "legal action").

When you are using a theory-driven analysis approach, the steps you take to develop your codebook are slightly different. In a theory-driven approach, the constructs of the theory or framework will be your main codes, and the subcodes of each code will emerge from the data. For example, in the same study of African-American women, we also used the theory of gender and power as a framework in our analyses and had "gender roles" as a code *a priori* to capture the theoretical construct of cathexis, but we found that for some of the women, "egalitarian" emerged as a subcode although contradictory to stereotypical gender roles. Even with a theoretical framework to guide you for your main codes, you would want to leave some flexibility for new main codes to emerge. In our example of the evaluation of a family planning program using the Bruce-Jain framework as the theoretical framework, all six constructs of this framework were used as theoretical main codes (the number of constructs you use from a framework will depend on your research questions). But imagine that as you are analyzing your data you notice that an important code is missing from the codebook. In this case, it would be appropriate for you to add the new main code that emerged from the data. An example of a theory-driven codebook with an additional new main code is provided in Table 16.3.

Coding Process

Intercoder Reliability. Once the two analysts have completed the first version of the codebook, the next step is to pretest the codebook by proceeding with the first round of coding of a subset of transcripts. Coding the data is a relatively simple task. As you read through the data, you systematically code with respect to the core concepts in your codebook. You can underline or highlight the units of data that apply to a particular

Table 16.3 Example of Main Codes and Subcodes Using a Theory-Driven Approach

Theoretical Main Codes	Subcode
1. **Choice methods**	• Availability of family planning methods
	• Limiting choice during family planning counseling
2. **Information given to clients**	• Availability of education materials
	• Family planning talks in waiting area
3. **Technical competence**	• Benefits of new equipment
	• Clinical difficulties when inserting IUDs
4. **Interpersonal relations**	• Scheduling system around provider needs
	• Increased communication between clinic departments
5. **Mechanisms to encourage continuity of care**	• Process of follow-up after IUD insertion
	• Referral procedures
6. **Appropriate constellation of services**	• STD testing available in the family planning clinic

Emergent Main Code	Subcode
7. **Perceived changes in quality (new code that emerged from the data)**	• Changes in scheduling procedures
	• Support from leadership

intercoder reliability
determined by comparing the application of the codes in each transcript and how the coders segmented the text

code while placing the assigned code in the margin (Sandelowski, 1995). In Box 16.2 we provide you with examples of two different transcripts that share the same code. This is coding by hand. It is important to note that there are myriad qualitative software packages available to facilitate the entire data-analysis process if desired (see the section on QDA software).

BOX 16.2. CODING EXAMPLE: EFFECTS OF ABUSE

Participant ID: 106

"Yeah like you just don't feel pretty and you don't feel like worth value or like nobody, I don't know like you're not worth—you know what I'm saying like maybe you deserved what is happening to you . . . "

Participant ID: 126

"It made me feel like, like I wasn't worth nothing like, for a second I'm just thinking like, I'm not worth nothing, if I sit here and a man, a boy hit me, I just thinking like, there's no point in me being here. So . . . then I try to leave, we tried not to be together, but wind up the same thing, we wind up getting back together."

---

percent agreement
a form of intercoder reliability that measures the percent of times that two coders agreed or disagreed in the coding of a text segment

After the first round of coding is completed, **intercoder reliability** analysis of the coded transcripts needs to be calculated. Intercoder reliability analysis entails comparing the application of the codes in each transcript and how the coders segmented the text (Carey and Gelaude, 2008; Carey, Morgan, and Oxtoby, 1996; Hruschka, Schwartz, Cobb St. John, Picone-Decaro, Jenkins, and Carey, 2004). It is extremely important to calculate intercoder reliability for an initial subset of transcripts because it measures the usefulness and validity of the codebook and helps the researcher accurately interpret the coded data. Clearly, you would not want to have the analysts code all of the transcripts only to find out the codebook was not valid and there was an unacceptable level of intercoder reliability.

Cohen's kappa
a form of intercoder reliability that accounts for agreement in coding that can occur due to chance

Although there are numerous measures or indices of intercoder reliability, the two most widely used measures for assessing intercoder reliability are **percent agreement** and **Cohen's kappa** (Cohen, 1960). Percent agreement is arrived at by simply calculating the number of times raters agree on a rating, then dividing by the total number of ratings. This measure can vary between 0 and 100 percent. Percent agreement is the most widely used measure because it is intuitively appealing and simple to calculate. However, we and other researchers recommend avoiding percent agreement to measure intercoder reliability; because it fails to account for agreement in coding that can occur due to chance, percent agreement may significantly miscalculate or inflate the true level of agreement (Carey, Morgan, and Oxtoby, 1996; Hruschka et al., 2004). Instead, we recommend using the *kappa statistic*, which takes into account agreement in coding that can occur due to chance and is a more stringent measure than percent agreement. If chance agreement is high, then the percent agreement will inflate the level of agreement that was actually due to a shared understanding of the codes and how they were applied. Kappa can be calculated by subtracting the estimated level of chance agreement from the observed level of agreement, then dividing by the maximum possible nonchance agreement. A level of agreement in the application of a code that is perfect or excellent would be equal to 1.00. Research by Hruschka and colleagues (2004) has demonstrated that a *kappa statistic* that is >.80 to .90 is an achievable target for intercoder reliability. Other research suggests that reaching a *kappa statistic* that is >.75 is also an acceptable target (Cicchetti, 1994; Fleiss, 1971).

It is to be expected that the first round of coding will produce low intercoder reliability; however, intercoder reliability can be significantly improved because, as mentioned previously, coding is an iterative process (Carey, Morgan, and Oxtoby, 1996; Hruschka et al., 2004). After intercoder reliability is performed, the coders meet to discuss discrepancies and questions about specific codes or text segments and to provide feedback on how to revise the codebook (for example, suggestions for new codes, clarifying a code definition) Any changes to the codebook need to be documented by saving the codebook as a new version; then the second round of coding proceeds. The same transcripts are recoded and an additional new subset of transcripts is selected so that the revised codebook can be tested with a fresh set of transcripts.

This process of coding, performing intercoder reliability, meeting with the coding team to review coded transcripts, and revising the codebook will likely occur many times until the team reaches a satisfactory level of intercoder reliability. For a manageable analysis and to facilitate intercoder reliability it is recommended that the number of codes be kept under 20 (Hruschka et al., 2004).

IN A NUTSHELL

This process of coding, performing intercoder reliability, meeting with the coding team to review coded transcripts, and revising the codebook will likely occur many times until the team reaches a satisfactory level of intercoder reliability.

Ultimately a high level of intercoder reliability can be achieved through this process as the coding team gains a better understanding of the data and the codebook (Carey and Gelaude, 2008; Hruschka et al., 2004; MacQueen et al., 2008; Patton, 2002).

As the researchers attempt to develop a reliable codebook and achieve a high level of intercoder reliability, it is essential that throughout this process the research question(s) being addressed be kept at the forefront. This may sound simple enough, but as researchers immerse themselves in qualitative data and coding meetings unfold, they can lose sight of the research question being addressed. To ensure that each code is relevant to the research questions, we recommend mapping your codebook in a spreadsheet to your research questions. This simple step can reveal the need to clarify codes, remove codes, or add new codes.

Using Memos

memos
written notes about data and the research process to provide additional context and insights documented during the course of the study

Memos—written notes about data and the research process—are extremely useful for the data analysis because they provide additional context and insights documented during the course of the study. Memos are different from field notes and annotated data. As mentioned previously in this chapter, annotations to the data are basic, additional factual information such as the interviewer's gender or the date the interview took place. Field notes are considered data that are collected during the course of the study; they refer to observations made specific to the research question and consist of descriptions of social interactions and the context in which they occurred (Roper and Shapira, 2000). For example, if a researcher was conducting interviews with commercial sex workers regarding their condom use behaviors with clients, the field notes would entail descriptions of the interaction with the sex worker during the interview, with details about the sex worker's responses to the questions and emotional reactions with possible interpretation of those reactions. Memos are not a description of the social context in which the research is taking place; rather, they are essentially the free-flowing thoughts of the researcher about what the data could mean, potential codes, possible relationships among different concepts or codes, notes about a theory or hypothesis, trends, or questions regarding the data (Glaser, 1998). Thus using memos should be a part of the coding process.

Field notes are data, whereas memos are an important tool to help researchers code and analyze the data; they should be used throughout the data analytic process. Researchers should write memos when they first start familiarizing themselves with the data by immersing themselves and reading and rereading. Memos can help researchers develop codes and the codebook and therefore should also be used during the coding process and interpretation of the data. Memos should always be linked to the appropriate data source. This can be done in the database that was created to manage and organize the data sources or with a QDA software package, if you are using one (see the following section). The analytic process can take months, so memos serve as important reminders of what the researcher was thinking at the beginning stages of analysis. Those initial memos can be compared to current memos and coded data, to help researchers piece together their conclusions or theory. Memos can vary in length and depth. They tend to start off with an idea or question and develop into more comprehensive narrative of what the data could mean. Memos can be written in a notebook, binders, word processing document, or QDA software. Whatever method you use to write your memos, just make sure that they are organized so that they are easily retrievable.

In our analysis process, we have found the following guidelines to be helpful when writing memos:

1. Label the memo. The label will depend on the intent of the memo and the complexity of your data. You can use a participant ID as the label; this helps if the participant said something very important or something that contradicts another participant. You can also use codes, when a memo relates or expands on a specific code.

2. Date your memo. This will help you keep track of your thought process during analysis and go back over your steps when needed.

3. Reference the transcript. Copy short quotes from transcripts into the memo and write a reflection on what potential new insights the excerpt has triggered or what concepts seem to be emerging.

4. Keep writing and revising memos. As you update your memos they should be getting more complex and closer to your results.

5. Relax! Memos are meant to be reflective; let your ideas flow.

In Box 16.3 we provide a couple of examples of memos written for a study that explores the relationship between gender-based violence and HIV infection.

BOX 16.3. EXAMPLE MEMOS

Initial memo	Memo during analysis
Date: 7/7/13	Date: 7/21/13
Topic: Partner's history of unfaithfulness	Topic: Partner's history of unfaithfulness
Did participants report that their partners were unfaithful? What (if anything) did participants do?	Most participants didn't do anything about their partner's cheating. In fact, they seem to just tolerate or cope with it . . . .
	Participant ID: 23
	"We talked about everything good, it was, you know, um, I guess when I became sober I could feel a lot of stuff, him going out, doing other stuff, when I'm high I don't pay that no attention. I don't notice that you got a girl across the street [laughs] you know?"

Qualitative Data Analysis Software

The first thing to know about QDA software is that it is a tool designed to help you manage and organize your coding and data analyses rather than a software package that *conducts* the analyses. You will not receive output that provides definitive results of a particular statistical test. In this context the researcher, rather than the QDA software, performs the analyses. Unlike the practice in much quantitative research—with a statistician brought in to conduct the analyses after data collection, who may or may not have been involved in the data collection or even other aspects of the design—qualitative analyses typically are performed by members of the research team who were involved from the beginning. Usually qualitative researchers are involved from the very start of the journey to the end, in that they develop the research question; decide on the strategy, data collection tools and methods, and codes; and write memos, develop diagrams, and find meaning in the data. A QDA software program cannot perform an analysis for you, but it can certainly help you with the coding process, as you can upload the codebook into the software along with your memos and then assign codes from your codebook to the selected text with a click of the mouse. A QDA software package can also easily help you to identify the major themes for your results by generating matrices of data by codes, creating models or diagrams, and showing overlapping themes. Moreover, many will calculate intercoder reliability and can also assist with the write-up by displaying all data assigned to certain codes so that illustrative quotes can be identified. Several QDA software packages have been developed and improved over the past couple of decades:

- **Paid QDA software**. QSR N6, ATLAS.ti 7, Ethnograph 6, QSR NVivo 10, MAXQDA, QDA Miner Lite, and others
- **Free QDA software**. CDC AnSWR, CDC EZ-Text, University of Pittsburgh CAT, and others

Although we do not compare each of these packages in terms of characteristics, we do delineate the pros and cons of using a QDA software package in Box 16.4, and as you can see, the pros outweigh the cons. The QDA software you choose will depend on your personal preference, budget, number of analysts, timeframe, sample size, and the complexity of the research. For instance, if your study has a small sample (fewer than 10 participants), your transcripts are short, and your timeframe is urgent, it probably makes more sense for you to code your data "old school" (by hand). On the other hand, if your sample size has more than 30 participants, your transcripts are long and complicated, and your team has more than three analysts, then we recommend using a QDA software package.

BOX 16.4. BENEFITS AND DISADVANTAGES OF USING A QDA SOFTWARE PACKAGE

Benefits:

- Provides a mechanism for organizing and managing large amounts of data
- Facilitates retrieval of coded data
- Makes it easy to modify raw data, codebook, and coding
- Supports the analysis of multiple types of data sources (such as Microsoft Word documents, PDFs, pictures)
- Creates professional diagrams
- Allows for transparency and replicability of analyses
- Can conduct word searches or queries to facilitate coding of text
- Facilitates team-based analysis (especially useful if analysts are in multiple locations)
- Can analyze multiple research questions
- Enables detailed systematic analysis
- Enables matrix comparisons by participant and code, or between two or more codes
- Allows the addition of attributions to data sources (such as city, type of participant)
- Performs intercoder reliability and percent analysis
- Allows incorporation of memos and links to codes or data sources
- Allows importing and coding of literature
- Includes support services from the vendor via email, phone, or social media

Disadvantages:

- Its use is time-consuming.
- Data could be vulnerable to computer and software glitches, so saving multiple copies each time is *key* to helping you keep your analysis on track.
- Licenses for paid software can be expensive.

Analysis Considerations for Triangulation

As we covered in Chapter Eight, **triangulation**—defined as the combination of multiple researchers, theories, methods, and data sources within a study—can be used to *confirm* results and have a more *complete* analysis.

triangulation
the combination of multiple researchers, theories, methods, and data sources within a study

Results can be confirmed when multiple data sources yield the same conclusions, and an analysis is more complete when it is studied from multiple perspectives. When conducting your analysis, it is important to keep in mind the purposes of triangulation so that you can create a clear plan that outlines your approach to triangulation when conducting your analyses. We recommend creating a table that maps research questions, methods, and data sources, and explains how the data will be triangulated (see Box 16.5). Returning to our "taking a trip" analogy, this table is akin to having a detailed roadmap that you can use to direct you along your research journey so that you can safely and efficiently arrive at your destination—which in this journey analogy represents analyzing the data and answering your research question.

IN A NUTSHELL

When conducting your analysis, it is important to keep in mind the purposes of triangulation so that you can create a clear plan that outlines your approach to triangulation when conducting your analyses.

BOX 16.5. EXAMPLE OF A TRIANGULATION PLAN

Research Question	Qualitative Data	Quantitative Data
What are the factors that facilitate and hinder collaboration between providers who are working to transition prisoners to HIV community care?	· Five focus groups with DOC staff · Thirty interviews with state services representatives and community HIV providers	Survey measuring demographics, case load, attitudes regarding HIV care, and so on

How will data be triangulated?

- Focus group data will be triangulated by comparing and contrasting across focus groups (confirmation) and quantitative data (completeness).

- Interview data will be triangulated by comparing and contrasting across interviews (confirmation) and quantitative data (completeness).

- Focus group data will be triangulated with interview data (confirmation and completeness).

How you set up your dataset is very important in your analysis process. Triangulation can be performed within one dataset for various types of data sources, theories, investigators, and qualitative methods (that is, interviews, focus groups, and the like). You can create data folders for different sites (space data triangulation) or data collection methods (interviews and focus groups) or even set up your codebook using constructs of multiple theories (theory triangulation). The key lies in organizing your data folders and code book in a manner that will facilitate the answers to your research questions.

For example, if you wanted to compare risk reduction programs with sex workers in three states, each data folder would represent a state. Transcripts within each data folder (state) could be designated to one or two coders. Once the data are coded, then you could begin running various QDA functions that allow the comparison of codes across sites and facilitate your interpretation. Here we would like to remind you that even though the QDA program provides you with an output, your analysis is far from complete. The next step in this process would be for you to read through the output(s), and identify the themes of the segments coded.

When you are conducting a between-methods triangulation (the use of both qualitative and quantitative approaches to answer the same research questions) your approach to triangulation will depend on whether data collection and analysis are **simultaneous triangulation** or **sequential triangulation**.

Simultaneous Data Analysis

In simultaneous analysis the data are merged through one of the following approaches:

- *Data transformation.* To make comparisons easier to perform, a qualitative dataset can be transformed into a quantitative dataset by reducing codes into numbers (for example, dichotomous variable of 0 and 1 identifying the presence or absence of a code). Even though most QDA programs have basic quantitative analysis features, we recommend you use a statistical package such as SPSS or SAS for your quantitative analysis so you can perform more complex statistical analyses.

- *Comparing the data using a matrix and team discussion.* A matrix is a useful tool when researchers need to determine if there are differences among participants or how coded text intersects. A matrix can be created by hand or by using the matrix query feature of your QDA software. If the aim is to determine differences in the use of codes among participants, a

simultaneous triangulation method in which both qualitative and quantitative data are collected and analyzed at the same time

sequential triangulation method in which the results of one approach are used to design and implement the other approach

matrix can be created in which rows represent codes and columns represent participants. This would give researchers a count of how many times the code was used among each participant. Alternatively, if the aim was to determine how the coded text intersects, then the rows and columns could be set up according to the type of code. Then the information on the matrix can easily be discussed among the research team (Creswell and Plano Clark, 2007). An example of a matrix that shows frequency of codes by participants is provided in Box 16.6.

BOX 16.6. EXAMPLE OF MATRIX BY MAIN CODES AND PARTICIPANTS

Main Code	Transcripts				
	A: Participant 110	B: Participant 105	C: Participant 106	D: Participant 111	E: Participant 113
1: Characteristics of Abuse	25	4	1	12	78
2: Negative Coping Strategies	0	0	0	2	3
3: Help Seeking	3	1	1	0	8
4: Sexual Relationship	9	3	4	10	28

Sequential Data Analysis

In sequential analysis the data are analyzed separately, and how they are analyzed depends on the type of data that are collected first. If quantitative data are collected first, then the qualitative data are used to supplement specific quantitative findings. Thus it is important to determine which quantitative findings will be explored further in the qualitative phase of that study before data collection begins. Likewise, when qualitative data are collected first, the findings from this phase are used as a foundation for the quantitative phase. For example, Bailey and Hutter (2008) conducted a study in Goa, India, in which they triangulated in-depth interviews and focus groups to develop and administer a survey. The researchers first conducted in-depth interviews with migrant men to increase their understanding of how these men perceive their risk of HIV infection. Data from the interviews were analyzed and used to develop vignettes for the focus group guide so as to stimulate discussion among participants regarding risk behaviors (it seems that participants found it easier to discuss risk behaviors of a fictitious individual). This triangulation of data allowed researchers to first validate the data collected in the interviews and then identify other risk behaviors. Afterward, qualitative findings were used to develop a quantitative survey that was locally informed.

Interpretation

In Chapter Eight we alluded to qualitative research being very much like a patchwork quilt, in that those seemingly small and disparate pieces of cloth, when stitched together, form something beautiful and demonstrate a greater meaning or purpose and cohesiveness. In this analogy, interpretation of the data represents the quilt. Interpretation of the data requires deriving a deeper and greater meaning from the main **themes**; their interconnections are then derived from a cursory printing of the most frequent codes and associated quotes. This is the point at which you move from codes to themes; however, before we continue, we want to avoid any confusion students and researchers alike may have regarding the difference between codes and themes. A theme emerges from the data, in the sense that you examine all of your data associated with a particular code and look for some underlying meaning to make sense of it all—in other words, to tell the story. Themes at this stage are the *result* of coding and deep reflective analysis of the coded data (try thinking like *The Thinker*). Whereas codes represent explicit observations of the concepts, themes represent more deeper, nuanced levels that are perhaps implied. For example, *social support* could be assigned as a code; however, *social support as a buffer of abuse* would be a theme. As mentioned previously, data analysis for qualitative research cannot be prescribed in the same way as quantitative analyses. Unfortunately, there is no *P*-value to examine or adjusted odds ratios to compare, so it is difficult to provide definitive procedures or one right method to come to an interpretation. The best we can do is provide guidance that may facilitate the process, but with the caveat that this process will depend, to a large degree, on the researcher's understanding of the sampled population, the issue or phenomenon under study, and their intimate relationship with the data.

themes
abstract constructs that investigators identify before, during, or after data collection

Conduct Coding Sorts

You may have interpreted the expression "The devil is in the details" as referring to some mysterious element hidden in the details; actually, it suggests that attending to the details is where the real challenge lies. This expression is appropriate for QDA, as at times it may feel like there is something hidden in all of the text (not a devil, we hope) and your task is to reveal it. Undergoing the lengthy process of coding, reading, rereading, and becoming intimate with the data, although not a certainty, should nonetheless produce several "aha!" moments when the main themes emerge from hiding. It is important to note that some of these themes, depending on the research question, may constitute a main theme, whereas others will be considered less important but nevertheless a part of the quilt.

coding sort

a compilation of similarly coded blocks of text from different sources into a single file or report

At this stage, it is very helpful to the interpretation to conduct a **coding sort** that initially focuses on the main themes. A coding sort is a "compilation of similarly coded blocks of text from different sources into a single file or report" (Ulin, Robinson, and Tolley, 2005, p. 142). If you can select, either copying and pasting if using a Microsoft Word document or through your QDA software, all the text associated with a particular code and put it all together in one document, then you will begin to grasp the more subtle nuances and implied underlying meaning and stitch it together.

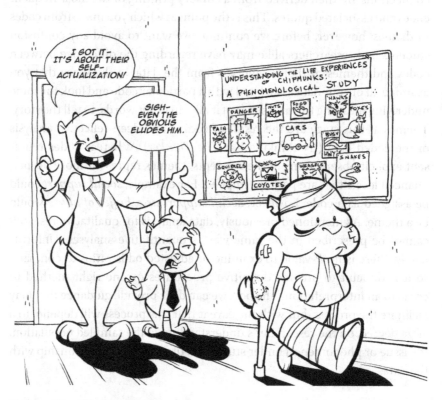

Dincus Has His "Aha!" Moment

Copyright 2014 by Justin Wagner; reprinted with permission.

The subtle nuances can be understood by examining whether the coded text reveals similar meanings or interpretations across all sets of focus groups and interviews, under different contexts, for all subgroups or by gender. Reading through the code sort, you may now begin to see subthemes emerging as well. For example, in the first two authors' study of African-American women who had experienced recent intimate partner violence, a code sort on the code "Social Support" showed social support was not simply having family and friends with whom they could discuss their abusive situations or partners. Initially, text that illustrated an expression of having a friend or family member to talk with about their abusive partner or ask for advice about what to do was coded as "Social Support"; however, once we performed a coding sort and reread all of the text, it became clear that social support had subtle nuances suggesting that it was not one-dimensional; rather, social support should be qualified as either negative or positive. We found that some women expressed that family or friends blamed them for the abuse they experienced—"What did you do to make him mad?"—or felt family or friends had pressured them to "just leave him." We deemed that these interactions were victim-blaming, trivializing, or expressions of frustration by the social support network and therefore were "negative" support. When women conveyed that a family member or friend provided emotional support along the lines of "My Mom said if I don't feel that the relationship is right for me, then I should get out of it," it was deemed "positive" social support. These two new subthemes revealed a new meaning that could be connected with other codes, such as "effects of abuse," to see how the "positive" social support subtheme might be less connected to "effects of abuse" than the "negative" social support, suggesting that positive social support may buffer women.

Other tactics to consider include looking for a particular context for what you are examining. Does the sociopolitical, cultural, or historical context provide a deeper level of understanding to the findings? Are there mixed or contradictory findings, and if so, how do they vary, and by what measures and other factors (such as different people involved, different locations) do they vary? The idea is to identify any variations in these factors (such as different subgroups) in addition to determining how some variations may subsequently constitute a subtheme that needs further exploration. Connecting themes to other themes or subthemes, although a complicated process, can be accomplished by generating matrices using QDA software.

Use Diagrams

Another way to examine relationships among themes that is key to the interpretation process is to generate a diagram or a **coding tree**. A coding tree is a specific type of diagram that shows the hierarchical connections among themes and the corresponding subthemes. Diagrams can help researchers organize the data in a visual way that can provide more of a bird's-eye view of the phenomenon being studied. Sometimes QDA can feel like you cannot see the forest for the trees, meaning that the analysis can become so overwhelming and detailed, due to the voluminous amount of data and codes, that it becomes difficult to see the bigger picture or the larger meaning. Diagrams trigger new insights and indicate areas that

coding tree
a diagram that shows the hierarchical connections among themes and the corresponding subthemes

warrant further thought or action (such as recoding, conducting additional interviews, asking different questions). Diagrams help researchers understand how themes function and coexist within a specific paradigm. Like memos, diagrams start off simple and develop into a more complex set of relationships. What is important is that you take the time to do them. Start off developing your diagrams on a white piece of paper, and then transfer that diagram into a Microsoft Word document or PowerPoint presentation (we have found PowerPoint to be very user-friendly in this task). As your analysis progresses, take the time to update your diagram. (We often update our diagrams by copying and pasting a diagram slide into the same PowerPoint file, so that we can view how the diagram has progressed within the same document and can go back if an update does not make sense.) Many QDA software packages also enable you to create diagrams of "nodes" and base them on thematic relationships or other characteristics of the participants, such as gender, race or ethnicity, or role, such as being a stakeholder.

For example, imagine that you are hired to conduct an evaluation of the level of collaborations between a Department of Corrections (DOC) and community and state services in providing services for recently released HIV-positive prisoners. In your initial attempt to understand these collaborations you create a simple diagram that depicts collaborations among the DOC, the community, and the state (see Figure 16.1). Your data collection methods include conducting key informant interviews and focus groups with DOC staff, community providers, and representatives of state programs. As your analysis of these transcripts progresses, your diagram evolves to a more complex analysis of collaborations (see Figure 16.2); now it depicts specific collaborations and lack of collaborations both among the DOC, community services, and state services and within each of these arenas.

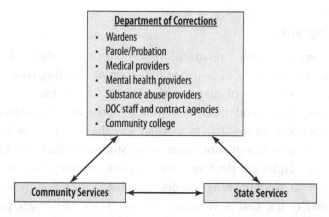

Figure 16.1 Initial Diagram on Collaborations

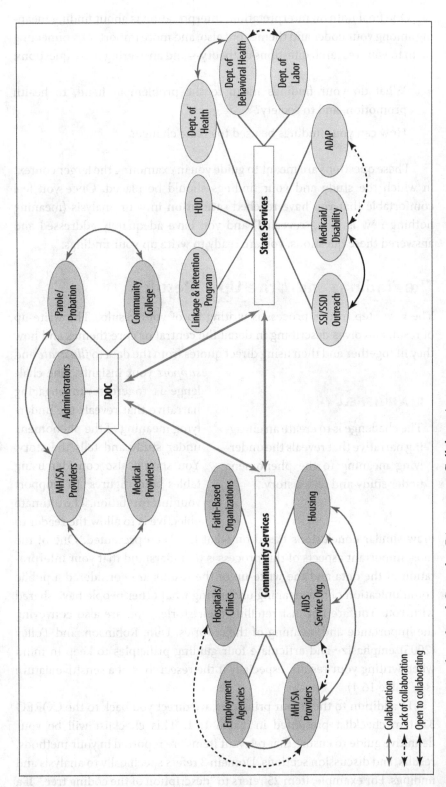

Figure 16.2 More Developed and Complex Diagram on Collaborations

Collaboration
Lack of collaboration
Open to collaborating

State Services
Dept. of Health
Dept. of Behavioral Health
Dept. of Labor
HUD
Linkage & Retention Program
Medicaid/Disability
ADAP
SSI/SSDI Outreach

DOC
Parole/Probation
Community College
Administrators
MH/SA Providers
Medical Providers

Community Services
Faith-Based Organizations
Hospitals/Clinics
Employment Agencies
MH/SA Providers
AIDS Service Org.
Housing

One final note on interpretation: Interpretation is about finding meaning among your codes and themes but also, and more important, connecting them to your research questions or theory—and answering these questions:

- What do your findings mean to the problem at hand, to health promotion, and to society?
- How can your findings be used to create change?

saturation
the point at which nothing new is being revealed in the data analysis

These questions are meant to guide you in examining the larger context in which the study and your findings should be placed. Once you feel comfortable that you have reached **saturation** in your analysis (meaning nothing new is being revealed) and you have adequately addressed and answered these questions, you are ready to write up your findings.

The Findings and Write-Up of Results

The next step in this process is writing up of your results. The write-up of results involves describing in detail the central or core themes and how they fit together and then using direct quotes from the data to *illustrate* and *support* your insights. The challenge is to create an engaging narrative that reveals the underlying meaning of the phenomena under study and tells the story. You should also consider using tables and figures to support your interpretation. The ultimate objective is to allow the reader to draw similar conclusions based on what has been presented. One of the most important aspects of this process is to understand that your interpretation of the data and the write-up of the results are considered a public communication of the meaning underlying what other people have shared with you. You are not just retelling their stories; you are also conveying the importance and meaning of their stories. Ulin, Robinson, and Tolley (2005) emphasize and articulate four guiding principles to keep in mind when writing your results, especially if the research is of a sensitive nature (see Table 16.4).

In addition to these four principles, we direct you back to the COREQ 32-item checklist presented in Table 16.1. This checklist will be your definitive guide to ensure that relevant items are reported in your methods, results, and discussion sections. Domain 3 refers specifically to analysis and findings. For example, item 25 refers to "description of the coding tree." If a

> **IN A NUTSHELL**
>
> The challenge is to create an engaging narrative that reveals the underlying meaning to the phenomena under study and tells a story.

Table 16.4 Four Basic Principles for Writing Qualitative Results

Principle	Description
Ensure balance and accuracy.	In reporting findings, aim for balance and accuracy, not neutrality. Present multiple sides of the particular issue being studied. Elicit the knowledge, understandings, and insights of the research participants, and represent their insights in context.
Ensure no harm to participants.	Ensure that no harm comes to those interviewed as a result of their participation and as a result of the publication, presentation, or dissemination of their views or experiences. Even when the published work does not give names, information could reveal the identity of some participants.
Give public voice to findings by sharing participants' own words.	Present participants' insights in their own words. Try to include quotes or even brief phrases (in participants' original language, along with translation).
Describe the context of your interactions and disclose your role.	Readers must have adequate details on when and how you gathered information, awareness of the nature of your relationship with those studied, and knowledge of your standpoint and motivation in carrying out the study. Also, state all sources of funding for the work.

Source: Adapted from Ulin, Robinson, and Tolley (2005), p. 176. With permission.

diagram of a coding tree was included in the results, then an accompanying description of the tree must also be included. We strongly suggest that you use this checklist when preparing your report or journal article, as it will assist you in preparing a comprehensive and logical presentation of the results.

Although there are myriad ways to approach the write-up of results, in health promotion research we generally use the research questions as a guide to organizing the choice of main themes to present. We typically present the themes sequentially using subheadings, followed by a description of the theme that provides its meaning, and then illustrative quote(s). Quotes should clearly reflect the theme but also convey the participants' emotions or feelings. Try to select quotes from a range of participants rather than pulling from one or two of the most articulate participants. Also, use pseudonyms rather than real names to protect identities and to personalize the quotes. Following the quotes, we also include an interpretation and provide context. For example, in the study we mentioned previously, on African-American women who experienced intimate partner violence, although many main codes emerged, initially our main codes were based on our theoretical framework (theory of gender and power), and our analysis revealed a main theme that paralleled the main code of one of the theoretical constructs, cathexis. We found that many women indicated that their male partner adhered to stereotypical gender roles. We further interpreted this finding in the context of HIV risk. This presentation is shown in Box 16.7. As indicated, you can see how the theme is presented first as a subheading. The theme is defined and corresponding quotes are provided. We also present how this theme relates to the concept of condom use negotiation in a context of a sexual double standard.

BOX 16.7. EXAMPLE OF A WRITE-UP OF A THEME

Presence of Cathexis

Across participants, the presence of cathexis—which theorizes that individuals perceive and conform to societally prescribed gender roles and behavioral norms that support women to behave or act as nurturing, passive, and obsequious and men as dominant, aggressive, and strong—emerged, as did a sexual double standard. Stereotypical gender roles may place a woman at increased risk for HIV by decreasing the amount of control she can exert in not only everyday contexts but also sexual contexts. Many women described their partner's adherence to stereotypical gender roles:

"Yes, he wants me to wait on him hand and foot. And wash his clothes, cook for him, serve him, you know, I do all the house cleaning, the ironing, and all of that stuff."

—Brenda

"He says that a woman's place is in the home. And that he should be the one that worked, and I [should] stay home and wait on the kids and wait on him."

—Sonia

Adherence to stereotypical gender roles is also congruent with maintaining a sexual double standard in which men are rewarded socially for their sexual promiscuity whereas women are punished and vilified. Women spoke of having to "prove their fidelity" by not asking their male partners to use a condom, thereby increasing their risk for HIV. One woman described this as follows:

"We didn't use a condom all this time, so why start now? [If I asked him to wear a condom] he'd probably get mad and probably say, 'Oh you must cheating on me.'"

—Donna

In this particular study of African-American women, because our sample was homogeneous, we could not examine variations of this theme by subgroups; however, if you explored the possibility of variations by subgroups during your data analysis, then you would want to present that as part of the results. Once you present your main themes in this manner, if appropriate, you could then provide a diagram that depicts the connections among the themes or other concepts along with an interpretation and contextual perspective.

In your write-up, you could also incorporate quantitative data that helps to support your qualitative findings. For example, when presenting your themes, it may be helpful for readers to know the prevalence of these themes occurring in your sample. For example, in our study of 48 African American women, we found that 33 women had reported a presence of stereotypical gender roles in their relationships. Although this is very useful information in that it provides additional evidence, it is critical to understand the purpose of presenting quantitative data in a qualitative research study. In this example, the majority of the study population (69 percent) reporting this theme provides support *only* for the idea that the main theme is relatively important; it is not meant to suggest that the results should be generalized to all African-American women or that the theme is representative of all African-American women. Thus we encourage the use of quantitative data to enhance the understanding of and add depth to the qualitative results rather than to suggest there is a higher level of generalizability of the data. When using quantitative data in this manner, you could weave it into the narrative when presenting each theme (for example, "Many of the women (69 percent) suggested that . . . "), or you could create a table that showcases the themes in one column and the frequencies of participants who reported the theme at least once in the other column. Returning to our quilt analogy, it may be helpful to view the inclusion of quantitative data as another square or piece of your quilt; although it should not be highlighted as a prominent piece or placed in the center, it nonetheless should be integral to the overall design—much like a border.

Finally, after your results have been written, in addition to the usual points made in the discussion section of a journal article (see Chapter Seventeen), for qualitative research, reflexivity should be a part of your write-up to acknowledge bias. If you refer back to Table 16.1, you can see that domain 1 involves providing content related to the research team and reflexivity. Some researchers suggest reporting how one's preconceptions, beliefs, values, assumptions, and position may have come into play during the research process. To provide an idea of how to report this, an example would be useful. Cohen and Crabtree (2008) conducted a content analysis of qualitative research in health care with the aim of establishing criteria to be used when evaluating qualitative research studies. The following text illustrates how biases can be acknowledged:

"Our perspectives affect this report. Both authors received doctoral training in qualitative methods in social science disciplines (sociology/communication and anthropology) and have assimilated these values into health care as reviewers, editors, and active participants in qualitative health care studies. Our training shapes our beliefs, so we feel most aligned with interpretivism. This grounding influences how we see qualitative research, as well as the perspectives and voices we examine in this analysis" (p. 335).

Summary

In the discipline of health promotion, the use of rigorous qualitative research methods has become much more commonplace, used either on their own or as part of mixed-methods studies, reflecting a need for a more in-depth understanding of community and clinical settings and the importance of context when implementing health promotion research and interventions. This chapter has presented an overview of basic strategies and methods used when approaching analysis of qualitative data, its interpretation, and the write-up of results. Because of the increased acceptance and uptake of qualitative research methods in more quantitative disciplines, we highlighted the consolidated criteria for reporting qualitative studies (COREQ), which was developed to guide both new and seasoned qualitative researchers and entails a 32-item checklist that is very useful when planning a qualitative study and in the reporting of the findings. We made a point of highlighting the importance of reflexivity during the process to ensure that researchers and consumers of research studies understand the researcher's perspective underlying the qualitative inquiry and how it may have affected the study and the results. Although analysis of qualitative data involves a lengthy process that is typically ongoing and begins during data collection rather than being the culmination, there are still systematic procedures that should be used for data management and codebook development. In addition, triangulation of data and intercoder reliability are two strategies that can enhance rigor and validity. A key theme that we hope emerged is that although qualitative data can assume many forms (audio, video, pictures, maps, text, words, and so on), there are usually commonalities that can be found and will become evident once an intimate relationship has been established between the data and the researcher(s). These commonalities begin as codes; once a deeper meaning has been derived, themes emerge. Presenting the connections among themes and subthemes through text, illustrative quotes, and diagrams will help convey the deeper meaning. The result should tell an engaging story within a historical, social, or political context while providing answers to research questions that could not be gleaned through quantitative methods or by describing a brand new theoretical framework.

KEY TERMS

Annotating the data	Percent agreement
Code	Reflexivity
Codebook	Saturation
Coding sort	Sequential triangulation
Coding tree	Simultaneous triangulation
Cohen's kappa	Themes
Concept	Theory-driven
Grounded theory	Triangulation
Intercoder reliability	Verbatim
Memos	

For Practice and Discussion

1. As obesity is a significant public health issue with multilevel determinants, researchers are interested in developing a new theory that will help explain the complex interrelationships among these determinants. A qualitative research study was conducted among 100 individuals who were considered obese according to their body mass index. The data collected included digital recordings of face-to-face semistructured interviews, interviewer notes, geospatial data, addresses of participants, and satellite photos of the neighborhoods where participants lived. You have been hired to be a part of the data analysis team. What would be your first order of business? How would you approach development of the codebook? What are the critical issues to take into consideration? As there were multiple interviewers and multiple data sources, what type of triangulation was implemented?

2. You are part of a qualitative research team that is investigating adolescents' perceptions of advertising for marketing of conventional cigarettes, electronic cigarettes, chewing tobacco, hookahs, snubs, flavored cigars, and dissolvable tobacco products (such as Camel strips). When you were a child, your grandfather died of lung cancer after smoking for 40 years (he started smoking at age 15). Discuss the importance of reflexivity in this study and what steps you think should have been taken to foster it. How would you approach the data analysis and the write-up?

3. As part of a research study that was a phenomenological study to assess what "safe sex" means to teenagers, you notice that a member of the data analysis team seems to be confused about the difference between a code and a theme. Discuss the differences between the two and make up examples for this research study. Prepare a sample write-up for one of the themes.

4. Read a journal article that involves an empirical qualitative study in public health. Using the COREQ (32-item checklist), see if you can identify how many of the items were reported in the article. Pull examples from the article to illustrate some of the items and report which items were not found.

References

Bailey, A., and Hutter, I. (2008). Qualitative to quantitative: Linked trajectory of method triangulation in a study on HIV/AIDS in Goa, India. *AIDS Care*, *20*(9), 1119–1124.

Bruce, J. (1990). Fundamental elements of the quality of care: A simple framework. *Studies in Family Planning*, *21*(2), 61–91.

Carey, J. W., and Gelaude, D. (2008). Systematic methods for collecting and analyzing multidisciplinary team-based qualitative data. In: G. Guest and K. M. MacQueen (Eds.), *Handbook for team-based qualitative research* (pp. 227–274). Plymouth, UK: Altamira Press.

Carey, J. W., Morgan, M., and Oxtoby, M. J. (1996). Intercoder agreement in analysis of responses to open-ended interview questions: Examples from tuberculosis research. *Cultural Anthropology Methods*, *8*(3), 1–5.

Cicchetti, D. V. (1994). Guidelines, criteria, and rules of thumb for evaluating normed and standardized assessment instruments in psychology. *Psychological Assessment*, *6*, 284–290.

Cohen, J. (1960). A coefficient of agreement for nominal scales. *Educational and Psychosocial Measurement*, *20*, 37–46.

Cohen, D. J., and Crabtree, B. (2008). Evaluative criteria for qualitative research in health care: controversies and recommendations. *Annals of Family Medicine*, *6*(4), 331–339.

Creswell, J. W., and Plano Clark, V. L. (2007). *Designing and conducting mixed methods research*. Thousand Oaks, CA: Sage.

Fleiss, J. L. (1971). Measuring nominal scale agreement among many raters. *Psychological Bulleting*, *76*(5), 378–382.

Glaser, B. G. (1998). *Doing grounded theory*. Mill Valley, CA: Sociology Press.

Hennink, M. M. (2007). *International focus group research*. New York: Cambridge University Press.

Hruschka, D. J., Schwartz, D., Cobb St. John, D., Picone-Decaro, E., Jenkins, R. A., and Carey, J. W. (2004). Reliability in coding open-ended data: Lessons learned from HIV Behavioral Research. *Field Methods, 16*(3), 307–331.

Hsiung, P.C. (2010). Lives and legacies: A guide to qualitative interviewing. Retrieved from http://www.utsc.utoronto.ca/~pchsiung/LAL/home

Lofland, J., and Lofland, L. (1995). *Analyzing social settings* (3rd ed.). Belmont, CA: Wadsworth.

MacQueen, K. M., McLellan-Lemal, E., Bartholow, K., and Milstein, B. (2008). Team-based codebook development: Structure, process, and agreement. In G. Guest and K. M. MacQueen (Eds.), *Handbook for team-based qualitative research* (pp. 119–136). Plymouth, UK: Altamira Press.

MacQueen, K. M., McLellan, E., Metzger, D., Kegeles, S., Strauss, R., Scotti, R., Trotter, R. T. II. (2001). What is community? An evidence-based definition for participatory public health. *American Journal of Public Health, 91*(12), 1929–1938.

Malterud, K. (2001). Qualitative research: Standards, challenges and guidelines. *The Lancet, 358*, 483–488.

Miles, M. B., and Huberman, A. M. (1984). *Qualitative data analysis: A sourcebook of new methods*. Thousand Oaks, CA: Sage.

Miles, M. B., and Huberman, A. M. (1994). *Qualitative data analysis: An expanded source book* (2nd ed.). Thousand Oaks, CA: Sage.

Miller, W. L., and Crabtree, B. F. (1999). The dance of interpretation. In B. F. Crabtree and W. L. Miller (Eds.), *Doing qualitative research* (2nd ed., pp. 127–144). Thousand Oaks, CA: Sage.

Onwuegbuzie, A. J., and Wilson, V. A. (2003). Statistics anxiety: Nature, etiology, antecedents, effects, and treatments—A comprehensive review of the literature. *Teaching in Higher Education, 8*(2), 195–209. doi:10.1080/13562510 32000052447

Patton, M. Q. (2002). *Qualitative research & evaluation methods*. Thousand Oaks, CA: Sage.

Roper, J. M., and Shapira, J. (2000). *Ethnography in nursing research*. Thousand Oaks, CA: Sage.

Sandelowski, M. (1995). Qualitative analysis: What it is and how to begin. *Research in Nursing and Health, 18*, 371–375.

Strauss, A. L., and Corbin, J. (1990). *Basics of qualitative research: Grounded theory procedures and techniques*. Thousand Oaks, CA: Sage.

Strauss, A., and Corbin, J. (1994). Grounded theory methodology: An overview. In N. K. Denzin and J. S. Lincoln (Eds.), *Handbook of qualitative research* (pp. 273–285). Thousand Oaks, CA: Sage.

Tong, A., Sainsbury, P., and Craig, J. (2007). Consolidated criteria for reporting qualitative research (COREQ): A 32-item checklist for interviews and focus groups. *International Journal for Quality in Health Care, 19*(6), 349–357. doi:10.1093/intqhc/mzm042

Ulin, P. R., Robinson, E. T., and Tolley, E. E. (2005). *Qualitative methods in public health: A field guide for applied research*. San Francisco: Jossey-Bass.

PART FIVE

CORE SKILLS RELATED TO HEALTH PROMOTION RESEARCH

CHAPTER 17

INTRODUCTION TO SCIENTIFIC WRITING

Richard A. Crosby
Ralph J. DiClemente
Laura F. Salazar

In many ways, the hallmark of a successful scholar is publication in peer-reviewed journals. In turn, journal editors have an obligation to publish only those reports of rigorous research that are written in a precise manner. In essence, having data from a rigorous study is not enough—it must be brought to life through skilled writing. Fortunately, academic tradition has created a fairly routine method of writing papers that report empirical findings. It is this method that must become a part of your acumen as a scholar. To that end, this chapter is devoted to teaching you the method known as scientific writing.

Students, practitioners, and researchers in the discipline of health promotion often experience a great deal of anxiety when they hear the admonition "publish or perish." Publishing should actually be thought of as an extension of the research enterprise—the necessary and logical endpoint of research efforts. Publishing is just one component of the larger and more important process of health promotion research. Nonetheless, the published report is indeed a critical piece of dissemination (see step nine of the nine-step model in Figure 1.5). Therefore researchers should be well versed in the art of scientific writing. We include the word "*art*" because there are few universal standards with respect to the construction of manuscripts that report findings from health promotion research. Publishing your work is not only a critical part of the scientific enterprise and a contribution to the knowledge base; scientific journal articles are essentially the "currency" by which all researchers

LEARNING OBJECTIVES

- Be able to skillfully select a journal that best matches your study findings.

- Be able to construct the abstract, introduction, methods, results, and discussion sections.

- Understand the complementary relationship of tables and figures to the written words of the results section.

- Differentiate between APA writing style and biomedical writing styles.

- Create conclusions that correspond directly to the stated research questions.

including health promotion researchers are judged. Without a record of publications, it is extremely difficult to obtain consideration for external federal funding.

One of the best strategies that will help you master scientific writing is to become an avid reader of journal articles. We recommend reading at least one journal article per day. Good readers become good writers who can also distinguish the quality of the research. Being a good consumer of research means you are able to expertly critique published articles so that you can understand the literature pertaining to your field of interest. Box 17.1 provides on overview of how to critique a research article that can also be used as a guide when writing your manuscript.

BOX 17.1. CRITERIA FOR CRITIQUING JOURNAL ARTICLES

General Criteria

Is the article well-written, meeting the following criteria?

- Concise
- Parsimonious
- Grammatically correct
- Well organized
- Logical
- Free of jargon
- Free of biased language

Is the topic timely and relevant to health promotion—that is, does the topic

- Have implications for practice?
- Have implications for research?
- Provide new insights into the problem?

Specific Criteria

Does the introduction provide the following?

- An overview that includes the extent of the problem and who is affected
- A theoretical framework for understanding the problem
- A review of the pertinent literature
- Identification of gaps
- An exact statement of the research question(s) and/or hypotheses if applicable

Does the methods section provide the following?

- A description of the study sample
- The sampling and recruitment methodology
- The research design employed
- Measures administered
- Data collection process and analytic procedures

Does the results section provide the following?

- A linkage to the research question(s)
- Necessary statistical information
- A clear description of finding
- Relevant tables and figures

Does the discussion section provide the following?

- A clear and concise overview of the findings
- A discussion of the findings in the context of the literature reviewed
- A potential and plausible explanation of the findings
- Implications for practice and future research
- A set of limitations for the research
- The significance and relevance of the findings to the field

Once you have become skilled and comfortable with critiquing others' work, you will be ready to create your own work and contribute to the body of scientific knowledge.

This chapter provides guidance in how researchers can tailor their work to "fit" the journal to which the manuscript will be submitted. It also introduces the basic structure of a manuscript and describes in detail how each section of the manuscript should be written and formatted to meet journal expectations of content and style. The chapter expands on the basic theme that publishing is essentially an extension of the research enterprise and is necessary and ethical. We emphasize that producing acceptable manuscripts from rigorous research does not need to be an overwhelming process. Of course, no matter how well the research manuscript is prepared, it is a challenge to publish findings based on research that is severely lacking in rigor. Hence the chapter assumes that the would-be author is summarizing a rigorous research process.

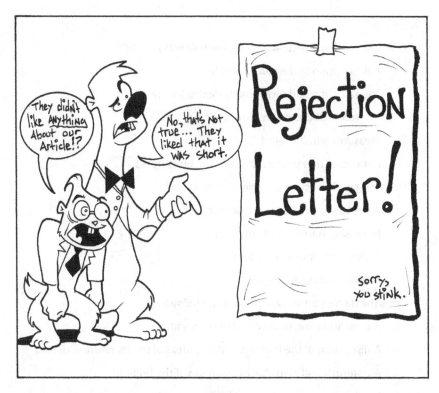

Mincus and Dincus Face Rejection

Copyright 2005 by Justin Wagner; reprinted with permission.

Finding the Right Fit

Three considerations are paramount when authors begin to assemble a research manuscript. First is choosing the best journal that aligns with the research topic, methodology, and perspective. Although at first this may appear to be a daunting task due to the myriad journal choices, authors should try to select the journal that will provide the *maximum impact* for both the topic and the practical significance of the study findings. The **impact factor** (IF) is a proxy for a journal's relative importance to the field; it is frequently determined, in any given year, by the average number of citations received per paper published in that journal during the two preceding years. For example, if a journal has an impact factor of 5 in 2013, that means its papers published in 2011 and 2012 received 5 citations each *on average* in 2013. The 2013 impact factor of a journal would be calculated as follows:

> **impact factor**
> a proxy of how valuable a journal is to its respective field or discipline

A = The number of times that articles published in that journal in 2011 and 2012 were cited by articles in indexed journals during 2013.

B = The total number of "citable items" published by that journal in 2011 and 2012. ("Citable items" are usually articles, reviews, proceedings, or notes, not editorials or letters to the editor.)

A/B = 2013 impact factor

Impact factors are typically located on a journal's website and can range dramatically, from 51.658 for a top-tier biomedical journal—for example, the *New England Journal of Medicine*—to 3.930 for a top-tier public health journal such as *American Journal of Public Health*.

Before we continue, you should have some basic knowledge about scientific journal formats and the business models behind them. Traditionally, journal publishers offered print-only versions. In recent years electronic publishing has become common in scientific publishing, as has been the case for most printed materials such as periodicals, newspapers, and books. Most print-only journals have expanded to online or electronic publications. This is true even for top-tier journals such as *Science* or the *Journal of the American Medical Association*. In fact, there is evidence that electronic publishing provides wider dissemination, hence greater impact factor. A number of journals have established electronic versions so that material can be disseminated more quickly, or have even moved entirely to electronic publication while still retaining their peer review process. Another interesting trend is that the number of scientific journals has proliferated in the past ten years. This trend is the result of a different type of subscription model, deemed "**open access**." Although the peer-review process is the same as with traditionally funded journals, open access journals use a funding model that does not charge readers or their institutions for access. To sustain this model and publish without charging subscription fees, up-front fees are charged and must be paid by the author once the article has been accepted. We want to emphasize, however, that paying the costs associated with publication of your article does not mean their requirements are less rigorous or their articles of lesser quality than those of journals that charge subscription fees. A distinct advantage to open access is that the user of the content is allowed to read, download, copy, distribute, print, search, or link to the full texts of these articles, because the author(s) are not required to transfer the copyright.

open access
journals that provide electronic copies of published articles to readers at no charge

Second, the journal should be selected for a readership that is interested and invested in the outcomes of your study. In a discipline as diverse as health promotion this consideration is particularly important, because the spectrum of health promotion research is vast, and therefore the findings of any given research effort seldom appeal to a general audience. The conclusions of the manuscript may have greater impact if the manuscript is targeted to a well-defined audience. Ideally, the audience should share a common interest in the research and its findings. For example, professionals in preventive medicine may benefit tremendously from a study conclusion that has implications for clinical practice (such as "Physicians and other health professionals who counsel pregnant adolescent females should be aware that marijuana use may be common among those in their first trimester"). Professionals who have dedicated their careers to improving health practices such as fostering exercise behavior may benefit from research that supports the efficacy of a novel approach (for example, "Findings suggest that changes to the physical environment of the workplace can have a favorable impact on the exercise behavior of employees").

Third, the nature of the study and the analyses should be understandable to the intended readership. Health promotion is multidisciplinary. Indeed, one measure of the growing strength of health promotion is the degree to which people from social sciences, behavioral sciences, law, education, nursing, and medical disciplines are collaboratively engaged in health promotion research. This diversity brings a welcome and critical mass of expertise to bear on a large number of disparate research questions. The drawback to this high level of diversity is that not all researchers "speak the same language." For example, psychologists often are well-versed in analysis of variance, whereas epidemiologists ply their trade with contingency table analyses. Sociologists may have a tremendous appreciation for community-level interventions, whereas physicians may be far more interested in clinic-based approaches to health promotion. One quick and efficient strategy for ensuring this fit is to know as much as possible about any professional organization sponsoring the journal (not all journals are sponsored by a professional organization).

Once the authors have agreed upon a journal, the next task is to locate the "Instructions for Authors" (also called "Author Guidelines" or "Submission Requirements") located on the journal's website or in a designated issue of the journal. These requirements usually change when the journal hires a new editor-in-chief; therefore authors should revisit the instructions immediately prior to writing. Box 17.2 displays a sample of journals that typically publish health promotion research.

BOX 17.2. EXAMPLES OF JOURNALS THAT PUBLISH ARTICLES RELEVANT TO HEALTH PROMOTION

Addiction

The American Journal of Health Behavior

The American Journal of Health Education

The American Journal of Health Promotion

American Journal of Preventive Medicine

American Journal of Public Health

Annals of Behavioral Medicine

Canadian Journal of Public Health

Ethnicity and Disease

Health Education and Behavior

Health Education Research

Health Promotion International

Health Psychology

Journal of Adolescent Health

Journal of Consulting and Clinical Psychology

Journal of Health Care for the Poor and Underserved

Journal of Men's Health

Journal of Women's Health

Journal of School Health

Journal of the American Medical Association

Patient Education and Counseling

Prevention Science

Public Health Reports

Social Science and Medicine

The journal instructions are explicit, providing authors with a number of manuscript categories for reporting empirical findings, such as a letter, a report, a brief report, or a full-length original article. Again, the authors must strive to find an ideal fit; selecting the wrong manuscript category may severely limit the odds of acceptance. Once the manuscript category has been identified, the authors should painstakingly adhere to the instructions that are specific to that category. Such instructions are typically broken down by section of the manuscript.

Sections of the Manuscript

The manuscript is typically divided into several discrete sections: abstract, introduction, methods, results, discussion, and references. We will examine each in detail.

Abstract

The abstract is your one and only chance to make a good first impression. Often the abstract is the only portion of an article that is widely disseminated and read in its entirety. In fact, most journals that publish health promotion research will make article abstracts freely available through online databases such as PubMed®. Accessing the abstract only is often the initial goal of readers, as doing so can usually give them enough information to determine whether or not they will benefit from reading the full article. Abstracts are also the medium for judging the quality of research that has been submitted for oral or poster presentations at professional conferences. Often the conference organizers will print the abstracts in the conference program and make them available on their website. As is true for any first impression, a good-quality abstract can greatly enhance the odds that readers will ultimately seek (and benefit from) the full article or attend the conference presentation.

Typically an abstract comprises 250 words or less. Within this limited number of words, the abstract must concisely describe the objective(s), methods, results, and conclusion(s) of the research. In addition, the abstract should convey essential information such as

- The research question(s)
- Sample size and sampling technique
- Participation rate
- Study design (retention rates, if applicable)
- Key measures
- Data collection methods
- Descriptive, bivariate, and multivariate findings (with test statistics)
- A one-sentence conclusion that addresses the research question(s)

Quick inspection of the items in this list suggests that the abstract is a stand-alone element of the manuscript. Indeed, the abstract should always be prepared as a digest of the complete story; it should *not* dilute the story through the use of vacuous phrases such as "implications will be discussed" or "a few examples of the findings will follow." Remember, space is limited, so make every word count!

The important and very demanding requirements of an abstract may at first seem impossible to meet, given a word limit of 250. However, the judicious selection of words and the elimination of any superfluous information can greatly aid the writer in bringing the word count within those limits. Traditionally, abstracts do not have to adhere to essential rules of grammar (see Box 17.3 for several examples). Of course, even with a stringent selection of words and thoughts, meeting the strict word limit may seem impossible. One way to achieve this is to reduce the number of findings presented. For example, it may be better to focus on the findings related to the primary research question. If space permits, then you can include the ancillary findings.

BOX 17.3. EXAMPLES OF ABRIDGED GRAMMAR IN ABSTRACTS

For the purposes of writing and submitting an abstract, the grammar in these examples is considered correct and acceptable.

A. Study Objectives

This study was designed to identify factors that may preclude people from accepting an AIDS vaccine when one is developed and approved for use.

or

To identify factors that that may preclude people from accepting an AIDS vaccine when one is developed and approved for use.

B. Study Design

The study used a prospective design with assessments at baseline, three months, six months, and twelve months.

or

A prospective study with assessments at baseline, three months, six months, and twelve months.

C. Study Sample

The sample comprised 679 adult volunteers recruited from cardiac outpatient units.

or

679 adult volunteers recruited from cardiac outpatient units.

D. Conclusion

The study findings provide support for the hypothesis that men are less likely than women to initiate cigarette use after the age of 21 years.

or

Findings suggest that men are less likely than women to initiate cigarette use after the age of 21 years.

Unfortunately, there are no universal standards for the structure of abstracts in the discipline of health promotion research. Some journals require that the abstract not have specific headings, but most journals specify which headings are mandatory and which are optional. Knowing these requirements (based on the published "Instructions to Authors") is therefore a prerequisite to creating an acceptable abstract.

Introduction

The scope and depth of a well-written introduction are a function of journal requirements. Typically, journals that cater to a largely medical audience (such as the *Journal of the American Medical Association*) prefer very short introductions (two to three paragraphs), whereas journals that fall under the umbrella of behavioral and social science disciplines (for example, *Health Education & Behavior*) prefer and encourage introductions that provide a great deal of detail and therefore allow more space for them. The difference between these two camps is a matter not only of degree but also of substance.

As described in Chapter One (steps two and nine), the research enterprise is focused on identifying and addressing key gaps in the existing literature. Thus one purpose of the introduction is to describe the chain of research that has led to the current study—this description sets the stage for the remainder of the manuscript and clearly prepares readers for a conclusion (or conclusions) that will represent the next link in this chain. An effective introduction has a predictable trajectory: you begin in broad terms and then narrow the focus to the specific research question.

Short introductions provide this information in summary form. Consider, for example, the following one-paragraph hypothetical introduction:

Although intensified HIV testing efforts and behavioral interventions may greatly contribute to reducing the incidence of HIV,[ref] the anticipated advent of a vaginal microbicide may represent a substantial turning point in the epidemic. Unfortunately, only two studies have investigated social and behavioral correlates pertaining to microbicide acceptance among female partners of injection-drug-using men, a population greatly at risk for HIV infection. The first study focused solely on the identification of demographic factors (such as race, ethnicity, and income),[ref] and the second investigated a large number of partner-related barriers to potential microbicide use.[ref] Related studies of other high-risk populations have found that self-efficacy for microbicide application and perceived threat of HIV infection were robustly associated with intent to use microbicides.[ref] As opposed to studies investigating intent (or actual participation) to enroll in randomized controlled trials of a microbicide,[ref] this study identified factors that may preclude women from using an HIV-preventive microbicide that was approved for use in western Kenya.

The introduction succinctly conveys the chain of research and notes the gap in the literature (in other words, no studies of women whose partners are injection-drug users and no studies of actual microbicide use). Each article is cited and described just enough to allow an interested reader to find out more by retrieving a specific article. The final sentence is the logical conclusion of the paragraph (and of the entire introduction).

Alternatively, longer introductions serve the same purpose, but they provide more depth to the literature reviewed. A longer version could describe each of the cited articles in greater detail. A long introduction, however, will nonetheless take on a general form that mimics the sample shown—that is, the chain of research is reviewed, a gap is identified, and the research question is stated.

One important caveat to writing an effective and targeted introduction is the judicious use of references. Given the ease of using search engines such as Google and accessing databases, it is tempting to excessively reference your introduction. Editors discourage citing a preponderance of articles because (1) it detracts from the quality and relevance of the reference list and (2) journal space is at a premium. A good reference list is a product of restraint in selection of articles; only those articles that are key to the research question should be cited. One good review article or meta-analysis should be cited, rather than citing the 8 or 10 articles that were reviewed. Also, citations should reflect research that is timely, meaning that it is current and provides the most recent findings. Moreover, your cited references should reflect quality versus quantity; the adage "less is more" certainly applies here. Occam's razor—"Admit no more causes of natural things than such as are both *true* and *sufficient* to explain their appearances"—should be your guiding principle for writing the introduction.

Methods: Study Sample

This subsection of the manuscript should provide details related to the generation of the study sample, such as the population from which the sample was drawn and the inclusion and exclusion criteria (as well as the number of otherwise eligible participants who were excluded based on these criteria). This section also should describe the sampling technique employed and provide the rationale for its selection. This rationale is critically important because it justifies the sampling technique (see Chapter Six). Consider the following hypothetical example:

To identify differences between low-income women who have and have not ever had a mammogram, we began with a sampling frame of women receiving WIC benefits in the state of Vermont. The sampling frame was a list of all women currently receiving benefits, with women receiving benefits for the longest period of time listed first through women receiving benefits for the shortest period of time listed last. Next, every twenty-fifth name on the list was selected; this created a systematic random sample. The sample therefore comprised women who had previously been categorized as low-income and it equally represented women regardless of how long they had been receiving WIC benefits.

The text states what sampling technique was used (systematic random sample) as well as the reasons the research team chose this approach.

Another requirement of this section is to report the participation rate, which is used as a gauge to judge the potential for *participation bias* (that is, whether volunteers were systematically different from those who refused to be in the study). Although a low participation rate does not necessarily mean that the sample was biased, it nonetheless suggests that this form of bias cannot be ruled out. Consider the following example:

> From December 2012 through April 2014, project recruiters screened 1,590 men attending health department clinics to assess eligibility for participating in a cancer prevention study. Of those screened, 685 were eligible to participate. Men were eligible if they were African American, 18 to 29 years old, unmarried, and had been previously diagnosed with cancer. Of those men not eligible to participate, the majority (83 percent) were either too young or too old. The current study consisted of 605 (88.3 percent) eligible men who volunteered and provided written informed consent. The majority (91.2 percent) of eligible men who did not participate in the study were unavailable due to conflicts with their employment schedules.

Note that the paragraph provides information pertaining to eligibility requirements and shows that age was the primary reason why screened men were not eligible. Lack of eligibility is *not* indicative of participation bias, because this is a reason for nonparticipation that is imposed by the research question rather than a self-selection phenomenon. The important numbers are 605 (the *n* for the study) and 685 (the number of eligible men who were asked to volunteer). By use of these numbers as the numerator and denominator, respectively, a participation rate was obtained and reported. Although universally accepted standards do not exist, participation rates in excess of 80 percent are widely considered acceptable (that is, the potential for a strong participation bias is considered sufficiently low).

In studies that have one or more planned follow-up assessments, you should also report the *retention rate* or the *attrition rate*. The retention rate is the percentage of participants who remained in the study and completed each of the follow-up assessments. Unfortunately, in prospective studies, retaining a high percentage of participants is a challenge. Consider, for example, an article that reports only a 51-percent retention rate. This information is important to report because it suggests a possibility for *attrition bias*. (Attrition bias can be assessed analytically, and these analyses should be reported in the results section—see Chapters Nine and Fifteen for analyses to assess attrition bias).

This section of the manuscript also meets several other obligations. The time period of data collection should be disclosed. This information lets readers judge whether the findings are dated and whether results are still relevant. For example, a study examining social media use by teens in the United States that was conducted in 2009 (but submitted for publication in 2014) would provide substantially different results from the same study conducted in 2013. The results would already be obsolete and not relevant. Also, because this is traditionally the first section of the manuscript that reports methodology, a sentence should be included informing readers that an Institutional Review Board approved the entire study protocol. (Indeed, journal editors will demand that this sentence be included.)

Methods: Data Collection

This section is designed to inform readers *how* the data were collected, not *what* data were collected. A subsequent section will provide readers with specific information about the measures or instruments used in the study. As described in Chapter Seven, data-collection modes span a broad range from paper-and-pencil assessments to electronic diaries. The mode of data collection must be a good match to the research question and study sample. A rationale for the selected method should be provided. Consider the following example:

> Based on studies suggesting decreased reporting bias,[ref] all self-reported measures were assessed using audio-computer-assisted self-interviewing (A-CASI). By providing a voice track that delivered each question to adolescents through headphones, A-CASI technology may have reduced problems that otherwise would have been posed by low literacy. The A-CASI technology also created a user-friendly interview method that automatically handled skip patterns in the questionnaire and provided adolescents with an interactive experience, possibly increasing their attention to the task. The private environment created by the A-CASI may also be useful with respect to the elicitation of honest responses for questions that

assessed sexual and drug-use behaviors.[ref] Adolescents' responses to the computer-delivered questions were automatically encrypted to ensure confidentiality. To help facilitate accuracy, a relatively short period of time was used when asking adolescents to recall past behaviors. Adolescents were assured that their names could not be linked to the codes used to identify documents containing their responses.

This example illustrates a good match between the research questions and the selected method of data collection. The study apparently asked adolescents to disclose information about their recent sexual behaviors and their recent drug-use behaviors. Complete with references to support their position, the authors justify their selection of A-CASI with respect to these research goals.

In addition to *how* the data were collected, this section should also provide information pertaining to the physical location *where* the data were collected. This information is important because the reader must have the necessary details to potentially replicate the study and because readers may want to make judgments regarding the potential effect of the setting on participants' responses. For example, collecting data from incarcerated men in prison may inadvertently affect how they respond to certain questions (for example, Have you had sex in the past seven days?) as opposed to interviewing men in a community center after their release. Finally, this section should also include a sentence that describes what compensation, if any, was provided to participants to encourage their participation.

Methods: Measures

The primary purpose of this section is to justify the constructs (for example, self-esteem) included and to describe the measures employed for assessing those constructs (such as the Rosenberg Self-Esteem Scale). See Chapter Seven for more details on constructs. If the study was guided by theory, then a sentence should be included in this section that articulates the particular theory used and that the chosen measures correspond to the theoretical constructs. This approach is mainly used in medical journals; for psychological or other social science journals, you may want to include a whole section on the theory in greater detail as part of the introduction. In the absence of a theoretical framework, authors should justify their selection of constructs based on previously conducted research.

Informing readers how the study constructs were measured is equally important. These constructs could be organized according to their role in the study. You could first describe the measures used to assess the X-variables (correlates in a cross-sectional study, predictors in a prospective study, or independent variables in an experimental study) followed by the measures used to assess the *Y*-variables (outcomes in observational research and dependent variables in experimental research). Within each category, authors may want to first describe single-item measures (such as measures of race or ethnicity, income, or geographic area) and then describe the use of scales or indices. For each scale or index, a rationale should be provided for the choice of that particular measure. Moreover, if previous psychometric data are available, these should be provided and referenced, as well as current psychometric findings. It is also important to provide a sample question from the scale or index. The number of items constituting each scale or index should also be reported. If this information is extensive, then a table can be used. Table 17.1 provides a sample of summary information that should be reported. These measures were used to assess eight constructs among a sample of high-risk adolescents. To conserve precious journal space, the table may also provide descriptive statistics for each measure. Readers can also be referred back to this table a second time when they are reading the results section of the manuscript.

When research questions necessitate the use of directly observed or biological measures, the nature and use of these measures should be described in great detail. Two samples follow:

(1) After the interview, men were asked to demonstrate the act of applying a condom to a penile model. Trained observers scored men's performance based on six criteria: correctly opens package, squeezes air from tip, places condom right side up on model, keeps tip pinched while unrolling, unrolls to base of model, and condom remains intact. Men received one point for each of the six steps they performed correctly. Those scoring three points or less and those scoring four points or more were classified as having lower and higher demonstrated ability, respectively.

(2) Two vaginal swab specimens were evaluated for *Neisseria gonorrhoeae, Chlamydia trachomatis,* and *Trichomonas vaginalis.* The first swab was placed in a specimen transport tube (Abbott LCx Probe System for *N. gonorrhoeae* and *C. trachomatis* assays) and tested for chlamydia and gonorrhea DNA by LCR. The second swab was used to inoculate a culture medium for *T. vaginalis* (InPouch TV test; BioMed Diagnostics, Inc., Santa Clara, California). A number of studies have established the high sensitivity (at least 97 percent) and specificity (at least 99 percent) of these assays.[ref]

For biological measures, the authors should disclose sensitivity and specificity estimates of the test used as well as provide references. Finally,

Table 17.1   Description of Scale Measures and Bivariate Correlations of These Measures with Self-Esteem among African-American Adolescent Females

Scale and Sample Item	# of Items	a	M	SD	Range
Body image[a] *I usually feel physically attractive.*	7	.73	27.2	4.8	12–35
Perceived family support[b] *My family really tries to help me.*	4	.86	15.2	4.3	4–20
Ethnic pride[c] *I feel good about Black culture.*	13	.74	42.3	4.6	20–52
Normative beliefs favoring males[d] *Your boyfriend gets angry when you don't do what he wants.*	8	.72	15.6	5.6	8–36
Perceived support from a special person[e] *I have a special person who is a source of comfort to me.*	4	.82	17.2	3.5	4–20
Traditional sex role beliefs[f] *Boys are better leaders than girls.*	7	.64	13.2	3.9	7–28
Religiosity[g] *How often do you attend religious or spiritual services?*	4	.68	10.4	2.7	4–16
Perceived support from friends[h] *My friends really try to help me.*	4	.87	15.3	4.4	4–20

[a] Higher scores represent a more favorable body image.
[b] Higher scores represent a greater perceived family support.
[c] Higher scores represent greater ethnic pride.
[d] Higher scores represent stronger beliefs favoring male decision making in a relationship.
[e] Higher scores represent greater perceived support from special persons.
[f] Higher scores represent more traditional sex-role beliefs.
[g] Higher scores represent greater religiosity.
[h] Higher scores represent greater perceived support from friends.

note that the name and location (city and state) of the company that produced the test should be disclosed. This practice is typically required by journals, and it also allows for replication by other researchers and possible comparison of findings across studies that use identical tests.

Methods: Data Analysis

This section should be brief yet informative. The authors have an obligation to compose a paragraph or two that informs readers about the specific statistical techniques that constituted the analytic procedures. Once described, these procedures should be followed without exception; introducing a new technique halfway through the results section creates confusion.

This section must describe the rationale and procedures used to transform any of the variables, if applicable. The use of descriptive statistics does not need to be included; however, the use of each kind of statistical test employed in the analyses should be disclosed at this point. A ratio-

IN A NUTSHELL

The authors have an obligation to compose a paragraph or two that informs readers about the specific statistical techniques that constituted the analytic procedures.

nale for the selection of every statistical test is *not* necessary; however, a rationale should be provided if one is not readily apparent or if the statistical test was complex. If appropriate references that support the selection of statistical tests, the rationale, or both are available, then they should be included. A manuscript may also benefit from succinct explanations of relatively novel tests or tests that are otherwise likely to be unfamiliar to readers of the journal. Finally, the authors should describe how they defined statistical significance. If statistical significance does not follow convention ($P < .05$), then a justification for choosing a different value should be provided.

When writing the methods section, it is important to provide sufficient detail to allow another research team to replicate the study. Indeed, achieving this level of descriptive detail is often considered a hallmark of well-written manuscripts.

Results: Characteristics of the Sample

This section is purely descriptive. The goal is to inform readers about the composition of the study sample. Common indices include race or ethnicity, sex, age, income level, and marital status. However, most indices reported should be selected based on the nature of the research question. For instance, if the research question concerns associations between family structure and teen pregnancy, then basic descriptive information regarding these variables should be provided. An example of this section follows:

> About one-third (34.2 percent) of the sample reported ever being pregnant, with 12.5 percent reporting a current pregnancy. The majority of participants reported residence with only their mother (59.3 percent) or with both their mother and father (32.1 percent). The remainder of the sample lived with friends (5.0 percent) or in their own apartment (3.6 percent).

When multiple sites are involved or participants are recruited from different venues, sample characteristics including number of participants can be provided for each of these different sites. Also, at this juncture, descriptive statistics for measures of key constructs should be reported. Table 17.1, for example, displays the range of scores, means, and standard deviations for each of eight assessed constructs. Referring readers to this table is therefore an important aspect of this opening part of the results section.

Results: Findings

This section is the heart of the manuscript. Describing the findings is not interpretive writing. Prose is not part of this section. The findings should be reported using technical writing; that is, using terse and precise language ("Just the facts, ma'am"). Your task is to report the final output from the statistical analyses. In reporting the final output using text appropriate for this section, you should present the statistical findings in terms of the research question or study hypotheses. This context is necessary for understanding the results. As an elementary example, consider output from a logistic regression analysis that yielded an odds ratio of 3.9 and an associated P level of .001. In the text, you would say, "Women who had a regular physician were almost four times more likely to get a pap test in the past year relative to those without a regular physician."

IN A NUTSHELL

Describing the findings is not interpretive writing. Prose is not part of this section. The findings should be reported using technical writing, that is, using terse and precise language.

Nearly all journals require that authors use tables and figures to extend the level of detail provided by the narrative used in the results section. The act of balancing text with these visuals, however, can be quite challenging. On one hand, the text must tell a complete story (as many readers will not inspect the visuals). On the other hand, the visuals must also tell a complete, stand-alone story that only extends and does not replicate the story told in words. This seemingly tall order can be simplified by using a few simple guidelines:

- Tables are a good place to report test statistics, confidence intervals, and P-values.

- Figures are an efficient way of displaying associations between two or three variables; for example, linear, quadratic, and cubic trends lend themselves to the use of figures.

- Tables and figures should have footnotes when these are needed to tell a complete story.
- Text should provide a bird's-eye view of the findings—nothing should be left out, but readers can be referred to visuals for details.

Discussion: General

Up to this point the manuscript has been guided by a blueprint that delineates the content and format of the sections. By convention, this entails a description of the research and thought processes underlying the research questions. Authors should not offer opinions or state implications of the research findings yet. The discussion section signals the beginning of a new set of rules and far fewer constraints with less structure. The discussion allows the authors (for the first time) to have their own voice! This voice, however, should not extend beyond the reach of the study findings. Stated differently, the study findings support the authors as they offer suggestions (albeit tempered by limitations of the study) to improve health promotion practice or policy.

Because the discussion is not driven by a rigid convention, it can be challenging to know how to proceed with the writing process for this section. However, several guidelines may prove quite useful:

- The opening paragraph is traditionally a place to summarize the findings. In this paragraph, avoid the use of statistics and jargon; instead strive for language that is comprehensible to the lay public.
- After the opening paragraph, it is useful to examine the findings in light of previous studies that have been reported. At this juncture authors should feel free to speculate as to why their findings may have differed from findings in other studies.
- Although the discussion should highlight findings that supported the study hypotheses, it should also offer explanations as to why any one hypothesis was *not* supported.
- Place the findings in a practice context. First and foremost, health promotion research should serve practitioners. Write each paragraph in a way that will put the findings to work in the field. Given that you've formulated research questions that are important to practitioners in the field, this task should be relatively easy.
- Offer the findings and describe their implications in humble language. There is no such thing as a definitive study. A study that is extremely high in rigor is still just one study—it has much more meaning if it corroborates and extends evidence from previous studies.

- To help find a balance between sufficient elaboration and too much elaboration, it is helpful to read several articles that appear in recent issues of the journal you have selected. Read the discussion sections in articles that have used a study design and analytic procedures similar to the study you have conducted.

Discussion: Limitations

This section is perhaps one of the most important and most difficult sections of the entire manuscript. Virtually every research study has limitations. Although a study's limitations are recognized weaknesses in the research that detract from the overall rigor, they nonetheless must be stated. Contrary to the instinct of some authors, limitations should be exhaustively identified. Authors should keep in mind that journal reviewers will readily spot limitations as they begin reading the manuscript—and begin forming a mental image of the limitations similar to Figure 17.1 as they progress through the manuscript.

IN A NUTSHELL

Virtually every research study has limitations. Although a study's limitations are recognized weaknesses in the research that detract from the overall rigor, they nonetheless must be stated.

It is good to know that because reviewers are themselves researchers, they seldom expect perfection; however, reviewers typically anticipate that authors will accurately and responsibly disclose the study limitations and their potential impact on the findings. In keeping with this expectation, authors need to show that they are indeed aware of each and every limitation. Providing an exhaustive list is simply a part of smart writing. Some common threats to internal validity were discussed in Chapter Five; in addition to those, Box 17.4 provides a display of common limitations that, if present, need to be addressed.

BOX 17.4. COMMON STUDY LIMITATIONS

Participation bias

Attrition bias

Social desirability bias, recall bias, and other problems inherent with self-reported measures

Limitations of the sampling technique

Limitations of the study design

Misclassification

Bias introduced by the transformation of variables

In experimental studies, bias introduced from lack of blinding and from contamination

Discussion: Conclusions

Conclusions are the pinnacle of the manuscript. To avoid diluting the message, the conclusions should be stated in a single paragraph—preferably a short one. In fact, two or three sentences can be sufficient for a well-written conclusion. Because being succinct is highly valued, authors must know exactly what to say and what not to say. The conclusions should be directly relevant to the research questions and provide a straightforward answer to each of the questions. Moreover, conclusions should not be definitive, as the research process entails ruling out alternative possibilities and providing

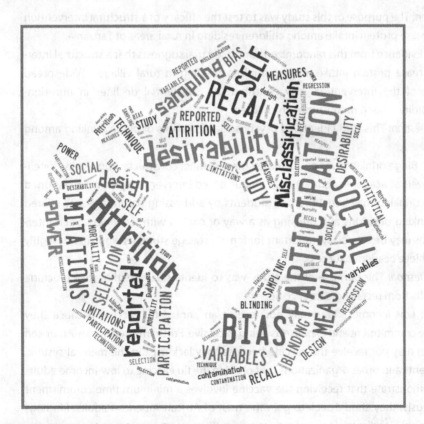

Figure 17.1 Reviewer's Mental Image of Limitations

support for hypotheses; it does not entail *proving* hypotheses. Authors should also avoid restating the findings or summarizing the research process.

One technique that may be helpful when constructing your conclusion is to imagine a news story based on your study. What would the headline say? How would the 30-second report on a local television channel sound? Indeed, few people may read the published article in its entirety, but massive numbers of people may read your three-sentence conclusion. Your conclusion should be strong and striking without being overly intellectual. For all practical purposes, it should be written for a lay audience and easy to understand. Finally, high-quality manuscripts are defined by the practical value of the conclusions. Indeed, health promotion research has value only when it informs health promotion practice and policy. You should be absolutely sure to place the findings squarely in the context of health promotion practice. Box 17.5 displays several sample conclusions.

BOX 17.5. EXAMPLES OF EFFECTIVE CONCLUSIONS

Research Question: The purpose of this study was to test the efficacy of a structural intervention designed to increase protein intake among children residing in rural areas of Tanzania.

Conclusion: Evidence from this randomized controlled trial suggests that a structural intervention can increase protein intake among children residing in rural villages. Widespread implementation of the intervention may contribute to substantial declines in nutrition-associated morbidity among rural Tanzanian children.

Research Question: This study identified psychosocial correlates of binge drinking among college females.

Conclusions: Binge drinking was predicted by three distinct constructs: impulsivity, loneliness, and low levels of academic motivation. Campus-based intervention programs designed to reduce binge drinking may benefit female students by addressing potential issues related to impulsive drinking decisions and drinking as a way of coping with loneliness. Such intervention programs may be especially important for female college students who are not highly motivated to achieve academic success.

Research Question: The purpose of the study was to identify barriers that may preclude low-income adults from receiving a flu vaccine.

Conclusions: Low-income adults may not receive an annual flu vaccine because they perceive the time commitment and expense as being excessive. Furthermore, African-American men and women may not receive the vaccine because they lack trust in the medical system. Health departments and other organizations that provide the flu vaccine to low-income adults may need to demonstrate that receiving the vaccine involves a minimum time commitment and, simultaneously, they should seek to gain the trust of African-American adults. Findings also suggest that policies directed toward reduced-price flu vaccines may promote acceptance.

References

A reference list is a mandatory section of any manuscript. The list may, however, be constructed using any one of a number of different styles. The selection of any given style is made by the journal editor and the editorial board. Although this lack of a universal system can appear confusing to new authors, most styles of referencing can be divided into two categories. Even within these two categories, some journals deviate from these styles; authors' instructions should always be consulted before compiling the reference list.

Numbered endnotes (biomedical referencing is one example) are probably the most common system used in journals that publish health promotion research. This system uses numbers in the text to denote corresponding references in a numbered reference or endnotes list. The other style used quite often is the author-date style; the American Psychological Association (APA) style (American Psychological Association, 2009) is one example. This style uses the authors' last names and the publication year for the text citation, and the reference list is alphabetized. Samples of the two styles as they would appear in the body of a manuscript follow:

Sample 1: Adolescents' lack of self-esteem has been associated with diverse health-compromising behaviors such as alcohol and cigarette use, the early onset of sexual activity, eating disorders, and general emotional distress.[1-4] Conversely, high levels of self-esteem have been identified as a protective factor against adolescents' engagement in these behaviors.[5-7]

Sample 2. Adolescents' lack of self-esteem has been associated with diverse health-compromising behaviors such as alcohol and cigarette use, the early onset of sexual activity, eating disorders, and general emotional distress (Brook, Rubenstone, Zhang, Morojele, & Brook, 2011; Kim, 2011; Portela de Santana, da Costa Ribeiro Junior, Mora Giral, & Raich, 2012; Youngblade, Theokas, Schulenberg, Curry, Huang, & Novak, 2007). Conversely, high levels of self-esteem have been identified as a protective factor against adolescents' engagement in these behaviors (Copeland-Linder, Lambert, Chen, & Ialongo, 2011; Dumas, Ellis, & Wolfe, 2012; Wheeler, 2010).

The citation style shown in Sample 2 is described in the *Publication Manual of the American Psychological Association, 6th edition* (2009). APA style is used by a large number of journals that publish health promotion research. Each citation gives the reader enough information to locate the reference in the alphabetized reference list—numbers (other than dates) are not used. By convention, the text citation usually comes at the end of the sentence (before the period), and multiple citations within any single set of parentheses are arranged alphabetically. For detailed instructions and other rules regarding APA style, consult the publication manual.

Before writing a manuscript, it is wise to learn the referencing style that will be required for the selected journal. Again, the endnote and author-date styles are basic categories; each has a number of variants that may be used. As a rule, a reference should have enough information that any reader could easily retrieve it from an electronic database. Rules for truncating the number of authors shown, placement of the publication year, abbreviation of journal names, and constructing other parts of the entry vary. Examples of how the reference should be written for the reference list in both endnote and author-date style follow:

1. Youngblade LM, Theokas C, Schulenberg J, Curry L, Huang IC, Novak M. Risk and promotive factors in families, schools, and communities: a contextual model of positive youth development in adolescence. *Pediatrics.* Feb 2007; 119 Suppl 1: S47–53.

2. Youngblade, L. M., Theokas, C., Schulenberg, J., Curry, L., Huang, I. C., & Novak, M. (2007). Risk and promotive factors in families, schools, and communities: a contextual model of positive youth development in adolescence. *Pediatrics, 119*(Suppl 1), S47–53.

Completing the Final Product

To apply the key concepts, a brief sample manuscript is shown in Box 17.6 in its entirety. Each main section will be presented separately and each will be annotated for teaching purposes.

BOX 17.6. SAMPLE MANUSCRIPT

Abstract

Background: The purpose of this study was to identify correlates of self-esteem among a sample of African-American female adolescents. *(Note that the research question is stated immediately.)*

Methods: A prospective study was conducted. As part of a larger HIV prevention study, a purposive sample (*n* = 522) of sexually active African-American female adolescents, ages 14 to 18, was recruited from low-income neighborhoods characterized by high rates of unemployment, substance abuse, violence, teen pregnancy, and STDs. Adolescents completed a self-administered questionnaire that contained the Rosenberg self-esteem scale (*α* = .79) and other scale measures that assessed constructs hypothesized to be associated with self-esteem.

(Key information includes sampling technique, the sample size [n], the inclusion criteria, assessment of the primary variable, and the study design.)

Results: The regression model explained 38 percent of the variance in adolescents' self-esteem scores. Significant correlates of higher self-esteem were having a more favorable body image (β = .35), greater perceived family support (β = .19), nontraditional sex role beliefs (β = .16), greater ethnic pride (β = .15), normative beliefs not favoring male decision making in a relationship (β = .12), and greater religiosity (β = .09). *(In a short amount of space the research question is answered using common statistical procedures.)*

Conclusion: Diverse psychosocial measures were associated with self-esteem among high-risk African-American female adolescents. Programs designed to enhance the self-esteem of this population may benefit by promoting more favorable body images, greater perceptions of family support, greater ethnic pride, and beliefs supporting egalitarian decision making. *(The conclusion is suggestive and practical, not definitive, and strongly related to health promotion.)*

Introduction

Self-esteem, an indicator of self-worth, has been defined as a critical index of mental health[1] and is an important construct often integrated in resiliency theories, where it has been conceptualized as a protective or buffering factor.[1,2] *(For purposes of brevity we have not included the reference list corresponding to these endnotes.)* Specifically, resiliency theories posit that adolescents in high-risk social environments may be protected from adopting health-compromising behaviors because of their high self-esteem, which is reflected in their desire and commitment to overcome negative circumstances. An important aspect of enhancing adolescents' self-esteem is tailoring program content to target those psychosocial influences associated with adolescents' high self-esteem. These influences are likely to vary depending on characteristics of the adolescents.[3-12] *(These opening sentences are based on twelve references—thus a chain of research is now available to the reader.)*

According to the U.S. Department of Health and Human Services report titled *Healthy People 2020*, minority adolescents are a priority population for health promotion interventions.[13] An especially important population is sexually active African-American adolescent girls residing in communities that predispose them to risk of infection with human immunodeficiency virus (HIV), other sexually transmitted diseases (STDs), pregnancy, delinquent behaviors, substance abuse, and a range of other risk behaviors and problems that negatively affect their quality of life.[13,14] *(This portion justifies the selected priority population.)* Research identifying the correlates of high self-esteem among this population could be a valuable source of information for developing and tailoring risk-reduction programs that include the enhancement of self-esteem as one objective. *(Here the practical value of the research is noted.)*

The purpose of this study was to identify the psychosocial correlates of high self-esteem among a sample of sexually active African-American female adolescents residing in a high-risk environment. *(The research question is concisely stated.)* Previous studies have suggested that social support,[15] particularly family support,[16] may be important to the self-esteem of adolescents. Based on a literature review, we also hypothesized that several other constructs would be positively correlated with self-esteem: favorable body image, religiosity, ethnic pride, and parental monitoring.[16–19] Additionally, we hypothesized that traditional sex role beliefs and having normative beliefs that favor male decision making in a relationship would be inversely correlated with self-esteem.[20] *(Study hypotheses and their basis are provided.)*

Methods

Study Sample. From December 2012 through April 2014, project recruiters screened 1,780 female teens in adolescent medicine clinics. Of those screened, 1,609 adolescents were eligible. Adolescents were eligible if they were female, African American, 14 to 18 years old, unmarried, and reported sexually activity in the previous 6 months. Of those adolescents not eligible to participate, the majority (98 percent) were not sexually active. Of those eligible, 1,457 (82 percent) were enrolled. *(Enough information is provided to let the reader make judgments about the potential for participation bias.)* The study protocol was approved by the University Institutional Review Board prior to implementation. *(This sentence, expressed in some form, is mandatory.)*

Data Collection. Data collection consisted of a self-administered questionnaire administered in a group setting, with monitors providing assistance to adolescents with limited literacy and helping to ensure confidentiality of responses. *(The readers are now aware of how the data were acquired.)* Adolescents were reimbursed $20.00 for their participation.

Measures

Criterion Variable. The Rosenberg self-esteem scale[21] was included as part of the assessment instrument. This scale has well-established psychometric properties and has been used widely with diverse populations to assess adolescents' self-esteem. The scale contained 10 items, scored using a 4-point Likert format, with responses ranging from "strongly agree" to "strongly disagree." Higher scores represented greater levels of self-esteem. Inter-item reliability of the scale was satisfactory ($\alpha = .79$). *(A great deal of attention is given to this variable because it is the outcome measure [Y].)*

Correlates. Two single-item measures of parental monitoring were assessed. One measure asked adolescents how often their parents or parental figure(s) knew where they were when not at home or in school. The other measure asked how often their parents or parental figure(s) knew whom they were with when not at home or in school. Eight scales were used to assess various constructs hypothesized to correlate with adolescents' self-esteem. Table 1 displays psychometric information for the 8 scales as well as a sample item for each. *(Note the use of a table [not shown here] to keep the text brief.)*

Data Analysis

Pearson product-moment correlations were calculated to assess strength and direction of the bivariate relationship between self-esteem and each of the hypothesized correlates. To assess the partial contribution of each of the hypothesized correlates working as a set in explaining the observed levels of self-esteem, multiple linear regression was used. Variables representing the correlates were entered into the regression model using a stepwise procedure with the alpha criteria set at .05 for entry and .10 for exit. The F-statistic was computed to test the overall significance of the final model. Acceptance of statistical significance was based on an alpha of .05. *(Enough information is provided that someone else could replicate the analysis.)*

Results

Characteristics of the Sample. The average age of the adolescents was 16.0 years (SD = 1.2). The majority (81.2 percent) were full-time students; 9.4 percent were part-time students, and the remainder were not enrolled in school. Nearly one-fifth of the adolescents reported that their family received welfare.

The Rosenberg self-esteem scale was completed by 98.6 percent of the adolescents (n = 515). Scores ranged from 16 to 40 (Md = 34.0, M = 33.4, SD = 4.8). Although the distribution of scores had a slight negative skew (skewness = 2.50), the degree of skewness was not sufficient to necessitate transforming the scores so that they more closely approximate a normal distribution. *(Note that a great deal of descriptive attention is given to outcome measure, including a consideration to transform the measure.)*

Bivariate Findings. Table 1 displays the Pearson product-moment correlations between each of the correlates and self-esteem. *(For brevity, the table is not shown in this example, but it should be noted that it serves dual purposes: (1) it describes the measures psychometrically, and (2) it provides bivariate correlation coefficients.)*

Each of the constructs was significantly correlated, in the hypothesized direction, with adolescents' self-esteem. In addition, positive correlations between the two single-item measures assessing parental monitoring and adolescents' self-esteem were observed. *(Text describes the table.)*

Adolescents' age was not significantly correlated with self-esteem (r = .07, P = .11). *(This text provides results that are not shown in the table.)*

Multivariate Findings. Table 2 displays the standardized partial regression coefficients and the proportion of unique variance accounted for by each correlate in the final model. Overall, the model explained 38 percent of the variance in adolescents' self-esteem (F = 49.3, df = (6,479), P < .0001). *(These values are rarely provided in tables.)* Body image was the most important correlate of self-esteem, followed by perceived family support. Ethnic pride was an important contributor to the overall model, and religiosity played a lesser but significant role in explaining the variance observed in adolescents' self-esteem. *(Text summarizes the values shown in Table 2.)*

Discussion

Findings suggest that African-American female adolescents' self-esteem may be associated with at least six relevant psychosocial constructs. The strong association between self-esteem and body image is not surprising, as some researchers have suggested that physical appearance is the most important factor in determining global self-worth for adolescents.[22] These findings also suggest that even among older adolescents, family support may be an important factor in contributing to their emotional well-being. *(Note that the text is speculative and no longer written in the past tense.)*

Influencing these six constructs may in turn promote higher levels of self-esteem, thereby providing high-risk adolescents with a valuable protective factor against health-compromising behaviors. Behavioral intervention programs may benefit African-American adolescent girls with low self-esteem by helping them improve their perceptions of body image and family support while affecting their ethnic pride. Additionally, programs may benefit this population by promoting more egalitarian beliefs about sex roles and decision making in the context of adolescent girls' relationships with male partners. *(The practical implications for health promotion are explored.)*

Limitations. These findings are limited by the validity of the measures *(Limitation 1)* and the inherent limitations of the cross-sectional design. *(Limitation 2)* In addition, the findings can be generalized only to sexually active African-American female adolescents. *(Limitation 3)* Finally, the sample was limited to economically disadvantaged African-American adolescents. Therefore the findings may not be generalized to other racial or ethnic groups or adolescents from different socioeconomic strata. *(Limitation 4).*

Conclusions. Diverse psychosocial constructs were found to be associated with self-esteem among a sample of high-risk African-American female adolescents. Several of the assessed constructs may be particularly amenable to behavioral intervention. *(Notice that the speculative language is couched as "may.")* Programs designed to increase high-risk African-American adolescent females' self-esteem may benefit from promoting more favorable body images, greater perceptions of family support, greater ethnic pride, and more egalitarian sex role beliefs. *(Again, a practical value of the research is noted.)*

Once you have your manuscript written and prepared, the last step is submitting it to the journal you have selected as the most appropriate. Figure 17.2 displays the process of taking the manuscript through the review process to become a published article.

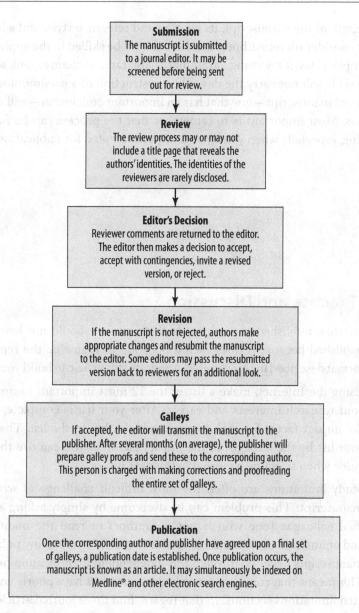

Submission
The manuscript is submitted to a journal editor. It may be screened before being sent out for review.

Review
The review process may or may not include a title page that reveals the authors' identities. The identities of the reviewers are rarely disclosed.

Editor's Decision
Reviewer comments are returned to the editor. The editor then makes a decision to accept, accept with contingencies, invite a revised version, or reject.

Revision
If the manuscript is not rejected, authors make appropriate changes and resubmit the manuscript to the editor. Some editors may pass the resubmitted version back to reviewers for an additional look.

Galleys
If accepted, the editor will transmit the manuscript to the publisher. After several months (on average), the publisher will prepare galley proofs and send these to the corresponding author. This person is charged with making corrections and proofreading the entire set of galleys.

Publication
Once the corresponding author and publisher have agreed upon a final set of galleys, a publication date is established. Once publication occurs, the manuscript is known as an article. It may simultaneously be indexed on Medline® and other electronic search engines.

Figure 17.2   How a Manuscript Becomes a Published Journal Article

Summary

A manuscript is a historical accounting of the entire research process. Success in publishing is therefore a direct function of success in conducting rigorous research. While there is an art to preparing this document, the majority of journals that publish health promotion research findings will give authors a very specific set of instructions for what should and should not be included in the manuscript, how the manuscript should be constructed, the length of the manuscript, its citation and reference style, and a host of other considerations. Although authors should be skilled in the application of simple rules for writing (grammar, paragraph structure, and so on), these skills will not carry the day. The construction of a parsimonious and pertinent manuscript—one that has an important conclusion—will ensure success. Most important is to remember that the process can be fun and exciting, especially when your manuscript is accepted for publication.

KEY TERMS

Impact factor   Open access

For Practice and Discussion

1. Locate a published journal article that you feel should not have been published because it does such a poor job of following the reporting format described in this chapter. Annotate this article to build your case.

2. Using the Internet, make a list of the 12 most important journals for your research interests and career. After your list is complete, locate the impact factor for each journal and add that to the list. Then sort your list by the strength of the impact factor so you can use this as a guide when selecting a journal in the near future.

3. Study limitations are often the most difficult challenge of writing a manuscript. This problem can be overcome by simply asking a qualified colleague (one who is not an author) to read the manuscript and enumerate the limitations. Unfortunately, far too many published manuscripts never go through this independent identification process. This means that countless published manuscripts have poorly enumerated limitations sections. In that regard, find three journal articles that report original investigations of a research question of interest to you. For each one, imagine that you are reviewing this (before publication) and you have been asked to make a list of all possible limitations. Use this chapter as guide to making these three lists.

4. In this chapter you learned about basic differences in citation and referencing styles (APA style versus biomedical style). To learn even more, go online and investigate software programs that manage citation and reference styles automatically. Learn as much as possible about each option and considered purchasing one of these for downloading and future use. As you investigate, please pay close attention to the

multiple options that are loosely classified as biomedical style; learn the names of these options so you can more efficiently use this software program as your career advances.

Reference

American Psychological Association. (2009). *Publication manual of the American Psychological Association* (6th ed.). Washington, DC: American Psychological Association.

CHAPTER 18

UNDERSTANDING THE GRANT PROCESS AND DEVELOPING AN EFFECTIVE RESEARCH GRANT APPLICATION

Ralph J. DiClemente
Laura F. Salazar
Richard A. Crosby

Health promotion research as a field is dependent upon funding. Obtaining funds requires submitting grant applications to a variety of funding agencies. Grant applications are often complex and require a high level of skill and perseverance on the part of researchers. Having an overview of the review process and an in-depth understanding of the typical components that comprise a grant application is critical.

Unlike the preceding chapters in this textbook, which have addressed an aspect of the research process, the overarching aim of this chapter is to describe the grant process and provide guidance in crafting an effective and successful research proposal. As mentioned in Chapter One, grantsmanship is a part of the research process; however, rather than being an explicit part of the research process, obtaining funding to conduct research is an implicit demand—and one that gives rise to the entire research enterprise.

First, we need to recognize that writing a research proposal to secure funding for a study is not mystical or magical. Anyone can learn the skills needed to be proficient at proposal writing. The caveat, of course, is that like most skills, grant writing requires a focused time commitment and practice. Becoming skilled in writing

LEARNING OBJECTIVES

- Understand the grant review process that is currently practiced by the National Institutes of Health.

- Describe the requirements for composing key sections of a typical grant application.

- Learn strategies for writing an effective proposal, with a particular emphasis on the approach section.

- Review a generalized template that can be used for composing a grant application.

grant proposals involves writing more than one proposal. In fact, most researchers do not get funded with their first proposal. For many, this process is incremental, iterative, and calibrated; it requires tenacity and is not for the faint of heart. We need to acknowledge that proposal writing, like any other skill—whether it be surfing, gymnastics, playing the piano, or playing baseball—requires extensive and focused practice to achieve proficiency. To emphasize: becoming a skilled proposal writer requires an investment of time and energy and a willingness to be receptive to constructive feedback. Once you become proficient, the returns on this investment will be intellectually satisfying, financially rewarding, and beneficial to the field of health promotion, the public's health, and society at large.

Although we talk of a "research proposal" as a generic product, it is useful to acknowledge that research proposals vary markedly depending on the source of funding. For example, a National Institutes of Health (NIH) proposal will have different requirements from, say, a Centers for Disease Control and Prevention (CDC) or private foundation proposal. Requirements differ even within an agency—NIH has an array of application types (R01, R03, R21, R34, U01, and so on) as well as varying research stages, purposes, and designs. This makes sense; a research proposal that would test the efficacy of a health promotion program (HPP) will differ in format, scope, and design from one that proposes to conduct an observational study or a qualitative research study that uses focus groups, elicitation interviews, or other qualitative methods. Notwithstanding the variability inherent in these myriad formats, proposals do share a common core of elements. Rather than attempting to address each variation, we will provide a template of the critical elements necessary for a successful research proposal.

The mission of the NIH is to support science in pursuit of knowledge about the biology and behavior of living systems and to apply that knowledge to extend healthy life and reduce the burdens of illness and disability. As part of this mission, applications submitted to the NIH for grants or cooperative agreements to support biomedical and behavioral research are evaluated for scientific and technical merit through the NIH peer review system. Of particular importance are changes within the past decade to the NIH peer review system. These changes are manifest in grant application review criteria, format, and scoring, so they are critically important to understanding how to be a proficient grant writer. Therefore we will devote considerable attention to describing these fundamental changes. To provide a framework for understanding these changes, we will contrast the new enhanced grant review criteria with the previous review criteria. The comparison between the two review criteria illustrates the new application format. Table 18.1 describes the five core criteria that reviewers use to score an application; we have added emphasis to some specific changes.

The NIH Grant Scoring System

Historically, reviewers assigned scores from 100 (exceptional) to 500 (poor—having major methodological weaknesses). However, in the past decade there has been a marked change in the NIH grant scoring system. In addition to an overall score, reviewers now provide a score for each of the five core criteria shown in Table 18.1. The scoring is also different: scores range from 1 through 9 for each criterion, with 1 being exceptional and 9 being poor.

Table 18.1   Comparison of Current and Previous NIH Review Criteria

	Previous Criteria	Current (Enhanced) Criteria
Significance	**Significance:** Does this study address an important problem? If the aims of the application are achieved, how will scientific knowledge be advanced? What will be the effect of these studies on the concepts or methods that drive this field?	**Significance:** Does this study address an important problem? If the aims of the application are achieved, how will scientific knowledge, **or public health practice, or clinical practice** be advanced? What will be the effect of these studies on the concepts, methods, **technologies, treatments, services, or preventative interventions** that drive this field?
Approach	**Approach:** Are the conceptual framework, design, methods, and analyses adequately developed, well-integrated, and appropriate to the aims of the project? Does the applicant acknowledge potential problem areas and consider alternative tactics?	**Approach:** Are the conceptual or clinical framework, design, methods, and analyses adequately developed, well-integrated, well-reasoned, and appropriate to the aims of the project? Does the applicant acknowledge potential problem areas and consider alternative tactics?
Innovation	**Innovation:** Does the project employ novel concepts, approaches or methods? Are the aims original and innovative? Does the project challenge existing paradigms or develop new methodologies or technologies?	**Innovation:** Is the project original and innovative? For example: **Does the project challenge existing paradigms or clinical practice**; address an innovative hypothesis or critical barrier to progress in the field? Does the project develop or **employ novel concepts, approaches, methodologies, tools, or technologies** for this area?
Investigator	**Investigator:** Is the investigator appropriately trained and well suited to carry out this work? Is the work proposed appropriate to the experience level of the investigator and other researchers (if any)?	**Investigators:** Are the investigators appropriately trained and well suited to carry out this work? Is the work proposed appropriate to the experience level of the principal investigator and other researchers? **Does the investigative team bring complementary and integrated expertise to the project (if applicable)?**
Environment	**Environment:** Does the scientific environment in which the work will be done contribute to the probability of success? Do the proposed experiments take advantage of unique features of the scientific environment or employ useful collaborative arrangements? Is there evidence of institutional support?	**Environment:** Does the scientific environment in which the work will be done contribute to the probability of success? Do the proposed studies benefit from unique features of the scientific environment, or subject populations, or employ useful collaborative arrangements? Is there evidence of institutional support?

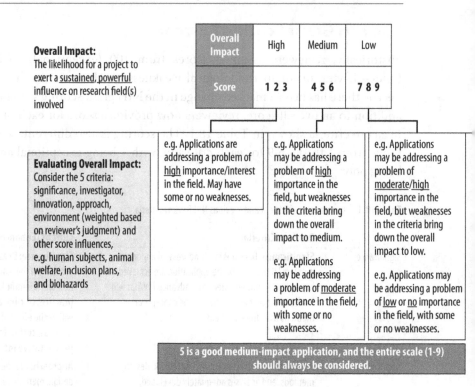

Figure 18.1   NIH Scoring System

Overall Impact. In addition to providing core criteria scores, reviewers also provide an **overall impact score**. Because this is the score that ultimately is used to determine funding, we describe it in greater detail.

overall impact score

the score used to determine whether a grant is in the fundable range

IN A NUTSHELL

Reviewers provide an overall impact score to reflect their assessment of the likelihood for the project to exert a sustained, powerful influence on the research field(s) involved, in consideration of the five core review criteria and additional review criteria (as applicable for the project proposed).

Reviewers provide an overall impact score to reflect their assessment of the likelihood for the project to exert a sustained, powerful influence on the research field(s) involved, in consideration of the five core review criteria and additional review criteria (as applicable for the project proposed). In one paragraph, reviewers briefly summarize the most important points of the critique, addressing the strengths and weaknesses of the application in terms of the five core review criteria. Reviewers recommend a score reflecting the overall impact of the project on the field, weighting the five core review criteria described in Table 18.1 as they feel appropriate for each application. An application does not need to be strong in all categories to be judged likely to have a major scientific impact and thus deserve a high merit rating. A **merit rating** is a score that is good enough to represent a proposal that has exceptional value to the field. For example, an investigator may propose to carry out important work that by its nature is not innovative but is essential to move a field forward or improve clinical decisions or outcomes.

merit rating
the score that represents
the value of a proposal

A Ghost in the Machine?

A "ghost in the machine" is the term applied by British philosopher Gilbert Ryle to a philosophical theory posited by René Descartes, who suggested a dualism between the mind (ghost) and the body (machine), each running in parallel. We apply this philosophical view to the NIH scoring system. Although the criteria-based scoring system seems, on the surface, to be reasonable, well-articulated, quantitatively based, and grounded, there is another dimension to this system that is not so transparent: the over-all impact score that is assigned to each proposal. Moreover, this overall impact score may not even be related to the scores assigned to the five core criteria. An illustration may be helpful. Suppose Investigator X submits a grant proposal to develop an HPP for Type 2 diabetics designed to reduce A1c (blood sugar level). The grant is reviewed by three members of the Scientific Review Group (SRG) and the resultant scores are as shown in Table 18.2.

Examine the scores in Table 18.2 very carefully. What do you notice? First and foremost, the grant proposal scored well on all of the five core criteria. Again, recall that the scoring system ranges from 1 to 9, with 1 being the ideal score. Examining the table of scores indicates that, by and large, the reviewers were very positive about each criterion. In fact, if you calculate a grand average score (meaning, each reviewer's average and then the average of these three averages), it equals 2.4. Now, what if we told you that the impact score for this grant was 37! How could this grant receive an impact score of 37 when the average of all the scores is 2.4? It might be reasonable to assume that the criterion scores would drive the impact

Table 18.2 Hypothetical Grant Application Scores

Core Review Criteria	Reviewer 1	Reviewer 2	Reviewer 3
Significance	2	3	2
Approach	3	4	4
Innovation	3	2	4
Investigator(s)	2	1	2
Environment	1	2	1

score. This is the dualism we mentioned earlier: the impact score does not necessarily reflect the criterion scores. The impact score reflects the cumulative scores from all SRG members (as many as 10 or more), not just the three members assigned to read and critique the grant proposal. Each SRG member submits an overall impact score that potentially can fall outside the range of the three reviewers' scores. Also, unlike the score for each of the five core criteria, the impact score must range from 10 to 90.

Additional Review Criteria

In addition to the five core review criteria specified in Table 18.1, other elements also factor into the SRG's determination of the scientific and technical merit of a grant application. Although these elements are not scored on a proposal, they can nevertheless influence whether the grant proposal will be funded. These additional elements are described in this section.

Protections for Human Subjects

For research that involves human subjects but does *not* involve one of the six categories of research that are exempt under 45 CFR Part 46, the SRG will evaluate the justification for involvement of human subjects and the proposed protections from research risk relating to their participation according to the following five review criteria: (1) risk to subjects, (2) adequacy of protection against risks, (3) potential benefits to the subjects and others, (4) importance of the knowledge to be gained, and (5) data and safety monitoring for clinical trials. For research that involves human subjects and meets the criteria for one or more of the six categories of research that are exempt under 45 CFR Part 46, the SRG will evaluate: (1) the justification for the exemption, (2) human subjects' involvement and characteristics, and (3) sources of materials. For more detail on how best to prepare this section, you may wish to review Chapter Three.

Inclusion of Women, Minorities, and Children

IN A NUTSHELL

When the proposed project involves clinical research (including behavioral research), the SRG will evaluate the proposed plans for inclusion of minorities and women, as well as the inclusion of children.

When the proposed project involves clinical research (including behavioral research), the SRG will evaluate the proposed plans for inclusion of minorities and women, as well as the inclusion of children. Of note, "children" are defined by NIH as persons under the age of 21. If the research does

PROGRAM CONTACT:
Redonna Chandler
301-443-4060
rchandle@mail.nih.gov

Release Date: 04/05/2013

Application Number: 1 U01 DA36233-01

Principal Investigators (Listed Alphabetically):
BRODY, GENE H PHD
DICLEMENTE, RALPH J PHD (Contact)

Applicant Organization: EMORY UNIVERSITY

Review Group: ZDA1 EXL-T (11)
National Institute on Drug Abuse Special Emphasis Panel
TRANSLATIONAL RESEARCH ON INTERVENTIONS FOR ADOLESCENTS IN THE
LEGAL SYSTEM: TRIALS (U01)

Meeting Date: 03/12/2013
Council: MAY 2013
Requested Start: 07/01/2013

RFA/PA: DA13-009
PCC: CM/RCB

Project Title: KIIDS: Knowing about intervention implementation in Detention Sites

SRG Action: Impact Score: 22
Next Steps: Visit http://grants.nih.gov/grants/next_steps.htm
Human Subjects: 30-Human subjects involved - Certified, no SRG concerns
Animal Subjects: 10-No live vertebrate animals involved for competing appl.
Gender: 1A-Both genders, scientifically acceptable
Minority: 1A-Minorities and non-minorities, scientifically acceptable
Children: 1A-Both Children and Adults, scientifically acceptable
Clinical Research - not NIH-defined Phase III Trial

Project Year	Direct Costs Requested	Estimated Total Cost
1	435,670	687,993
2	444,504	701,943
3	449,978	710,587
4	440,368	695,412
5	417,326	659,025
TOTAL	2,187,846	3,454,960

ADMINISTRATIVE BUDGET NOTE: The budget shown is the requested budget and has not been adjusted to reflect any recommendations made by reviewers. If an award is planned, the costs will be calculated by Institute grants management staff based on the recommendations outlined below in the COMMITTEE BUDGET RECOMMENDATIONS section.

Figure 18.2 Summary Statement of Grant Application Scientific Review

not include women, minorities, or children, you must provide a compelling justification for why each group is excluded. For example, a study that involves an HPP intervention for men who have sex with men (MSM) would justify the exclusion of women by stating that MSM is a priority population for HIV prevention and the intervention would not necessarily be appropriate for women. The important point is that if you are excluding women or children, you must provide a justification showing that the exclusion is necessary and warranted.

Vertebrate Animals

In health promotion research, animals will rarely if ever be involved. If your study does involve live vertebrate animals, the SRG will evaluate their involvement as part of the scientific assessment according to the following five points:

1. Proposed use of the animals, and species, strains, ages, sex, and numbers to be used

2. Justifications for the use of animals and for the appropriateness of the species and numbers proposed

3. Adequacy of veterinary care

4. Procedures for limiting discomfort, distress, pain, and injury to that which is unavoidable in the conduct of scientifically sound research, including the use of analgesic, anesthetic, and tranquilizing drugs and/or comfortable restraining devices

5. Methods of euthanasia and reason for selection if not consistent with the American Veterinary Medical Association guidelines on euthanasia

Resubmission Applications

When reviewing a resubmission application (formerly called an amended application), the SRG will evaluate the application as now presented, taking into consideration the responses to comments from the previous SRG and changes made to the project.

Renewal Applications

When reviewing a renewal application (formerly called a competing continuation application), the SRG will consider the progress made in the last funding period.

Revision Applications

When reviewing a revision application (formerly called a competing supplement application), the SRG will consider the appropriateness of the proposed expansion of the scope of the project. If the revision application relates to a specific line of investigation presented in the original application that was not recommended for approval by the committee, then the committee will consider whether the responses to comments from the previous SRG are adequate and whether substantial changes are clearly evident.

Biohazards

Reviewers will assess whether materials or procedures proposed are potentially hazardous to research personnel and/or the environment and, if needed, determine whether adequate protection is proposed.

Budget and Period Support

Reviewers will consider whether the budget and the requested period of support are fully justified and reasonable in relation to the proposed research. Reasonable in this context means that the scope of activities, the time commitment, and other direct costs are critical to the implementation of the research. You do not want to inflate your budget just to reach the maximum budget allowed, as reviewers will not view that favorably. On the other hand, you do not want to underestimate your budget. If the scope of work exceeds the funds requested, you will have a difficult time fulfilling the specific aims of the research.

Select Agent Research

Select agents refer to pathogens or biological toxins. Again, in health promotion research this is a category that you are unlikely to use. Nonetheless, reviewers will assess the information provided in this section of the application, including (1) the select agent(s) to be used in the proposed research, (2) the registration status of all entities where select agent(s) will be used, (3) the procedures that will be used to monitor possession, use, and transfer of select agent(s), and (4) plans for appropriate biosafety, biocontainment, and security of the select agent(s).

Applications from Foreign Organizations

Reviewers will assess whether the project presents special opportunities for furthering research programs through the use of unusual talent, resources, populations, or environmental conditions that exist in other countries and either are not readily available in the United States or augment existing U.S. resources.

Resource Sharing Plans

Reviewers will evaluate the following Resource Sharing Plans: (1) Data Sharing Plan; (2) Sharing Model Organisms; and (3) Genome Wide Association Studies. Resource sharing is part of

IN A NUTSHELL

Resource sharing is part of NIH's mission and scope because it allows for further dissemination and analyses to be performed by others not involved in the original research after the grant ends.

NIH's mission and scope because it allows for further dissemination and analyses to be performed by others not involved in the original research after the grant ends. The Data Sharing Plan will be most relevant to health promotion. Box 18.1 provides an example of a Data Sharing Plan.

BOX 18.1. SAMPLE DATA SHARING PLAN FOR NIH PROPOSAL

Data Sharing Plan

The proposed study will include data collection from (1) a community-based intervention featuring a Diffusion of Innovations model, standard reflective clinical practice critique (RCPC) outreach methods, and academic detailing for health care providers—tested using a nonequivalent comparison design; this trial will end when 500 fecal immunochemical test (FIT) specimens have been returned in the intervention health district; (2) a social network analysis ($n = 64$) used to provide interim feedback regarding key characteristics of effective change agents used in the diffusion model, (3) a navigation program (based on current RCPC practices for cervical cancer) that will be applied to people testing FIT-positive ($n = 60$), and (4) an internet-based program designed to foster annual repeat FIT screening—tested using a randomized controlled trial design ($n = 220$). All study data will be stored on secure, password-protected computers. The project team will make their data available as widely and as freely as possible while safeguarding the privacy of participants and protecting confidential and proprietary data. Intellectual property and data generated as part of this project will be governed by University and NIH policies, including the Final NIH Statement of Sharing Research Data, February 26, 2003. These policies cover data generated from basic research, clinical studies, surveys, and other types of research involving human subjects and laboratory work. Furthermore, any research resources that were developed primarily with non-NIH funds will be shared in line with NIH policy for the purposes of this grant. Data and resources that are suitable for publication in peer-reviewed journals (that is, have been validated and are of sufficient merit and quality) will be published in a timely manner in the scientific literature. The information will also be presented at national meetings in poster or platform sessions. Individual requests for data will be honored on a case-by-case basis as appropriate to the research protocol. Other means of archiving and providing a safe data enclave are provided as part of the University information technology infrastructure efforts. No limits or caveats for coauthorship will be required as a precondition for receiving data. Furthermore, all requested data will be provided with appropriate documentation to prevent misuse, misinterpretation, or confusion. Other policies, including local, state, and federal laws and the Privacy Rule under the Health Insurance Portability and Accountability Act (HIPAA) will be adhered to when providing such data. All project data will be retained for a minimum of 3 years following closeout of the project, in accordance with NIH policy.

The Scientific Review Group

Now that you understand the scoring and review criteria, we would like to describe the actual review process. This is the point when the reviewers serving on the SRG assemble in a room, ready to begin reading their grant application critiques, to engage in constructive discussions about the grants, and to begin deliberations for assigning impact scores (see Figure 18.3). This is, as the saying goes, "where the rubber meets the road." Here is where grants receive an impact score that will be used to determine their likelihood of funding.

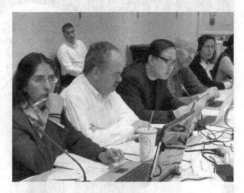

Figure 18.3 Scientific Review Group Meeting

Assuming that not many readers have been on an SRG, it may be useful to conceptualize this section with a flow chart, identifying the sequence of steps taken during the SRG meeting. Recall that usually there are three reviewers for each grant application, who are assigned to read and critique each grant. They are termed the primary and secondary reviewers. Figure 18.4 describes the sequence of activities during an SRG.

It is important to note that although consensus is not required, reviewers are asked to carefully consider all points of view during the SRG discussion and, keeping an open mind, find common ground and compromise where appropriate.

Selecting Your Research Topic

Now that you have insight into the criteria used to evaluate a grant, the scoring system, and how the actual review is conducted, we would like to turn your attention to selecting the research topic that will be the focus of your grant proposal. The desire to write a research proposal is not driven by whim. Indeed, the rationale for writing a grant proposal to do research, whether it is qualitative, observational, or interventional, exists in the context of research priorities often set by funding agencies. These priorities typically relate back to

IN A NUTSHELL

The rationale for writing a grant proposal to do research, whether it is qualitative, observational, or interventional, exists in the context of research priorities often set by funding agencies.

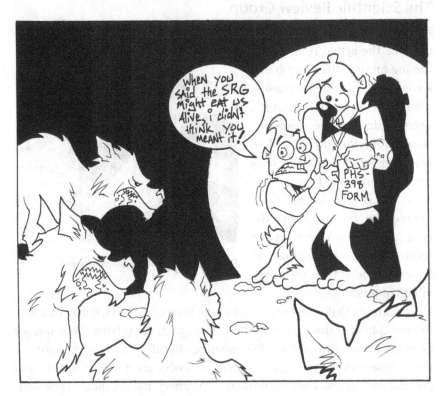

Mincus and Dincus's Grant Is Reviewed

Copyright 2005 by Justin Wagner; reprinted with permission.

the goals and objectives articulated in Healthy People 2020. The research priorities can range from enhancing vegetable consumption among adolescents, to enhancing mammography-seeking behavior among elder women, to promoting safer sex behavior among MSM, to mention just a few examples. In health promotion, the range of priorities is as limitless as our imagination. You should elect to conduct research in an area and on a topic for which you feel passion, that needs additional research (which excludes almost nothing), and that, if your study is done well, could have an important impact on a segment of society and health promotion research and practice.

To be effective as a health promotion researcher requires an intrinsic interest in the subject matter. The first criterion in selecting your research topic is to choose one that is of great interest to you. A few ground rules may help to identify potential research topics. The first rule is to not select a research topic only because it is fashionable or trendy. Fashion in health promotion research, as in clothes or music, changes with time—each has a limited shelf life. The second criterion is to select a topic that is most salient

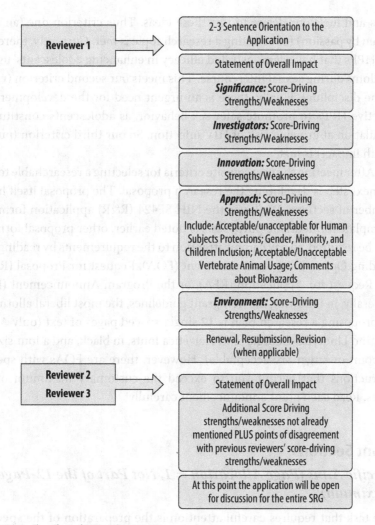

Figure 18.4 Flow Chart of Critique Presentation

to the field, that the field is wrestling with in terms of understanding how best to address the issue. The third criterion is to select a topic that has the potential for public health impact. This criterion suggests that the research be applied (in other words, it should be research with a practical, real-world application). In health promotion research, our mission is not one of basic science—that is, it is not research that may not have immediate or direct application to real-world issues.

We will illustrate these concepts with an example from our own research. We have a strong interest in and commitment to designing interventions to promote adolescents' adoption of condom use during sexual intercourse as a way to reduce their risk of becoming infected with STDs, including HIV. This interest allows us to identify potential research ideas and fuels our desire to test these ideas. Thus criterion one (an idea driven by passion) for selecting a research topic is met. Currently, there are few HPPs that have demonstrated efficacy in enhancing adolescents' use of condoms during sexual intercourse. This meets our second criterion (value to the discipline). Finally, there is an urgent need for the development of effective HPPs to promote safer sex behavior, as adolescents constitute a population at growing risk of HIV infection. So our third criterion (public health impact) is met.

After meeting the prerequisite criteria for selecting a researchable topic, the next step is developing the research proposal. The proposal itself has a number of sections. We'll use the NIH SF424 (R&R) application forms as a template for heuristic purposes. As noted earlier, other proposal formats may be required, so pay careful attention to the requirements by reading the Funding Opportunity Announcement (FOA), Request for Proposal (RFP), and Request for Application (RFA), or the Program Announcement (PA). Generally, in following the new grant guidelines, the most liberal allotment for proposing a research plan is 12 single-spaced pages of text (only Arial, Palatino Linotype, Georgia, and Helvetica fonts, in black, and a font size of 11-point or larger are acceptable). However, there are FOAs with special instructions that permit you to exceed the customary maximum of 12 pages. Read each grant announcement carefully!

specific aims
a concise and realistic description of what the proposed research is intended to accomplish

research strategy
the 12 pages for R01s, comprising three main parts: significance, innovation, and approach

Grant Sections

Specific Aims (Page Allocation = 1, Not Part of the 12-Page Maximum)

One task that requires careful attention is the preparation of the **specific aims**. The importance of this single page cannot be overstated. The specific aims page will be the readers' first impression of your proposal, as it represents a summary of the entire **research strategy**. The research strategy is essentially the three components of the grant proposal: **significance**, **innovation**, and **approach**. It is critical that your specific aims section is *targeted*, well-written, and clear and does a good job of selling your research. In essence, the specific aims section is your sales pitch to the reviewers. The specific aims section should be written only after the entire research strategy has been developed, reviewed, modified, and finalized, as at that point you will have described your approach succinctly, and you can use phrases and sentences from your research strategy in your specific aims.

There are usually five elements to a well-crafted and dynamic specific aims section:

significance
the importance of the application to the field

innovation
what is new and unique about the study; for example, explores new scientific avenues, has a novel hypothesis, will create new knowledge

approach
what you plan to do and how you plan to do it

1. A brief paragraph describing the problem to be investigated

2. A brief summary of why your approach will solve the problem and how it is innovative

3. A brief description of your approach

4. The aims and associated hypotheses of the research, if applicable

5. The long-term impact or significance of the findings for enhancing public health.

Because this section is named "Specific Aims," many researchers, young and old, often think the fourth element (the aims and associated hypotheses) is the only element to include in this section; however, this section requires much more information.

Significance Section (Page Allocation = 2 to 3)

The Significance section explicitly describes the public health significance and scope of the problem and answers these questions: If the aims of the application are achieved, how will scientific knowledge or public health practice or clinical practice be advanced? What will be the effect of these studies on the

IN A NUTSHELL

The Significance section should examine and frame existing empirical research relevant to the study and also show how your study will advance the field and what the effects will be.

concepts, methods, technologies, treatments, services, or preventative interventions that drive this field? Thus the significance section should examine and frame existing empirical research relevant to the study and also show how your study will advance the field and what the effects will be. It is an opportunity to carefully consider data from diverse sources.

A word of caution is in order. Although the research literature may be replete with numerous studies, this section should be a targeted and synthesized review. It is not a term paper, a master's thesis, or a dissertation. The goal of this section is to develop a rationale for the proposed study, for its conceptualization, and for its importance. Avoid getting mired in an extensive and lengthy review of the literature. In fact, the NIH has removed the term "background" formerly found in this section; accordingly, it should *not* be included, as it is distinctly different from the significance of what you propose to do.

In constructing this section, it is important to understand the research literature—its strengths and weaknesses—so that you can make a compelling argument for the proposed study. Indeed, if a satisfactory argument for the proposed study cannot be formulated, then the logical question arises: Why do the study? As you review the research literature, you should begin to make distinctions among studies. Some of these studies are well done and others are not. Some are observational and others are interventions. Not all studies are equally well designed, implemented, or analyzed. Studies will use different populations. You, as a health promotion scientist, bring your unique skills to bear in synthesizing the existing literature. Start to look through the literature, identifying studies that may directly address your specific aims, studies that may tangentially address your specific aims, and studies that are unrelated to your aims but may have relevance to your intervention strategy or HPP approaches by virtue of having been used in other health promotion studies.

With the need to study the proposed population established, the Significance section should provide a platform on which to build your HPP. First, however, you need to demonstrate competence with different behavior change strategies, and show that they are relevant to your proposed HPP. This is where many investigators falter. They can summarize the research literature with respect to identifying the problem, but they fail to provide an adequate discussion of the rationale for the underlying theories, principles, strategies, and techniques that they propose in their approach section. We cannot overstate the importance of clearly demonstrating a thorough understanding of the literature and the application of underlying theories, principles, strategies, and techniques and how they are relevant to your proposed research. SRG members are often overburdened with having to read and critique many proposals in a relatively short period of time.

IN A NUTSHELL

Keep in mind that SRG members may not be intimately familiar with all facets of your proposed research. *When in doubt, write it out!*

Keep in mind that they may not be intimately familiar with all facets of your proposed research. *When in doubt, write it out!* In this instance, it is better to err on the side of redundancy than to make an error of omission by not including relevant information that is critical to building an argument to support funding your proposed study.

Finally, this section requires closure. Having cleared a path through the morass of research literature, now you are ready for a conclusion. How you conclude the section is critical, as the conclusion may be what the members of the SRG remember most prominently. So you should write this last part of the Significance section with great attention to punctuating key points that will sell the value of your proposal to even the most skeptical reviewers. What should be included in this last part?

The objective is to enumerate and describe how the proposed study can significantly contribute to the field. Be brief, but be comprehensive. Also, here is an opportunity to express your passion and excitement. Research should not be a dispassionate enterprise. Quite the contrary—research is brimming with passion. You should include statements about how this study creates an exciting opportunity to interact with others from diverse scientific disciplines in a multidisciplinary approach; to develop new and innovative HP intervention strategies or lay the groundwork via observational research for future HP interventions; and to apply HP strategies observed to be effective in other fields of health promotion research to your proposed study, population, and venue. Finally, add one statement that reiterates the clear, cogent, and compelling clinical and public health significance of your proposal.

> **IN A NUTSHELL**
>
> Research should not be a dispassionate enterprise. Quite the contrary—research is brimming with passion.

Innovation (Page Allocation = No More Than 1)

The primary objective of your grant proposal is to emphasize the innovation of your research; the HPP, the measures, or other facets that differentiate your study from others. Key questions that you need to address have to do with whether the proposed project is original or innovative. In this context innovation, rather than conveying its literal meaning of novelty, refers to whether or not the project challenges existing research or clinical paradigms or clinical practice. Does your proposal address an innovative hypothesis or critical barrier to progress in the field? Does it use new methodological or theoretical frameworks in a new way that will advance the field? One example could be if you were proposing a new HPP that combined theoretical approaches or had adapted it for a completely new or high-risk population. Does the project develop or employ novel concepts, approaches, methodologies, tools, or technologies for this area? An example here would be to articulate the use of new sampling methodologies or new measurement instruments that advance the field and have not been applied in the same way before.

A word of caution: although innovation is highly valued, its value is dependent on how well the approach is articulated and executed. Indeed, the Approach section is the single most influential factor affecting the impact score; however, reviewers will need to see that your innovation is feasible. The message here is simple: be innovative, but not at the cost of sacrificing scientific rigor.

Approach (Page Allocation = 8 to 9)

approach
section describing the
proposed research plan,
methodology, and data
analysis

The next section of the proposal is the **approach**; this is by far the largest section in your proposal. Although all the elements of a research proposal are important, this section is the most critical. This section describes the proposed research plan, methodology, and data analysis. There is no standard format for this section. However, we provide a template, using an example of our own intervention research, which you can modify to suit your particular needs.

Part 1: Overview of the Research Plan or Design　The overview should contain the following elements:

1. The overarching aim
2. The type of study (qualitative, cross-sectional, longitudinal, or intervention)
3. The primary outcome
4. The sample selection
5. The number of study participants
6. A brief enumeration of the study's assessment procedures
7. Randomization procedures, if an intervention
8. The theory underlying the study
9. A brief description of the HPP, if an intervention
10. The length of the follow-up period
11. Data analysis

Even with the elements articulated, what exactly constitutes an overview is often not intuitively clear. To aid you, we have provided an example of an overview in Box 18.2.

BOX 18.2.　SAMPLE OVERVIEW OF THE RESEARCH DESIGN

Overview of the Research Design

This study is a Phase III randomized controlled trial designed to evaluate the efficacy of an HIV intervention relative to receiving the standard-of-care counseling that accompanies the treatment of STDs at the County Health Department. A random sample of 960 African-American females, 15 to 19 years of age, will be recruited at the County Health Department STD Program following receipt of treatment and standard-of-care preventive counseling for STDs. At baseline, eligible adolescents will complete an audio-computer-assisted self-interview

(A-CASI) and provide a urine specimen that will be analyzed using newly developed nucleic acid amplification assays to detect three prevalent STDs (chlamydia, gonorrhea, and trichomoniasis). Adolescents randomized to the control condition will view a brief video about the importance of proper nutrition. Those randomized to the HIV intervention will participate in a group-format HIV intervention implemented over three consecutive Saturdays (four hours each day). Adolescents will be asked to return at 6 and 12 months post-intervention to complete an A-CASI-administered psychosocial interview that is similar to the baseline interview and to provide urine specimens for STD assay. An intent-to-treat analysis, controlling for baseline assessments, will determine the efficacy of the HIV intervention, relative to standard-of-care STD counseling only, in reducing HIV-associated sexual behaviors and incident STDs over a 12-month follow-up period. Secondary analyses will evaluate the impact of the intervention condition, relative to the control condition, on hypothesized mediators of HIV-preventive behaviors.

Although a succinct overview of the study provides a foundation on which to build this section, it is usually helpful to also present a schematic representation of the proposed research design. A well-designed visual is worth a thousand words, as it provides a snapshot of the entire project that the SRG can keep in mind as you begin to enumerate and describe each element more fully. In Figure 18.5 we present an example of a figure outlining the research design.

Part 2: Description of the Study Site and Population The next element in this section is often a description of the study site and population.

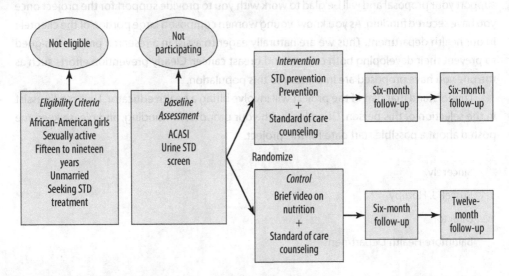

Figure 18.5 Example of a Schematic Diagram Outlining the Research Design

This is an opportunity to demonstrate your familiarity with both the proposed study site and the population in which you propose to conduct your study. Be succinct, but provide ample information about the site and population that is directly relevant to the proposed study. Here it is important to provide letters from site administrators that describe their support and enthusiasm for the proposed study, their willingness to commit site resources, and their willingness to provide access to the study population. Letters are included as an appendix to the proposal. Box 18.3 provides a sample letter of support.

BOX 18.3. SAMPLE LETTER OF SUPPORT

September 21, 2014

Doctor H. Noitall, Ph.D.

College of Public Health

1547 Baxter Road, NE, Room 542

Baltimore, MD 30322

RE: A Cancer Prevention Program for Young Women

Dear Dr. Noitall:

It was great to meet with you recently and learn about your proposal to test the feasibility of a three-session intervention designed for young women residing in Baltimore. Your idea to also test the efficacy of using support groups to promote behavior change is excellent. I fully support your proposal and will be glad to work with you to provide support for the project once you have secured funding. As you know, young women compose a large portion of the clientele in our health department. Thus we are naturally eager to assist in a research project designed to prevent their developing both cervical and breast cancer. Clearly prevention efforts such as the one you have proposed are important to this population.

I understand that part of the project will involve hiring a health educator. I will gladly assist in the selection of this person. Good luck with your proposal for funding, and please keep me posted about a possible start date for this project.

Sincerely,

Russell J. Hornby

Director

Baltimore Health Department

Part 3: Eligibility Criteria for Study Participation   In this section, precisely articulate the inclusion and exclusion criteria for the proposed study. This typically includes criteria such as age, race or ethnicity, gender, marital status, and presence or absence of a specific disease or risk behavior. The inclusion criteria should be tailored to correspond to the aims of the study. In addition to specifying the inclusion criteria, it is often helpful to explicitly specify the exclusion criteria.

Part 4: Research Design and Methods   At this juncture, let's review for a moment what you have accomplished in the Approach section of the proposal. You have (1) provided a succinct overview of the proposed study, including a graphical representation of the research design; (2) described the study site and population; and (3) specified the eligibility (inclusion and exclusion) criteria. Your next step is to begin describing the research plan.

Organizing and Designing the Research Plan

There are countless ways in which you could organize and present the research plan. We will show you one way, which we think provides a logical approach that the SRG can easily understand. We recommend presenting the research plan in three sequential phases. Each phase represents a unique set of research activities and tasks that need to be completed to successfully develop, implement, and evaluate the proposed study. In this way we provide a systematic, logical, and chronological sequence of research tasks and activities. The idea is for the research proposal to be an integrated whole, with each section of the proposal building on and informing subsequent sections. The more integrated the proposal, the easier it is to understand its flow and logic.

IN A NUTSHELL

The idea is for the research proposal to be an integrated whole, with each section of the proposal building on and informing subsequent sections. The more integrated the proposal, the easier it is to understand its flow and logic.

We can categorize the research plan into three phases. Phase I describes program development, Phase II describes program implementation, and Phase III describes program evaluation. In the following sections, we review the elements commonly identified in each phase of the research plan. Not all of the activities in these phases may be appropriate for all research studies; however, we describe a research plan designed specifically to develop, implement, and evaluate an HPP. Of course, this plan is readily modifiable for observation studies (for cross-sectional or longitudinal studies).

Phase I: Program Development   The primary Phase I activities include:

- Hiring staff
- Conducting formative research
- Describing the underlying theoretical framework guiding the study
- Creating a community advisory board
- Developing the theoretically based HPP
- Training the health educators to implement the HPP
- Pilot testing the HPP
- Specifying the data collection procedures
- Selecting measures for inclusion on the assessment instrument
- Pilot testing the data collection instrument
- Training staff to administer the data collection instrument

In this section, we provide a brief description of each of the components included in Phase I.

Hiring Staff. In this section, you specify the names or position titles of staff to be hired. To facilitate the SRG's understanding of whether your staffing plan is appropriate to the research tasks and activities, it is useful to list the project year in which staff members are brought in (that is, added to the project payroll). This demonstrates a degree of sophistication with respect to allocating staff time to complete project-related tasks. Unfortunately, this skill is rarely taught in graduate courses. Experience and having conducted a feasibility study will be instrumental in guiding the allocation of staff effort across each year of the proposed study.

Conducting Formative Research. In many studies, front loading (building research activities at the beginning of the project) includes formative research to assist in tailoring the HPP. This is a sound research methodology. It's appropriate to specify the time period during which you propose to conduct formative research; for example, "During months 02 to 04 we will conduct a series of eight focus groups." Specify the purpose of the formative research, such as "Focus groups will be conducted to examine relevant causal factors potentially missing in our theoretical models." Next, it is useful to cite any prior experience by team members in conducting

IN A NUTSHELL

As a rule, if you propose a research activity, there should be someone specified in the research proposal with the requisite skills and experience to conduct that activity.

formative research; in this case, focus groups as well as those who will be designated to conduct the focus groups and analyze the data. As a rule, if you propose a research activity, there should be someone specified in the research proposal with the requisite skills and experience to conduct that activity.

Describing the Underlying Theoretical or Conceptual Framework. As in the previous sections, specify the time frame in which this activity or task is to be accomplished and describe the project staff dedicated to accomplishing the activity or task. Next, define the theoretical or conceptual models that underlie the HPP. Briefly summarize model components and their relevance to the proposed HPP. At this point, it is appropriate to cite prior or preliminary research with these theories or models and their relevance and utility for explaining the phenomenon under study.

Creating a Community Advisory Board (CAB). Much of health promotion research is conducted in community settings. Thus it is advantageous to propose a community advisory board (CAB) as part of the study. Specify the number and composition of the CAB members and how they will be identified, recruited, and compensated. Also, note the meeting schedule of the CAB and its scope of activities. One activity may be to review any project materials, such as the research survey, to ensure that they are culturally competent, comprehensive, and readable. Another activity is to ensure that the proposed HPP is culturally competent, addresses key concerns as identified by members of the target community, and is acceptable to community standards. Again, it is valuable to enclose letters of support from prospective CAB members. These letters are typically scanned and saved as one attachment to the proposal in an appendix.

Developing the Theoretically Based HPP. Here is an opportunity to shine! You have read the empirical literature, you have conducted qualitative and preliminary research and proposed additional research in this proposal, and you have conducted a feasibility study. Begin this section by specifying the time frame in which the HPP will be developed (for example, during months 03 through 09) and the personnel who will develop the HPP (for example, "Drs. DiClemente, Salazar, and Crosby will develop the HPP in conjunction with the project health educators and peer educators and with input from the CAB").

Once you have described the "when" and "who," it is time to describe the HPP itself. A word of advice: be sure to tightly integrate the HPP with the underlying conceptual model or theory. The conceptual model and theory is designed to guide the development and implementation of the HPP—use them accordingly. It is critical to demonstrate a clear and obvious linkage between the underlying conceptual model or theory and your HPP activities.

IN A NUTSHELL

It is critical to demonstrate a clear and obvious linkage between the underlying conceptual model or theory and your HPP activities.

Describing the content of the HPP requires specifying each of the intervention elements. In a multisession HPP, describe the sessions in the sequence in which they are offered. Although 12 pages may seem like a lot of space, you will find that being succinct is critical in preparing a coherent and comprehensive description of the HPP. A table that specifies HPP activities and the mediator(s) targeted by these activities can be useful as a summary. As an illustration, in Box 18.4 we provide an example of how to describe the theoretical linkages to an STD-preventive HPP.

BOX 18.4. THEORETICAL LINKAGES TO A HEALTH PROMOTION PROGRAM

Social cognitive theory (SCT) will guide the design of the STD prevention intervention. According to SCT, behavior is the result of interactions among personal factors, environmental factors, and behavior. Personal factors include an individual's confidence in performing a certain behavior (self-efficacy), the individual's expectations about the outcomes associated with performing that specific behavior (outcome expectancies), and the individual's goals related to the behavior. Environmental factors include normative influences (peer norms) and the support that an individual may receive from others.

The aim of the proposed study is to enhance adolescents' confidence in their ability to self-regulate their sexual behavior. The STD prevention intervention will teach adolescents about safe and unsafe sexual practices as well as the outcomes associated with each. Given that the teens in the proposed study were treated for an STD, the intervention will teach youth about the link between having an STD and the increased risk of HIV infection. The STD prevention intervention will also teach teens skills such as (1) goal setting; (2) engaging in safer sexual behaviors (such as using condoms correctly and consistently, abstaining from sex, and limiting their number of sexual partners); and (3) communicating effectively with one's sexual partner (that is, differentiating among passive, assertive, and aggressive communication styles and communicating the need for one's partner to be tested for STDs). The STD prevention intervention will also be designed to create a normative atmosphere supportive of safer sex practices and self-protective communication styles. By supplying much-needed information and skills, we hope to enhance adolescents' self-efficacy to refuse risky sex and their ability to insist on condom use during sexual intercourse.

To reiterate, the goal of this specific section is to make the connection between the underlying theory and the HPP activities or components transparent to the SRG. Intervention mapping—enumerating each activity of the proposed HPP and linking it to one of the underlying conceptual model or theory constructs—is critical to demonstrating your depth of understanding of the model or theory and how it is applied in building your HPP.

Training the Health Educators to Administer the HPP. An important element often overlooked in research proposals by new and established investigators alike is specifying *who* will implement the HPP and *how* they will be trained. Now that you've carefully crafted your HPP, describe the personnel who will implement it: their professional training (for example, MPH in behavioral sciences or health education), their sociodemographic characteristics, if relevant to the effective implementation of the HPP, and their background experiences.

Once the personnel have been briefly described, it is useful to describe the training they will receive prior to implementing the HPP. This can be a brief paragraph that articulates the training procedures used to train staff to proficiency. These could include any of the following: viewing videos, role-playing the HPP, role reversal in which the health educator may be asked to play the part of a study participant, group discussions, direct instruction, and so on. It is important to evaluate implementation personnel prior to their interacting with study participants. Also, have a plan available for corrective training and termination, should an implementation staff member be unable or unwilling to conduct the HPP as designed. It is beneficial to note that quality assurance procedures will be used to monitor implementation fidelity. Identifying the possibility of drift in interventions is also important, as this requires remedial training of project staff.

Pilot Testing the HPP. Be sure to include language in your proposal assuring the SRG that the proposed HPP will be pilot tested. When the HPP is completed, the staff trained, and modifications made to both the HPP and training protocols, a pilot test of the entire protocol is vital. In a pilot test, it is valuable to select participants from the target population who meet the eligibility criteria. The HPP will be assessed for feasibility and participant satisfaction; any problems identified can be rectified, and the HPP will be modified as necessary. Similarly, any difficulties encountered in implementing the HPP can be identified and rectified prior to actually starting the trial. A word of advice: build in adequate time to conduct the pilot study and make modifications to the staff training protocol and HPP itself; you should also specify the time frame in which the pilot study will be implemented and modifications made.

IN A NUTSHELL

Build in adequate time to conduct the pilot study and make modifications to the staff training protocol and HPP itself; you should also specify the time frame in which the pilot study will be implemented and modifications made.

Specifying the Data Collection Procedures. This section is devoted to articulating the data collection procedures used in the proposed study. If there are multiple procedures, it is critical to adequately describe each procedure. For example, "We will use three data collection procedures: (1) a web-based survey, (2) a urine specimen, and (3) a retrospective review of clinic records." Describe the first data element with respect to time to completion: "The web-based interview is approximately 60 minutes in length." Describe where the data collection procedure will be conducted: "The web-based survey will be self-administered and completed at a time convenient for the participant." Finally, describe what type of data this procedure will yield: "The web-based survey is designed to assess potential moderators, psychosocial beliefs, and sexual behaviors at baseline and 6- and 12-month follow-up." Basically, describe each data collection procedure in sufficient detail. Then proceed to describe the remaining data elements in a similar and systematic fashion.

Selecting Measures for Inclusion in the Assessment Instrument. A critical aspect of any study is selecting measures (for example, scales, indexes, single-item measures) used to assess the constructs articulated in the proposal. Furthermore, selection of constructs for assessment should be guided by several factors:

- The underlying conceptual or theoretical model guiding the proposed study
- A thorough review of the research literature examining potential moderators, mediators, and outcomes among the target population
- The research team's prior experience
- Input from the CAB
- Prior formative or qualitative research
- Results of the pilot study

Once you have selected the constructs, select measures to assess them. Whenever feasible, these measures should have demonstrated reliability and validity with the target population (see Chapter Seven for a more detailed discussion of reliability and validity).

Pilot Testing the Data Collection Instrument. As noted previously with respect to the HPP and staff training, a pilot test can be very useful. Likewise, pilot testing the data collection instrument(s) allows the research team to assess their psychometrics and comprehension, as well as cultural, developmental, and gender relevance for the target population. This section should be brief. It should state that during a specified time period (for example, during months 08 through 10) the assessment instrument(s) will be pilot tested with a small sample selected from the target population. The pilot sample should be selected so that the individuals meet the proposed study eligibility criteria.

Training Staff to Administer the Data Collection Instrument(s). Training is critical to avoid ambiguity with respect to implementing study protocols. Given the amount of time, energy, and emphasis placed on the results obtained from HPPs, staff training should be an integral component of any research plan. Depending on the data collection instruments, it is useful to articulate the protocols that will be followed as well as the qualifications of the personnel involved

IN A NUTSHELL

Given the amount of time, energy, and emphasis placed on the results obtained from HPPs, staff training should be an integral component of any research plan.

in data collection (in other words, a trained research associate with experience in collecting similar data from the target population). Specify any training protocols that will ensure standardized data collection. This is increasingly important if there are multiple data collectors and the data will be collected using personal interviews, which are more susceptible to interviewer bias and socially desirable responding by participants.

Phase II: Program Implementation   Phase II activities include:

*   Recruiting the study sample
*   Screening and sampling procedures
*   Administering the baseline assessment
*   Randomizing participants to the study conditions
*   Selecting and implementing the control condition
*   Conducting quality assurance process evaluations

- Specifying follow-up procedures
- Defining strategies for enhancing retention

Recruitment. In this section of your proposal, it is critical to specify key elements related to the recruitment of your sample, such as:

- Sampling method (for example, convenience, random sampling, venue-day-time sampling)
- Procedures for recruitment
- Projected sample size
- Time period during which the sample will be recruited
- Rate of recruitment (such as number recruited per week)
- The population from which the sample will be recruited

A variety of recruitment strategies can be used to attract people to participate in HPP studies. Using recruitment procedures that have proven effective in other studies with the target population is invaluable. Again, experience with the target population will be useful in evaluating the strategies that may be most effective. Who is conducting the screening? Where is it being conducted? How will it be conducted? How will the person conducting the screening be trained? What previous relevant experience recommends the person proposed to conduct the project screening activities? All of this information is relevant for the SRG.

Likewise, describe the sampling procedures. For example, "The recruitment-retention coordinator will use a random numbers table to identify potential participants to approach and screen for eligibility. This process will continue until the targeted number of participants has been recruited. The recruitment-retention coordinator will also collect sociodemographic information from those who elect not to participate as well as their rationale for not participating in the study for later comparison with those who elect to participate."

If feasible, and not in violation of IRB regulations, collecting sociodemographic data from those potential and eligible participants who decline to participate in the study can provide a useful gauge of the representativeness of the final sample recruited. As in other aspects of the study, extensive training of the personnel responsible for screening and sampling is critical.

Administering the Baseline Assessment. In this section, describe the protocols and procedure for administering the baseline assessment. Again, it is vitally important to be specific in this description. The SRG is interested in knowing who will invite participants to complete the baseline assessment and where the assessment will be conducted.

Randomizing Participants to the Study Conditions. A central concern in any HPP randomized trial design is the randomization protocol. It could be as simple as a coin toss—however, although a coin toss is considered a random event by some, your randomization protocol should entail much more sophisticated procedures. See Chapter Ten for more detailed information on different randomization procedures. This section on randomization should specify who will determine the randomization sequence, who will conduct randomization, and how randomization will be executed.

Selecting and Implementing the Control Condition. Selecting and implementing the control condition is also a vital concern when the HPP involves a between-groups design. Therefore it is important to explain the rationale for selecting a particular control condition. Regardless of the type of control condition (for example, placebo-attention, wait-list), like the HPP, this section requires specification of who, what, when, and where. Describe the qualifications or relevant sociodemographic characteristics of the personnel responsible for implementing the control condition, the control condition content, and when and where the control condition will be implemented.

Quality Assurance Process Evaluation Procedures. As discussed in Chapters Five and Ten, one threat to the internal validity of any HPP study is variability in administering either the intervention or, in the case of a placebo-controlled trial, the placebo-control condition. Even though a protocol has been developed to promote standardization of HPP delivery, designed to enhance implementation fidelity, there is the potential for health educators or program facilitators to "drift," that is, to change the way they administer the HPP over time. The SRG will want to know what procedures are in place to detect and minimize the threat of differential implementation of the intervention. In this part, you will describe the process you will implement to ensure fidelity to HPP protocols. For example, "participants will be asked to rate anonymously each session attended for the facilitators/implementers' adherence to session protocols." In combination, you could also include, "independent raters will be assigned to evaluate 50% of HPP sessions for facilitators/implementers' adherence to session protocols."

Specifying Follow-Up Procedures. The aim of this section is to delineate the follow-up assessment procedures. The procedures should be well articulated, specifying who will conduct the follow-up assessments, when, and where. If participants are compensated for completing follow-up assessments, specify the type (for example, gift cards, monetary compensation, movie tickets) and amount of compensation and when it is provided to participants. Also of importance, specify who will contact participants, when, and how, and whether transportation will be provided to facilitate participants' ability to access the data collection venue.

IN A NUTSHELL

A major concern in any longitudinal study, which includes intervention trials, is the maintenance of the study cohort.

Defining Strategies for Enhancing Retention. A major concern in any longitudinal study that includes intervention trials is the maintenance of the study cohort. Although a number of tracking procedures have proven effective, a pilot study or previous research with the target population is invaluable in determining the optimal set of tracking protocols and procedures that will facilitate maintenance of the cohort in the proposed study. See Chapter Nine for a more thorough discussion of possible protocols and procedures.

Phase III: Program Evaluation (Describe How You Will Assess Whether the HPP Was Effective)

Phase III activities should describe:

- Data management and verification checks
- The data analytic plan
- The power analysis
- The project timeline

It is important to clearly convey to the SRG that you have thoughtfully planned each of these activities. Also, be sure that the planned analyses exactly match the aims and associated hypotheses. In developing the data analytic plan, it is essential to have extensive input and guidance from a statistician. In this section we provide some guidance in preparing this part of the research plan.

Data Management and Verification Checks. Describe how the data will be managed so that reduction, cleaning, entry, and verification of participants' responses for analysis will be performed. Typically, data management should fall under the direction of the data analyst, usually a statistician with expertise in relevant statistical techniques. In some cases studies hire a data manager. You should specify who your data manager will be and that person's qualifications.

The Data Analytic Plan. In this section, the data analytic plan will need to describe who will perform the data analyses and how the aims will be fulfilled statistically, and if applicable, how the hypotheses are tested. You must describe the specific statistical techniques that will be used for each aim or hypothesis and also the software package that will be used. For specific statistical analyses that are appropriate in health promotion, we refer you to Chapters Fourteen and Fifteen; however, your statistician should write this section if you are not qualified. Increasingly, statistical analyses have become much more complex and sophisticated; thus reviewers expect a high level of detail and sophistication in this section.

The Power Analysis. One other aspect integrally related to the determination of the study sample is the power analysis (see Chapter Fourteen for a more detailed description of the power analysis.). The power analysis needs to be described to justify the targeted sample size, accounting for attrition. To determine the proposed study's sample size, the investigator usually examines an analysis for the primary hypothesis. Using other studies or previous research by the investigative team, the principal investigator posits an estimated effect size. A thorough rationale for the estimated effect size should be provided; for example, "To estimate our effect size, we relied on the most recent intervention research that incorporated STDs as a measure of program efficacy. We estimated a conservative effect size of 30-percent difference for STD re-infection rates between the STD prevention condition and the control condition. We used a one-tail test, setting alpha at $P = .05$, with power of 0.80 to calculate the sample size necessary under these conditions." Always take attrition into account. If the sample size needed is estimated to be 800, and you assume 20-percent attrition, then be sure to recruit 1,000 participants (this includes the projected 20-percent loss to follow-up), which will yield an effective analytic sample size of 800 participants.

> **IN A NUTSHELL**
>
> Using other studies or previous research by the investigative team, the principal investigator posits an estimated effect size. A thorough rationale for the estimated effect size should be provided.

Outlining the Project Timeline. The project timeline is one of the final components of any proposal, and an important one. The timeline is your estimation of the start and termination of specific research activities. Again, in the absence of experience, it is difficult to construct an accurate timeline. However, pilot research and others' published experiences can be

Table 18.3 Template for a Five-Year Project Timeline

Activities	Project Month												
	1	5	10	15	20	25	30	35	40	45	50	55	60
Awarded funds	X												
Hire and train staff		XXXX											
Conduct focus groups		XXXX											
Develop HIV intervention			XXXX										
Pilot HIV intervention			XXX										
Develop the interview			XXXXXX										
Pilot the interview			XXXX										
Transfer and pilot the ACASI			XXXX										
Recruit for baseline assessments					XXXXXXXXXXXXXXXXXXXXXXXXX								
Begin four-month follow-up assessments					XXXXXXXXXXXXXXXXXXXXXXXX								
Begin eight-month follow-up assessments						XXXXXXXXXXXXXXXXXXXXXXXX							
Begin twelve-month follow-up assessments						XXXXXXXXXXXXXXXXXXXXXXXX							
Data analysis and manuscript preparation											XXXXX		

invaluable in developing a realistic timeline. Table 18.3 is a template using a Gantt chart format that provides a visual overview of research activities over the five-year duration of a project.

Time to Electronically Send in Your Grant: Write a Cover Letter

Now that your grant is written, it is time to have it submitted. This process is handled by your institution's office of sponsored programs through Grants.gov. But before that button is pushed, you should increase your chance of success by including a cover letter that will facilitate your grant application's being reviewed by the most qualified reviewers. Reviewers with expertise in your area will best recognize the potential for your research to advance the field and contribute to public health. Applicants may request particular study sections (and even a particular institute or center) in a cover letter submitted with the application. The letter is stored in a separate location and not forwarded to reviewers. Review the rosters of the SRGs to locate the study section where members have the appropriate expertise to review your project. This is an opportunity to also provide names of any reviewers who may have a conflict of interest and should *not* be considered as reviewers of your application. It is important to match your area of research with the areas reviewed by the study section.

Summary

This chapter has provided a blueprint for crafting a research proposal, including the critical aspect of understanding the review process. We have described a number of elements that are critical to a successful proposal as well as to a valid study. We want to remind you, however, that proposal writing is an incremental, iterative, and calibrated learning process. The suggestions presented in this chapter will be an asset to you once you begin this learning process. As you become engaged in the research enterprise, we suggest that you consult the brief list of tips that we provide in Box 18.5, with a helpful mnemonic for hitting your proposal out of the ballpark!

BOX 18.5. TIPS FOR CRAFTING A SUCCESSFUL PROPOSAL

H Have all instructions for assembling the application been carefully followed?

O On time (the deadline is not a suggestion or flexible!)

M Make sure your budget corresponds to the personnel allocation for each project year.

E Exchange ideas with investigators of funded studies that may be similar to yours.

R Realize that there is no substitute for unwavering determination!

U Understand the importance of carefully choosing the research team (this could be the beginning of a long and productive relationship).

N Never, ever give up!!!

We also encourage readers to complement the knowledge and skills acquired from reading this chapter with more detailed texts (Pequegnat, Stover, and Boyce, 2011; Chapin, 2004). Foremost, we encourage readers to carefully consider the time, labor, and monetary resources necessary for designing, implementing, and evaluating an HPP. Given the importance of identifying effective HPPs, it is worth a considerable expenditure of energy and resources to design the most rigorous study feasible. Ultimately, a prerequisite to success in any field or endeavor is dedicating ample time and effort. Furthermore, it is often helpful to involve other colleagues in the proposal process. Selecting colleagues with the requisite skills needed to develop, implement, and evaluate the proposed study is one of the most important decisions you will make. Finally, keep in mind that constructing a great proposal is "1 percent inspiration and 99 percent perspiration."

If your career were an Olympic event it would be a marathon, not a sprint. You will experience failure and disappointment, but you can still achieve success. As Winston Churchill so aptly stated, "Success is the ability to go from one failure to another with no loss of enthusiasm." Remember that perseverance and fortitude pay off in the long run.

KEY TERMS

Approach

Innovation

Merit rating

Overall impact score

Research strategy

Significance

Specific aims

For Practice and Discussion

1. Give some thought to a grant proposal that you would like to write to secure funding. Create a detailed outline of the grant proposal, using the template in this chapter as a guide. Modify your outline as needed for your proposed study, then write up a draft specific aims section.

2. After concluding the preceding exercise, share your grant outline with another classmate and have her share her grant outline with you. Review and critique the outlines according to what should be included in each section and whether enough attention was given to significance, innovation, and approach. Be constructive in your feedback.

3. Ask your instructor to obtain a grant proposal (their proposal or a colleague's). Again, form two or three SRGs; each SRG will independently review, discuss, and score the grant. After all scoring is complete, a representative from each SRG will present their rationale for the final overall impact score. Summarize the weaknesses and strengths for each of the relevant sections.

4. You and your colleagues are going to submit a grant proposal that will assess the risk and protective factors associated with prescription drug abuse among adolescents. The design will be a prospective cohort design in which you will recruit adolescents online and follow them

over the course of 12 months. Discuss what the significant risks would be. What are the main points you would want to make in your Human Subjects Protection section? How will you handle the data and protect their privacy? How will you handle parental consent?

References

Chapin, P. G. (2004). *Research projects and research proposals: A guide for scientists seeking funding*. New York: Cambridge University Press.

Pequegnat, W., Stover, E., and Boyce, C. A. (Eds). (2011). *How to write a successful research grant application: A guide for social and behavioral scientists*. New York: Springer.